# Nursing and COVID-19 I

# Nursing and COVID-19 I

Editors

**Richard Gray**
**Sonia Udod**

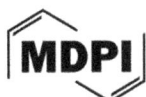

Basel • Beijing • Wuhan • Barcelona • Belgrade • Novi Sad • Cluj • Manchester

*Editors*

Richard Gray
School of Nursing and
Midwifery, La Trobe
University
Melbourne, Australia

Sonia Udod
College of Nursing,
University of Manitoba
Winnipeg
Winnipeg, Canada

*Editorial Office*
MDPI
St. Alban-Anlage 66
4052 Basel, Switzerland

This is a reprint of articles from the Special Issue published online in the open access journal *Nursing Reports* (ISSN 2039-4403) (available at: https://www.mdpi.com/journal/nursrep/special_issues/nursing_COVID-19).

For citation purposes, cite each article independently as indicated on the article page online and as indicated below:

Lastname, A.A.; Lastname, B.B. Article Title. *Journal Name* **Year**, *Volume Number*, Page Range.

**ISBN 978-3-0365-9070-7 (Hbk)**
**ISBN 978-3-0365-9071-4 (PDF)**
doi.org/10.3390/books978-3-0365-9071-4

© 2023 by the authors. Articles in this book are Open Access and distributed under the Creative Commons Attribution (CC BY) license. The book as a whole is distributed by MDPI under the terms and conditions of the Creative Commons Attribution-NonCommercial-NoDerivs (CC BY-NC-ND) license.

# Contents

**About the Editors** . . . . . . . . . . . . . . . . . . . . . . . . . . . . . . . . . . . . . . . . . . . . . . . . **vii**

**Catarina Lobão, Adriana Coelho, Vitor Parola, Hugo Neves, Joana Pereira Sousa and Rui Gonçalves**
Changes in Clinical Training for Nursing Students during the COVID-19 Pandemic: A Scoping Review
Reprinted from: *Nursing Reports* **2023**, *13*, 378–388, doi:10.3390/nursrep13010035 . . . . . . . . . **1**

**Kholofelo Lorraine Matlhaba**
Virtual Practical Examination for Student Nurse Educators in Health Sciences Education during the COVID-19 Pandemic: A Narrative Review
Reprinted from: *Nursing Reports* **2023**, *13*, 214–229, doi:10.3390/nursrep13010021 . . . . . . . . . **13**

**Mwila Kabwe, Jennifer L. Dittmer, Jaimee Oxford, Catina Eyres, Ancara Thomas, Andrew Mahony and et al.**
A Novel Approach to Managing a COVID-19 Outbreak at a Farm in Outer Regional Victoria, Australia
Reprinted from: *Nursing Reports* **2022**, *12*, 717–725, doi:10.3390/nursrep12040071 . . . . . . . . . **29**

**Diego Serrano-Gómez, Verónica Velasco-González, Ana Rosa Alconero-Camarero, José Rafael González-López, Montserrat Antonín-Martín, Alicia Borras-Santos and et al.**
COVID-19 Infection among Nursing Students in Spain: The Risk Perception, Perceived Risk Factors, Coping Style, Preventive Knowledge of the Disease and Sense of Coherence as Psychological Predictor Variables: A Cross Sectional Survey
Reprinted from: *Nursing Reports* **2022**, *12*, 661–673, doi:10.3390/nursrep12030066 . . . . . . . . . **39**

**Mohammed Gh. Alzahrani, Nazik M. A. Zakari, Dina I. Abuabah, Mona S. Ousman, Jing Xu and Hanadi Y. Hamadi**
Examining Healthcare Professionals' Telehealth Usability before and during COVID-19 in Saudi Arabia: A Cross-Sectional Study
Reprinted from: *Nursing Reports* **2022**, *12*, 648–654, doi:10.3390/nursrep12030064 . . . . . . . . . **53**

**Catarina Lobão, Adriana Coelho, Rui Gonçalves, Vitor Parola, Hugo Neves and Joana Pereira Sousa**
Changes in Clinical Training for Nursing Students during the COVID-19 Pandemic: A Scoping Review Protocol
Reprinted from: *Nursing Reports* **2022**, *12*, 210–216, doi:10.3390/nursrep12010021 . . . . . . . . . **61**

**Alan M. Beck, Amy J. Piontek, Eric M. Wiedenman and Amanda Gilbert**
Perceptions of COVID-19 Mitigation Strategies between Rural and Non-Rural Adults in the US: How Public Health Nurses Can Fill the Gap
Reprinted from: *Nursing Reports* **2022**, *12*, 188–197, doi:10.3390/nursrep12010019 . . . . . . . . . **69**

**Hanadi Y Hamadi, Nazik M. A. Zakari, Ebtesam Jibreel, Faisal N. AL Nami, Jamel A. S. Smida and Hedi H. Ben Haddad**
Stress and Coping Strategies among Nursing Students in Clinical Practice during COVID-19
Reprinted from: *Nursing Reports* **2021**, *11*, 629–639, doi:10.3390/nursrep11030060 . . . . . . . . . **79**

**Patricia Torrent-Ramos, Víctor M. González-Chordá, Desirée Mena-Tudela, Laura Andreu Pejó, Celia Roig-Marti, María Jesús Valero-Chillerón and et al.**
Healthcare Management and Quality during the First COVID-19 Wave in a Sample of Spanish Healthcare Professionals
Reprinted from: *Nursing Reports* **2021**, *11*, 536–546, doi:10.3390/nursrep11030051 . . . . . . . . . **91**

**Aisha Majrashi, Asmaa Khalil, Elham Al Nagshabandi and Abdulrahman Majrashi**
Stressors and Coping Strategies among Nursing Students during the COVID-19 Pandemic: Scoping Review
Reprinted from: *Nursing Reports* 2021, *11*, 444–459, doi:10.3390/nursrep11020042 . . . . . . . . . **103**

**Heather Naylor, Cynthia Hadenfeldt and Patricia Timmons**
Novice Nurses' Experiences Caring for Acutely Ill Patients during a Pandemic
Reprinted from: *Nursing Reports* 2021, *11*, 382–394, doi:10.3390/nursrep11020037 . . . . . . . . . **119**

**Gasmelseed Ahmed, Zainab Almoosa, Dalia Mohamed, Janepple Rapal, Ofelia Minguez, Issam Abu Khurma and et al.**
Healthcare Provider Attitudes toward the Newly Developed COVID-19 Vaccine: Cross-Sectional Study
Reprinted from: *Nursing Reports* 2021, *11*, 187–194, doi:10.3390/nursrep11010018 . . . . . . . . . **133**

**Son Chae Kim, Christine Sloan, Anna Montejano and Carlota Quiban**
Impacts of Coping Mechanisms on Nursing Students' Mental Health during COVID-19 Lockdown: A Cross-Sectional Survey
Reprinted from: *Nursing Reports* 2021, *11*, 36–44, doi:10.3390/nursrep11010004 . . . . . . . . . . . **141**

**Phillip Joy, Megan Aston, Sheri Price, Meaghan Sim, Rachel Ollivier, Britney Benoit and et al.**
Blessings and Curses: Exploring the Experiences of New Mothers during the COVID-19 Pandemic
Reprinted from: *Nursing Reports* 2020, *10*, 207–219, doi:10.3390/nursrep10020023 . . . . . . . . . **151**

**Athina E. Patelarou, Theocharis Konstantinidis, Evangelia Kartsoni, Enkeleint A. Mechili, Petros Galanis, Michail Zografakis-Sfakianakis and et al.**
Development and Validation of a Questionnaire to Measure Knowledge of and Attitude toward COVID-19 among Nursing Students in Greece
Reprinted from: *Nursing Reports* 2020, *10*, 82–94, doi:10.3390/nursrep10020012 . . . . . . . . . . . **165**

**Carlo V. Bellieni**
Nurses and Doctors Heroes? A Risky Myth of the COVID19 Era
Reprinted from: *Nursing Reports* 2020, *10*, 37–40, doi:10.3390/nursrep10020006 . . . . . . . . . . . **179**

**Abbas Al Mutair, Anas Amr, Zainab Ambani, Khulud Al Salman and Deborah Schwebius**
Nursing Surge Capacity Strategies for Management of Critically Ill Adults with COVID-19
Reprinted from: *Nursing Reports* 2020, *10*, 23–32, doi:10.3390/nursrep10010004 . . . . . . . . . . . **183**

# About the Editors

**Richard Gray**

Professor Richard Gray has been working at La Trobe University since 2017, becoming Theme Lead (Healthy Peoples Families and Communities) in 2021. He provides research leadership across La Trobe University, with an overall responsibility over the research theme of "Healthy People Families and Communities", facilitating research and industry opportunities in consultation and collaboration with Deans, Associate Deans, and Research Center Directors. Prof. Gray supports the Deputy Vice-Chancellor in the leadership and management of research at La Trobe University. He originally trained and worked as a Mental Health Nurse at the Maudsley Hospital in London before training in epidemiology and public health at the London School of Hygiene and Tropic Medicine. Subsequently, he has worked as a mental health services researcher focused on improving physical health outcomes for people experiencing mental ill-health, initially at the Institute of Psychiatry, King's College London, and later at the University of East Anglia and finally, La Trobe University. He is an Elsevier highly cited researcher, and his work has directly impacted the care and treatment of people experiencing mental ill-health in Australia and internationally. He is the Editor-in-Chief of Nursing Reports and is actively involved in the open science movement. He is a Fellow of the Royal Society of Public Health.

**Sonia Udod**

Dr. Sonia Udod has an active program of research in organizational leadership, the role of the nurse leader and nurse work environments. Her research focuses on nurse leader development, important for the creation of high-quality healthcare workplaces, leading to quality nurse, patient, and organizational outcomes. She is passionate about enhancing nurse leader capacity in the workplace and teaching students to be effective leaders. She has teaching expertise in leadership and management and advanced qualitative methods. She is committed to knowledge dissemination through peer-reviewed publications.

She has received numerous awards and scholarships, including the following: the Professional Nursing Award of Excellence in Research from the Association of Regulated Nurses of Manitoba, Top Researcher in Socio-Health, New Investigator Establishment Grant Award, Saskatchewan Health Research Foundation, Gail Donner Fellowship in Nursing, and Rosenstadt Doctoral Dissertation Award from the Faculty of Nursing, University of Toronto.

She has held several positions in service as Chair of the Leadership, Management and Policy Interest Group, Canadian Association Schools of Nursing, and International Director for the Association of Leadership Science in Nursing, and she is an inaugural member of the Leadership Institute in the Asper School of Business, University of Manitoba.

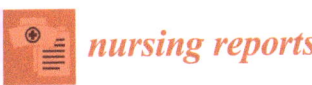 

Review

# Changes in Clinical Training for Nursing Students during the COVID-19 Pandemic: A Scoping Review

Catarina Lobão [1,*], Adriana Coelho [1,2], Vitor Parola [1,2], Hugo Neves [1,2], Joana Pereira Sousa [2,3] and Rui Gonçalves [1]

1. Health Sciences Research Unit: Nursing (UICISA: E), Nursing School of Coimbra (ESEnfC), 3000 Coimbra, Portugal
2. Portugal Centre for Evidence-Based Practice: A Joanna Briggs Institute Centre of Excellence (PCEBP), 3000 Coimbra, Portugal
3. School of Health Sciences—Polytechnic of Leiria, Center for Innovative Care and Health Technology—ciTechCare, 2411-901 Leiria, Portugal
* Correspondence: catarinalobao@esenfc.pt

**Abstract:** (1) Background: The COVID-19 pandemic has cost social, economic, cultural, and educational life, distressing nursing training and practice. This study aimed to map the literature on changes in clinical training for nursing students during the COVID-19 pandemic. (2) Methods: A scoping review was conducted according to JBI methodology's latest guidance. A set of relevant electronic databases and grey literature was searched to report results published in English, Spanish, and Portuguese. (3) Results: A total of 12 studies were included in the study, addressing changes in clinical training in undergraduate nursing students due to COVID-19 pandemic activity, published between 2020 and 2022. (4) Conclusions: Nursing schools made an effort to replace traditional clinical training with several activities, primarily based on simulation or virtual activities. However, contact with others is essential, and simulation programs or scenarios cannot provide it.

**Keywords:** changes; clinical training; COVID-19; nursing students; review

## 1. Introduction

The emergence and effect of the SARS-CoV-2 coronavirus transformed educational approaches, as clinical settings were no longer available for internship, and nursing schools had to replace and reshape clinical scenarios [1] by reinventing strategies and adjusting teaching, learning, and assessment methods in nursing education [2,3].

It created unprecedented opportunities for nursing education as it required creative teaching techniques to promote students' clinical learning, ensuring that the necessary learning outcomes and professional competencies were achieved [4,5].

The traditional clinical practice and face-to-face experiences were replaced by technological environments, for both students and faculty, with screen-based simulation [4], remote or virtual simulated learning experiences using commercial products or telehealth [6], and technology-enhanced storyboard techniques [7]. Moreover, nursing schools were unprepared for remote instruction transition during the COVID-19 pandemic, which challenged their curricula [5].

The discipline of nursing focuses on human reactions to health disease occurrences and life processes, where face-to-face nursing care is vital [8]. Thus, training students who will be qualified nurses caring for people involves developing specific skills, reflecting on role-playing discussions, exchanging clinical experiences, professional and multidiscipline relationships, and critical thinking [8].

The pandemic raised numerous challenges in teaching nursing students, specifically in the clinical context. This new reality allowed [9] students to achieve the required clinical hours and therefore complete their degrees if they were senior students. On the other hand,

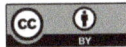

young nursing students had their clinical placements delayed due to rapid changes in the clinical environment. Conversely, lock-in policies forced junior students to discontinue or delay clinical education [9]. What alternatives were offered to these students?

According to JBI methodology and the previously published review protocol [10], we conducted a scoping review to map the changes in clinical training for undergraduate nursing students during the COVID-19 pandemic.

Moreover, it would be relevant to do this mapping at any level of education. The focus on undergraduate students is because the fundamentals of nursing are acquired in this period. During training, when undergraduate students receive the information and abilities that set nurses apart from laypeople as professional healthcare providers, it is a crucial time in the professional development of nursing students [11]. If it is compromised, the repercussions will manifest from the base of the nursing profession.

This review aims to understand how faculties adapted curricula to face the problem of inaccessibility to clinical settings and how academics developed programs to target clinical teaching, learning, and assessment strategies for nursing students in similar contexts. This map identified relevant topics on nursing education strategies to improve nursing students' knowledge development and helped identify potential research gaps. This mapping will support, in the near future, comparison studies between changes in teaching before and after the pandemic, and comparison studies between changes implemented temporarily and those which "came to stay".

An initial search of MEDLINE (PubMed), the J.B.I. Evidence Synthesis, the Cochrane Database of Systematic Reviews, PROSPERO, and Open Science Framework (O.S.F.) revealed that, currently, there are no scoping reviews or systematic reviews (published or in progress) about this subject [12–14].

This scoping review was developed to answer the following questions:

- What are the changes in clinical practice training for nursing students during the COVID-19 pandemic? (By change it means an alternative to clinical practice in context).
- What is the context of clinical practice training for nursing students where the changes are described? (By context it means the level/year of training).
- What are the academic and personal implications in the nursing student learning process? (By implications, it is intended to map the consequences of the training changes on a personal or academic level).

## 2. Materials and Methods

The JBI latest guidance methodology guided this scoping review [12–14], and was reported following the Preferred Reporting Items for Systematic Reviews and Meta-Analyses Extension for Scoping Reviews (PRISMA-ScR) guidelines [15]. This review protocol has been previously published [10].

### 2.1. Inclusion Criteria

According to the JBI recommendations mnemonic "P.C.C." for scoping reviews, the inclusion criteria were: **Participants**—Undergraduate nursing students. **Concept**—Studies exploring nursing students' clinical training changes during the COVID-19 pandemic. **Context**—Any clinical practice setting, independent of the country of the study. **Types of sources**—Studies with quantitative, qualitative, and mixed methods study design. In addition to these, all types of systematic review were considered.

### 2.2. Search Strategy

The search strategy was used to identify published and unpublished primary studies and reviews.

Two reviewers developed the search strategy and peer-review by an expert third reviewer who considered the Peer Review of Electronic Search Strategies (PRESS) checklist [16]. The JBI recommended that three-step search strategy was applied [12,14]. Records in English,

Spanish, and Portuguese were included to ensure a suitable selection procedure and data extraction.

The search strategy was adapted to the specificities of each information source. The databases searched included MEDLINE (via PubMed); CINAHL Complete (EBSCOhost); Cochrane Central Register of Controlled Trials; Cochrane Database of Systematic Reviews; LILACS; Scopus; and SciELO. The search for unpublished studies included DART-Europe and OpenGrey. As an example, the search strategy used for MEDLINE (via PubMed) is presented in Table 1. The search was structured in both Medical Subject Headings (MeSH) and text words shown in the literature. The terms were combined using truncation symbols and Boolean operators ("OR" and "AND"). Lastly, the reference lists of the articles included in the review were screened for supplementary papers.

**Table 1.** Search strategy for MEDLINE (via Pubmed) conducted on 28 March 2022.

| Search | Query | Record Retrieved |
|---|---|---|
| #1 | "students, nursing"[MeSH Terms] OR ("nurs*"[All Fields] AND "student*"[Title/Abstract]) | 59,061 |
| #2 | "clinical training"[Title/Abstract] OR "clinical learning"[Title/Abstract] OR "clinical placement"[Title/Abstract] OR "clinical practice"[Title/Abstract] OR "preceptorship"[MeSH Terms] | 232,745 |
| #3 | "covid 19"[MeSH Terms] OR "SARS-CoV-2"[MeSH Terms] OR "covid*"[Title/Abstract] OR "SARS-CoV-2"[Title/Abstract] | 237,488 |
| #4 | ("students, nursing"[MeSH Terms] OR ("nurs*"[All Fields] AND "student*"[Title/Abstract])) AND ("clinical training"[Title/Abstract] OR "clinical learning"[Title/Abstract] OR "clinical placement"[Title/Abstract] OR "clinical practice"[Title/Abstract] OR "preceptorship"[MeSH Terms]) AND ("covid 19"[MeSH Terms] OR "SARS-CoV-2"[MeSH Terms] OR "covid*"[Title/Abstract] OR "SARS-CoV-2"[Title/Abstract]) | 111 |

Study languages were restricted to those mastered by the authors—English, Spanish, and Portuguese—to ensure a good-quality selection procedure and data extraction. No time limit was considered in this review. However, the research has considered the COVID-19 pandemic; as such, all the studies included were dated equal to or greater than 2019.

Furthermore, since this scoping review aims to map the changes in clinical training for undergraduate nursing students during the COVID-19 pandemic, no rating of the methodological quality was provided, according to the JBI methodology, and as a result, practice recommendations were provided with caution. As mentioned by JBI "no assessment of methodological quality and formal synthesis takes place as part of a scoping review" [12].

*2.3. Study Selection and Screening Process*

All the records identified over database searching were retrieved and kept in Mendeley® V1.19.4 (Mendeley Ltd., Elsevier, Amsterdam, The Netherlands) and duplicates were removed. Two reviewers independently screened the titles and abstracts. A pilot test was made to verify whether inclusion criteria were met. The two independent reviewers assessed the full text of selected citations in detail against the inclusion criteria. The references of the included studies in the review were hand-searched. Disagreements among the two reviewers were solved through discussion or with a third reviewer. In the case of the inaccessible full article, the author was contacted [15].

## 3. Results

The data total of two hundred and fifty-nine studies were identified from the databases. After removing eighty-three duplicates, one hundred and seventy-six references remained. The titles and abstracts of these articles were reviewed, resulting in a total of sixty-six eligible records. After the complete reading of these records and application of the previously defined inclusion criteria, two were excluded because they were in a language different from those the research team spoke. Additionally, nine did not comply with the requirements referring to the population, six did not comply with the selected context, and thirty-seven were excluded due to the concept not being stipulated by the inclusion criteria.

As such, after the identification and screening phases of the review procedure (Figure 1), 12 studies were included in this review.

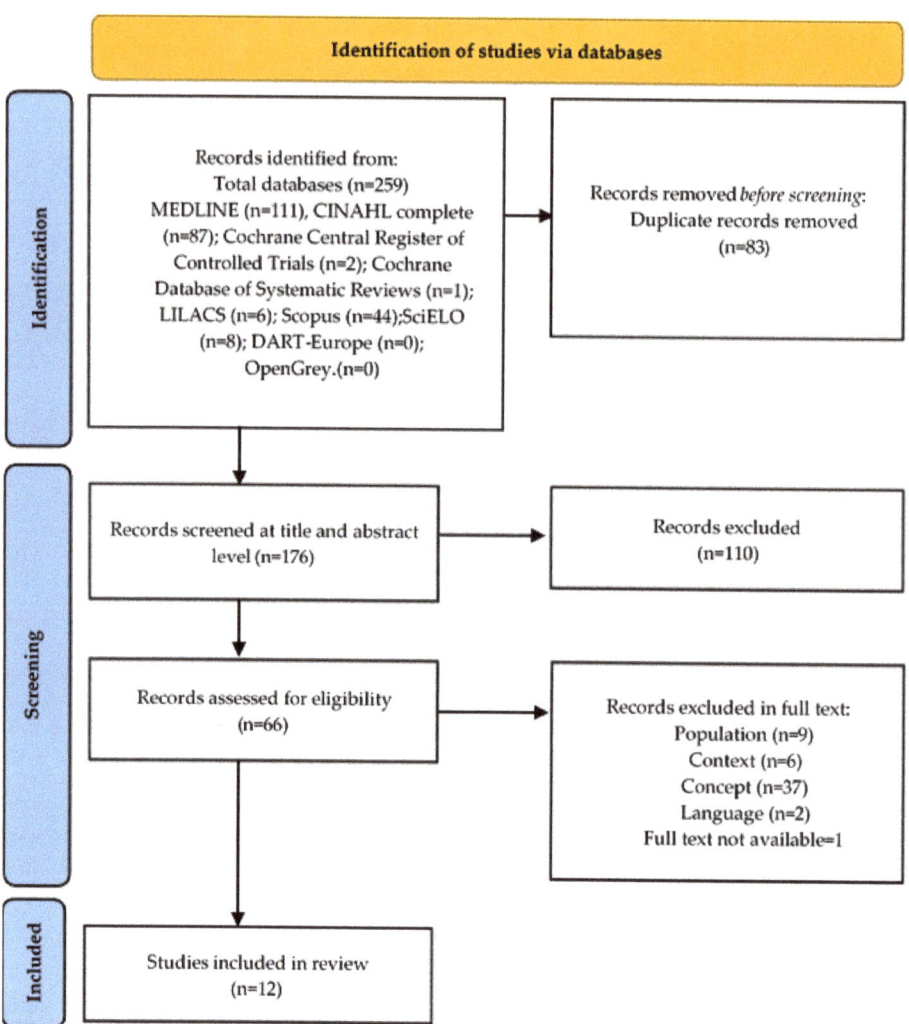

**Figure 1.** PRISMA Flowchart.

*Data Analysis and Presentation*

The characteristics of the included studies and the answers to the review question are summarised in Table 2. Of the twelve studies included in this review, one was conducted in Indonesia, six in the USA, one in Germany, one in Colombia, one in Hong Kong, and two in the Republic of Korea. The studies were published in the years 2020 ($n = 2$), 2021 ($n = 8$), and 2022 ($n = 2$).

**Table 2.** Articles included in the scoping review.

| Author Year Country | Population | Changes in Clinical Training | Context of Clinical Training | Implications |
|---|---|---|---|---|
| Anggraini, S., Chrisnawati, C. & Warjiman, W., 2022 Indonésia [17] | 30 nursing students | Applying the Hospital Clinical Practice Based Simulation (HCPBS) Model to the practical learning outcomes of nursing profession students. This model provides a practical experience close to hospital conditions in which professional nursing students gain experience in caring for patients, communicating with patients and families in role-play, and case management. | Nursing Profession stage | It was effective in increasing the practical learning achievement of nursing profession students. It was beneficial to review the theories that had been obtained previously. They have carried practice out in the form of practice both with friends and with phantoms so that they can still apply their expertise/skills according to theory. An effective learning strategy cannot replace real life but must be used as an addition to the learning process. |
| Banjo-Ogunnowo, S. & Chisholm, L., 2022 USA [18] | Nursing students (Licensed Vocational Nurses (LVN) to Associate Degree Nursing (ADN) students) | Uses virtual learning as an alternative to in-hospital clinic. Group 1 (traditional learning): students participated in four-hour classroom lectures, two 2-h labs, and one 12-h clinical experience per week for 8 weeks during the Spring 2019 semester. Group 2 (virtual learning): students participated in 4-h virtual lectures, two 2-h virtual lab sessions, and 12 h of virtual simulation using i-Human cases each week for 8 weeks during the COVID-19 pandemic. Group 1 and Group 2 participated in pre-conference and post-conference (debriefing) for each clinical or virtual simulation experience. | Maternal–pediatric course | No statistically significant difference was observed between the traditional and virtual learning groups. |
| Bode, S. et al., 2021 Germany [19] | 6 pediatric nursing students | 2 week-week rotation on the Interprofessional Training Ward in Pediatrics (IPAPAED) was replaced by the Interprofessional COVID-19 Replacement Program (I-reCovEr) in four 60-min face-to-face sessions. | Interprofessional training ward in pediatrics | No differences were observed. |
| Bradford, H. et al., 2021 Columbia [20] | Midwifery and Women's Health Nurse Practitioner | It used synchronous and asynchronous simulations for formative learning. A majority of students accessed one or more of these simulations: Adapted simulation opportunities: objective structured clinical examinations (synchronous), IUD—intrauterine device training (synchronous), trigger films (synchronous or asynchronous), bilateral learning tools (asynchronous), and suturing skills simulations (synchronous). | Women's health nursing | These simulation opportunities serve as valuable adjuncts to traditional learning and provide a levelling of experience to students with variable accessibility and capability to engage in the clinical setting. Some virtual opportunities may be implemented before entry to the clinical setting to promote skill acquisition, use of person-centered language, and student confidence. Simulated clinical experiences are an evidence-based approach for developing and enhancing the acquisition of clinical and communication skills, decision-making, and self-confidence. Provides readiness to begin or return to the clinical setting. |
| Cowperthwait, A., et al., 2021 USA [21] | 80 senior undergraduate students | Clinical practice was replaced by simulation. | Psychiatric mental health | It was valued as a reflective pause in the middle of the simulation was possible; students learned by watching other colleagues interact with the same patient; the ability to discuss following responses or important lines; receiving feedback. |
| Fung, J. et al., 2021 Hong Kong [22] | 188 final-year nursing undergraduate students | A virtual simulation education program with debriefing replaces the traditional clinical practicum in the COVID-19 situation. | Medical and surgical cases | A significant improvement was perceived by students in clinical competence and the nursing process. Self-efficacy has also been boosted. Communication and critical thinking were applied better in the traditional clinical environment. |
| Hassler, L. et al., 2021 USA [23] | 98 s-degree nursing students and 11 clinical groups | Flipped clinical practice: synchronized remote clinical experience to simulate the experience of the traditional hospital setting | Students had to choose one clinical specialty: adult health, mental health, pediatrics or obstetrics. | The flipped clinical experience was a successful methodology to reinforce clinical concepts. |
| Hwang, H. & Chun, Y., 2021 Republic of Korea [24] | 59 randomly expressed nursing students: ($n = 30$) experimental group; ($n = 29$) control group | Clinical practice education using virtual reality. The experimental group used the vSim of a nursing program, and the control group of nursing students did not use the vSim of a nursing program as an alternative practice for clinical practice. | | Applying and not applying simulation clinical practice education using virtual reality positively affected critical thinking disposition and clinical practice performance, but it was not statistically significant. |
| Kim, M., Kang, H. & Gagne, J., 2021 Republic of Korea [25] | 20 nursing students | Use of virtual simulation as an alternative to clinical practice for nursing with six steps: (a) suggested reading, (b) pre-simulation quizzes that provide students with an overview of the contents, (c) interactive clinical nursing scenarios authorized by the NLN, (d) post-simulation quizzes, (e) documentation assignments, and (f) guided reflection questions. | "Unspecified information" | Difficulties were encountered in using the virtual simulation because students needed to use English, which was not their native language and some specific cultural differences; Benefits to student confidence and competence in providing patient-centered care: it allowed the user to care for patients from admission to discharge by themselves, and they were able to self-assess and strengthen their skills through repeated questionnaires, a feedback log, and reflection. Gaps in satisfaction due to a need for improvement: some students reported a lack of reality and the limited function of the vs. and stated that the vs. differs fundamentally from reality. The care is given by pressing buttons rather than by communicating directly with, and providing nursing care to, patients, thus allowing certain essential activities to be ignored. |
| Revell, S. et al., 2022 USA [26] | 93 undergraduate nurse students | Traditional clinical hours were supplemented with 18 h of on-campus simulation experiences, 6 self-paced case studies, participation in COVID-19 vaccination and/or testing clinic activities, and two 2-h synchronous online seminars. The students developed 2 scholarly journals focused on reflection and application of knowledge to clinical practice as well as a self-reflection paper. | Medical–surgical | Transformative learning was evident in the writing of the students. Students demonstrated response to change, discovering resilience, developing confidence, finding gratitude, embracing advocacy, and transforming and becoming a nurse. Students recognized the opportunities mentorship afforded them, despite challenges. |

**Table 2.** Cont.

| Author Year Country | Population | Changes in Clinical Training | Context of Clinical Training | Implications |
|---|---|---|---|---|
| Shea, K. & Rovera, E., 2020 USA [27] | 244 nursing students | Using virtual simulations and remote simulations as telehealth with standardized patients provided an alternative for 50% of the required direct patient care hours during the COVID-19 pandemic and campus closure. | Nursing Fundamentals and Community Health Promotion and Wellness Reproductive Health and Mental Health Medical/Surgical and Pediatrics Advanced Medical/Surgical and Community Health | The inability to complete the required clinical hours can delay the graduation dates of some students, disrupting the new nurses entering the workforce. Finding ways to replace clinical practice hours with simulation activities has become a priority. |
| Wands, L., Geller, D., & Hallman, M., 2020 USA [28] | 42 senior nursing students | Over 4 weeks, students collectively logged over 1200 h of simulation time, attending approximately 100 sessions. Students used 4 free online simulation programs to substitute in-person clinical experiences:<br>- Canadian Alliance of Nurse Educators Using Simulation (CAN-Sim). High-quality video-based virtual simulations focus on adult acute care scenarios involving medical diagnoses of urosepsis, diabetic ketoacidosis, and respiratory distress;<br>- The Virtual Healthcare Experience with an opportunity to explore a virtual hospital with five different departments: emergency, pediatrics, medical–surgical, maternal and child, and mental;<br>- National League for Nursing's (NLN) Advancing Care Excellence Series in the form of clinical scenarios with six vulnerable populations: pediatrics, veterans, seniors, individuals with disabilities, Alzheimer's patients, and caregivers of individuals with Alzheimer's;<br>- Augmented Reality Integrated Simulation Education (ARISE) included simulation scenarios containing real-life storylines with four levels that increase in complexity from basic assessment to crisis. Scenarios cover the topics of chest pain, heart failure, wound management, pediatric asthma, obstetrics, therapeutic communication, and end-of-life. | "Unspecified information" | The students reported experiencing positive growth in confidence in their assessment skills, ability to prioritise care and interventions, communication with patients and their families and the health care team, and providing interventions that foster patient safety. Less positive aspects included difficulties encountered when trying to manage multiple technological devices to display videos or other materials from websites, sessions being cancelled on short notice, and the inability to ensure student engagement if the student did not turn on or keep their camera on |

The first study analysed was conducted by Anggraini, Chrisnawati, and Warjiman (2022) [17] in Indonesia, targeting 30 nursing students during clinical nursing training. To continue the training of those students, they used a simulation program that proved beneficial in reviewing the theories obtained previously (Table 2).

The study by Banjo-Ogunnowo and Chisholm (2022) [18] was conducted on nursing students who were developing their learning in the maternal–pediatric course. They used virtual learning as an alternative to clinical practice in hospital settings (Table 2).

The third study [19] analyzed was developed by a team of researchers from Germany. In this study, nursing students received the interprofessional COVID-19 substitution program (I-reCovEr) during clinical teaching in a pediatric setting (Table 2).

Another study included [20] was conducted in Columbia (U.S.A.) by Bradford et al. (2021) with midwifery and women's health nurse practitioner students. Synchronous and asynchronous simulation sessions were offered for their formative learning. These simulation opportunities served as valuable adjuncts to traditional learning and provided a level of experiences to students with unequal access and capability to engage in the clinical setting (Table 2).

In the study developed by Cowperthwait et al. (2021) [21], during clinical training in psychiatric mental health nursing, eighty senior undergraduate students were allocated to a simulation that replaced the physical clinical context. The main benefits emphasized by the students were the reflection developed during the simulation sessions, the opportunity to receive feedback, and the learning acquired through the observation of other colleagues in the interaction with the same patients (Table 2).

Fung et al. (2021) [22] conducted a study in Hong Kong with 188 final-year undergraduate nursing students. In this study, a virtual simulation educational program replaced traditional clinical practice in medical and surgical cases with debriefing. In the students' perception, this educational program was beneficial in developing clinical competence and the nursing process. However, communication and critical thinking were better applied in the traditional clinical setting (Table 2).

In a study by Hassler et al. (2021) [23], flipped clinical practice was analysed through a synchronized remote clinical experience in one clinical specialty chosen by 98 s-year nursing students. Students emphasized that they saw the methodology as successful to reinforce clinical concepts to simulate the experiences of the traditional hospital setting's clinical training (Table 2).

Another study included in this scoping review and developed by Hwang and Chun (2021) [24] put into evidence the use of clinical practice education with virtual reality in the Republic of Korea (Table 2). Fifty-nine nursing students were divided into two groups. In this study, the experimental group was exposed to the vSim nursing program as an alternative practice to the traditional clinical practice using virtual reality. Their results showed positive benefits in clinical thinking and clinical practice performance but without wide statistical significance.

From the Republic of Korea arrived the study of Kim, Kang, and Gagne (2021) [25], which highlighted the use of a six step virtual simulation alternative program to the traditional nursing clinical practice (Table 2). The proposed six step virtual simulation alternative program evidenced the difficulties perceived by the students in using a non-native language and the impact of the specific cultural differences shown in the scenarios. On the other hand, the developed confidence and competence in providing patient-centered care were shown as benefits of virtual simulation.

The study by Revell et al. (2022) [26] disclosed the results of supplementing the traditional clinical period with an 18-h simulated experiences pack (Table 2). The authors revealed the evidence of transformative learning expressed by students. The sample of undergraduate nursing students demonstrated an evident response to the change and challenges, discovering and developing other professional competencies and skills.

In 2020, Shea and Rovera [27] developed a study with two hundred and forty-four nursing students exposed to virtual and remote simulations as telehealth with standardized patients as an alternative of half of the clinical practice hours (Table 2). During the health emergency period and the university campus closure, every effort was needed to replace clinical practice hours and stop the interruption of the nursing graduation process with simulation activities in different clinical areas.

The last analyzed study, developed by Wands, Geller, and Hallman (2020) [28], presents to the scientific community a four-week simulation program with forty-two nursing students to substitute their in-person clinical experiences (Table 2). By using four free online simulation programs, logged over 1200 h, the students referred to experiencing positive growth in different professional competencies and skills despite difficulties when trying to manage multiple devices to access the virtual sessions and materials.

Our findings show that nursing schools made an effort to replace traditional clinical training with several activities, primarily based on simulation or virtual activities, allowing students to improve their abilities in caretaking [17,18,21,24,25,27,28]. Simulation sessions were structured in steps, with suggested reading, pre- and post-simulation quizzes, interactive clinical scenarios, and reflection [25,26]. They improved communication skills by role-playing, gaining experience in practical activities, and flipping clinical practice to replicate traditional care [17,20,23]. Scholarly journals were also proposed to enhance reflection and knowledge acquisition by virtual clinical practice [26].

After simulation sessions, debriefing moments were taken where simulation and case management were analyzed [18,22] or replaced by online seminars [26].

One of the included articles, Banjo-Ogunnowo and Chisholm (2022) [18], mention as a strategy the use of a virtual platform—the i-Human platform was widely used to assess case scenarios, including patient history, physical assessment, defining nursing diagnoses, and prioritizing interventions [18,29], although other virtual platforms were used by universities [30,31].

The primary contexts varied from maternal–pediatric [18,19,23,27], women's health [20], psychiatric mental health [21,23,27], medical–surgical health [22,26,27], adult health [23], nursing fundamentals/profession stage [17,27], and community health promotion and wellness reproductive health [27].

## 4. Discussion

In this scoping review, we identified twelve primary studies, mainly from the U.S.A., addressing changes in clinical training in undergraduate nursing students due to COVID-19 pandemic activity, published between 2020 and 2022.

Concerning the simulation time, the included articles varied in context and ranged from 18 h to 8 weeks of rotation [18,19,26,28].

The adoption of virtual lessons allowed each nursing school to define clinical training replacement time, letting students progress at their graduation level. At the end of the program, students reported that this learning methodology enabled them to continue clinical training, with advantages in reviewing concepts, nursing theories, and applying them in simulation scenarios or later engaging in clinical settings [17,20]. Reflective and debriefing periods were viewed as positive. Professor–student and student–student interaction encouraged discussion, feedback, and interchange of opinions [21,22], analysis of clinical competencies and information to include in the nursing process [22,24], and clinical concepts reinforcement [23]. A positive modification in students' attitudes was also noticed, such as confidence, resilience, gratitude, or embracing advocacy [20,25,26,28]. On the other hand, managing multiple technological devices for videos or website material was more challenging. Additionally, simulation widgets in the English language were hard to understand for those whose native language was not English and simulations were not adapted to cultural users' differences [25]. The lack of understanding of simulation widgets in English among non-native speakers could be attributed to language barriers, where individuals may not have a good command of the English language, making it challenging for them to understand technical terms and concepts. Additionally, cultural differences could play a role, as certain phrases or expressions may not be familiar to individuals from different cultures. To address these challenges, it may be necessary to provide language and cultural adaptations to simulation widgets. As technology advances, the need for technical skills and understanding will likely increase, making it even more critical to bridging language and cultural barriers.

The Pandemic made it challenging for nursing schools to adapt their curricula to allow students to continue their practice and advance at their graduation level. Each school sets a different program, adjusting to its needs, making its comparison difficult. Overall, synchronous or hybrid virtual classes narrowed relations between professors and students. Narrowed relations refer to the potentially reduced level of interaction and engagement between professors and students in virtual or hybrid learning environments compared to face-to-face classes. In a virtual or hybrid setting, students may feel more disconnected from their professors and peers, which can decrease the quality of interaction, collaboration, and feedback. Depending on each context, setting specific scenarios allowed a deeper reflection on practice, connecting concepts and theories. However, users also had to invest time in acquiring technological competencies, which could be time-consuming and challenge the learning process. The interaction between users and simulation programs was centered on pressing buttons rather than the natural interaction between carer and cared [25].

The results were similar when comparing clinical practice education with virtual reality and traditional learning. There were no observed differences between these two learning approaches [18,19,24], although both improved learning abilities, mainly on previous practice before clinical training, in conjunction with reflection on person-centered needs, developing communication skills, and performing decision-making in a controlled environment [17,20].

The simulation was not new in nursing, where specific practices were already used, such as resuscitation or technical training before clinical practice [32]. The pandemic set a new view for the patient through the usage of technological widgets. Clinical practice was replaced by virtual scenarios, in which the interaction between participants (students and professors) promoted a richness of sharing.

A potential limitation of this scoping review was that only studies published in English, Portuguese, and Spanish were included. Articles published in other languages may potentially add information to this review's results. Furthermore, since the objective of this scoping review was to map, no rating of the methodological quality was used. In contrast to systematic reviews where implications or recommendations for practice are a key feature, scoping reviews are not designed to underpin clinical practice decisions; therefore, the assessment of methodological quality or risk of bias of included studies (which is critical when reporting effect size estimates) does not occur [33].

Finally, the concept "changes" was not included in the search strategy in order not to exclude potential studies relevant to the present review.

## 5. Conclusions

The impact of the coronavirus pandemic created the need to reinvent strategies and readjust teaching, learning, and assessment processes in nursing education, namely in a clinical context. This scoping review identified twelve primary studies about changes in clinical training for nursing students during the COVID-19 pandemic published between 2020 and 2022. This mapping shows that the pandemic made it challenging for nursing schools to adapt their curricula to allow students to continue their practice and advance at their graduation level.

In this sense, nursing schools tried to replace traditional clinical training with several activities based on simulation or virtual activities. However, contact with others is essential, and simulation programs or scenarios cannot provide it. Simulation is essential for skill development, however, developing technical and non-technical skills simultaneously requires direct contact with patients.

More studies should be carried out within the scope of the long-term consequences of adopting these methodologies in nursing practice.

**Author Contributions:** Conceptualization: C.L., A.C., R.G., V.P., H.N., and J.P.S.; Validation: V.P. and H.N.; Writing—initial draft preparation: C.L., A.C., R.G., V.P., H.N., and J.P.S.; Writing—review and editing: C.L., A.C., R.G., V.P., H.N., and J.P.S. All authors have read and agreed to the published version of the manuscript.

**Funding:** This research received no external funding.

**Institutional Review Board Statement:** Not applicable.

**Informed Consent Statement:** Not applicable.

**Data Availability Statement:** Not applicable.

**Acknowledgments:** The authors wish to acknowledge the Health Sciences Research Unit: Nursing, Nursing School of Coimbra, Portugal and the Portugal Centre for Evidence-Based Practice: a Joanna Briggs Institute Centre of Excellence, Portugal.

**Conflicts of Interest:** The authors declare no conflict of interest.

## References

1. Silva, F.T.M.; Kubrusly, M.; Peixoto Junior, A.A.; Vieira, L.X.S.D.S.; Augusto, K.L. Adaptations and Repercussions in the Experiences in a Hybrid Education University during the Sars-CoV-2 Pandemic TT-Adaptações e Repercussões Nas Vivências Em Escola de Ensino Híbrido Durante a Pandemia Por Sars-CoV-2. *Rev. Bras. Educ. Med.* **2021**, *45*, e068. [CrossRef]
2. Agu, C.F.; Stewart, J.; McFarlane-Stewart, N.; Rae, T. COVID-19 Pandemic Effects on Nursing Education: Looking through the Lens of a Developing Country. *Int. Nurs. Rev.* **2021**, 1–6. [CrossRef]
3. dos Santos Ferreira, A.M.; Príncipe, F.; Pereira, H.; Oliveira, I.; Mota, L. COVimpact: Pandemia COVID-19 Nos Estudantes Do Ensino Superior Da Saúde. *Rev. Investig. Inovação em Saúde* **2020**, *3*, 7–16. [CrossRef]

4. Leighton, K.; Kardong-Edgren, S.; Schneidereith, T.; Foisy-Doll, C.; Wuestney, K.A. Meeting Undergraduate Nursing Students' Clinical Needs: A Comparison of Traditional Clinical, Face-to-Face Simulation, and Screen-Based Simulation Learning Environments. *Nurse Educ.* **2021**, *46*, 349–354. [CrossRef]
5. Bourgault, A.; Mayerson, E.; Nai, M.; Orsini-Garry, A.; Alexander, I.M. Implications of the COVID-19 Pandemic: Virtual Nursing Education for Delirium Care. *J. Prof. Nurs.* **2022**, *38*, 54–64. [CrossRef] [PubMed]
6. Kazawa, K.; Teramoto, C.; Azechi, A.; Satake, H.; Moriyama, M. Undergraduate Nursing Students' Learning Experiences of a Telehealth Clinical Practice Program during the COVID-19 Pandemic: A Qualitative Study. *Nurse Educ. Today* **2022**, *111*. [CrossRef]
7. Roberts, M.L.; Mazurak, J.O.E. Virtual Clinical Experiences in Nursing Education: Applying a Technology-Enhanced Storyboard Technique to Facilitate Contextual Learning in Remote Environments. *Nurs. Educ. Perspect.* **2021**. [CrossRef] [PubMed]
8. Lira, A.L.B.D.C.; Adamy, E.K.; Teixeira, E.; Silva, F.V.D. Educação Em Enfermagem: Desafios e Perspectivas Em Tempos Da Pandemia COVID-19. *Rev. Bras. Enferm.* **2020**, *73*, e20200683. [CrossRef] [PubMed]
9. Swift, A.; Banks, L.; Baleswaran, A.; Cooke, N.; Little, C.; McGrath, L.; Meechan-Rogers, R.; Neve, A.; Rees, H.; Tomlinson, A.; et al. COVID-19 and Student Nurses: A View from England. *J. Clin. Nurs.* **2020**, *29*, 3111–3114. [CrossRef]
10. Lobão, C.; Coelho, A.; Gonçalves, R.; Parola, V.; Neves, H.; Sousa, J.P. Changes in Clinical Training for Nursing Students during the COVID-19 Pandemic: A Scoping Review Protocol. *Nurs. Rep.* **2022**, *12*, 210–216. [CrossRef] [PubMed]
11. Lundell Rudberg, S.; Westerbotn, M.; Sormunen, T.; Scheja, M.; Lachmann, H. Undergraduate Nursing Students' Experiences of Becoming a Professional Nurse: A Longitudinal Study. *BMC Nurs.* **2022**, *21*, 1–10. [CrossRef] [PubMed]
12. Peters, M.D.J.; Godfrey, C.; Mcinerney, P.; Munn, Z.; Tricco, A.C.; Khalil, H. Chapter 11: Scoping Reviews. In *JBI Manual for Evidence Synthesis*; Aromataris, E., Munn, Z., Eds.; JBI: Adelaide, Australia, 2020.
13. Khalil, H.; Peters, M.; Godfrey, C.M.; McInerney, P.; Soares, C.B.; Parker, D. An Evidence-Based Approach to Scoping Reviews. *Worldviews Evid.-Based Nurs.* **2016**, *13*, 118–123. [CrossRef]
14. Peters, M.D.J.; Marnie, C.; Tricco, A.C.; Pollock, D.; Munn, Z.; Alexander, L.; McInerney, P.; Godfrey, C.M.; Khalil, H. Updated Methodological Guidance for the Conduct of Scoping Reviews. *JBI Evid. Synth.* **2020**, *18*, 2119–2126. [CrossRef] [PubMed]
15. Tricco, A.C.; Lillie, E.; Zarin, W.; Brien, K.K.O.; Colquhoun, H.; Levac, D.; Moher, D.; Peters, M.D.J.; Ma, Q.; Horsley, T.; et al. PRISMA Extension for Scoping Reviews (PRISMA-ScR): Checklist and Explanation. *Ann. Intern. Med.* **2018**. [CrossRef]
16. McGowan, J.; Sampson, M.; Salzwedel, D.M.; Cogo, E.; Foerster, V.; Lefebvre, C. PRESS Peer Review of Electronic Search Strategies: 2015 Guideline Statement. *J. Clin. Epidemiol.* **2016**, *75*, 40–46. [CrossRef]
17. Anggraini, S.; Chrisnawati, C.; Warjiman, W. The Effectiveness of the Implementation of the Hospital Clinical Practice Based Simulation Model on the Practice Learning Outcomes of Nurse Profession Students During the Covid-19. *Indones. Nurs. J. Educ. Clin.* **2021**, *6*, 185–191. [CrossRef]
18. Banjo-Ogunnowo, S.; Chisholm, L. Virtual versus Traditional Learning during COVID-19: Quantitative Comparison of Outcomes for Two Articulating ADN Cohorts. *Teach. Learn. Nurs.* **2022**. [CrossRef]
19. Bode, S.; Dürkop, A.; Wilcken, H.; Peters, S.; Straub, C. Interprofessional Learning during Sars-Cov-2 (Covid-19) Pandemic Conditions: The Learning Project i-Recover as a Substitute for a Rotation on an Interprofessional Training Ward. *GMS J. Med. Educ.* **2021**, *38*, 1–8. [CrossRef]
20. Bradford, H.M.; Farley, C.L.; Escobar, M.; Heitzler, E.T.; Tringali, T.; Walker, K.C. Rapid Curricular Innovations During COVID-19 Clinical Suspension: Maintaining Student Engagement with Simulation Experiences. *J. Midwifery Womens. Health* **2021**, *66*, 366–371. [CrossRef]
21. Cowperthwait, A.; Graber, J.; Carlsen, A.; Cowperthwait, M.; Mekulski, H. Innovations in Virtual Education for Clinical and Simulation Learning. *J. Prof. Nurs.* **2021**, *37*, 1011–1017. [CrossRef] [PubMed]
22. Fung, J.T.C.; Zhang, W.; Yeung, M.N.; Pang, M.T.H.; Lam, V.S.F.; Chan, B.K.Y.; Wong, J.Y.-H. Evaluation of Students' Perceived Clinical Competence and Learning Needs Following an Online Virtual Simulation Education Programme with Debriefing during the COVID-19 Pandemic. *Nurs. Open* **2021**, *8*, 3045–3054. [CrossRef] [PubMed]
23. Hassler, L.J.; Moscarella, D.; Easley, L.; Olaode, S. Flipped Clinical Teaching: Battling COVID-19 With Creative and Active Pedagogy. *J. Nurs. Educ.* **2021**, *60*, 534–537. [CrossRef] [PubMed]
24. Hwang, H.-Y.; Chun, Y.-E. Simulation Clinical Practice Education That Combines Virtual Reality Effects on Clinical Thinking Disposition and Clinical Practice Performance. *Rev. Int. Geogr. Educ. Online* **2021**, *11*, 246–253.
25. Kim, M.J.; Kang, H.S.; De Gagne, J.C. Nursing Students' Perceptions and Experiences of Using Virtual Simulation During the COVID-19 Pandemic. *Clin. Simul. Nurs.* **2021**, *60*, 11–17. [CrossRef] [PubMed]
26. Revell, S.M.H.; Sethares, K.A.; Chin, E.D.; Kellogg, M.B.; Armstrong, D.; Reynolds, T. A Transformative Learning Experience for Senior Nursing Students. *Nurse Educ.* **2022**, *47*, 161–167. [CrossRef]
27. Shea, K.L.; Rovera, E.J. Preparing for the COVID-19 Pandemic and Its Impact on a Nursing Simulation Curriculum. *J. Nurs. Educ.* **2021**, *60*, 52–55. [CrossRef]
28. Wands, L.; Geller, D.E.; Hallman, M. Positive Outcomes of Rapid Freeware Implementation to Replace Baccalaureate Student Clinical Experiences. *J. Nurs. Educ.* **2020**, *59*, 701–704. [CrossRef]
29. Weston, J.; Zauche, L.H. Comparison of Virtual Simulation to Clinical Practice for Prelicensure Nursing Students in Pediatrics. *Nurse Educ.* **2021**, *46*, E95–E98. [CrossRef] [PubMed]

30. Verkuyl, M.; Lapum, J.L.; St-Amant, O.; Hughes, M.; Romaniuk, D. Curricular Uptake of Virtual Gaming Simulation in Nursing Education. *Nurse Educ. Pract.* **2021**, *50*, 102967. [CrossRef]
31. Callender, L.F.; LuValle Johnson, A.; Clark, J.N.; Terrero de la Osa, A. Coordinating Clinical Rotations During the Novel Corona Virus 2 Pandemic. *J. Nurs. Educ.* **2021**, *60*, 394–396. [CrossRef]
32. Glasper, A. Simulation and Student Learning: Will NMC Policy Lead to Lasting Change? *Br. J. Nurs.* **2021**, *30*, 498–499. [CrossRef] [PubMed]
33. Peters, M.D.J.; Marnie, C.; Colquhoun, H.; Garritty, C.M.; Hempel, S.; Horsley, T.; Langlois, E.V.; Lillie, E.; O'Brien, K.K.; Tunçalp, Ö.; et al. Scoping Reviews: Reinforcing and Advancing the Methodology and Application. *Syst. Rev.* **2021**, *10*, 263. [CrossRef] [PubMed]

**Disclaimer/Publisher's Note:** The statements, opinions and data contained in all publications are solely those of the individual author(s) and contributor(s) and not of MDPI and/or the editor(s). MDPI and/or the editor(s) disclaim responsibility for any injury to people or property resulting from any ideas, methods, instructions or products referred to in the content.

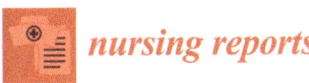 

*Review*

# Virtual Practical Examination for Student Nurse Educators in Health Sciences Education during the COVID-19 Pandemic: A Narrative Review

**Kholofelo Lorraine Matlhaba**

Department of Health Studies, University of South Africa, Pretoria 0002, South Africa; matlhkl@unisa.ac.za; Tel.: +27-12-429-2073

**Abstract:** (1) Background: There is a gap in the literature that explores challenges and opportunities relating to virtual or e-assessment health science education with particular relevance to the Health Sciences Education practical examination for student nurse educators. Therefore, this review aimed to address this gap and provide recommendations for enhancing identified opportunities and for overcoming identified challenges.; (2) Methods: The review was conducted across Google Scholar, PubMed/MEDLINE, Science Direct, Directory of Open Access Journals, Complementary Index, SCOPUS, and the Cumulative Index to Nursing and Allied Health Literature (CINAHL) with the intention of identifying opportunities and challenges presented by e-assessment in the HSE practical examination for student nurse educators during the COVID-19 pandemic.; (3) Results: The following aspects are discussed: (1) opportunities, including benefits, for both student nurse educators and facilitators and opportunities for Nursing Education; and (2) challenges, including issues with accessibility and connectivity as well as the attitudes of both students and facilitators.; (4) Conclusions: Despite challenges which included connectivity issues that led to frustration and stress, the unpreparedness and attitudes of students and facilitators, there are some opportunities that have emerged from e-assessment that can be beneficial to both the students and the facilitators, as well as the institutions. These include a reduced administrative burden, improved teaching and learning, and immediate feedback from facilitators to students and from students to facilitators.

**Keywords:** student nurse educators; e-assessment; virtual practical examination; health sciences education

**Citation:** Matlhaba, K.L. Virtual Practical Examination for Student Nurse Educators in Health Sciences Education during the COVID-19 Pandemic: A Narrative Review. *Nurs. Rep.* **2023**, *13*, 214–229. https://doi.org/10.3390/nursrep13010021

**Academic Editors:** Richard Gray and Sonia Udod

Received: 10 December 2022
Revised: 2 February 2023
Accepted: 3 February 2023
Published: 8 February 2023

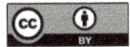

**Copyright:** © 2023 by the author. Licensee MDPI, Basel, Switzerland. This article is an open access article distributed under the terms and conditions of the Creative Commons Attribution (CC BY) license (https://creativecommons.org/licenses/by/4.0/).

## 1. Introduction

Assessment is a crucial element of any effective teaching and learning strategy [1] at all stages of education, particularly in higher education in the Human and Health Sciences. Within teaching and learning in the Health Sciences, physical examination skills are essential to the practice of clinical care, and students traditionally study and practice their physical skills in person in a particular setting, because this involves considerable time spent on hands-on learning [2]. The same notion is shared with Nursing Education, whereby student nurse educators practice their teaching skills and are assessed on those skills.

In March 2020, the World Health Organization (WHO) declared the highly infectious and deadly COVID-19 disease to be a worldwide pandemic. The COVID-19 pandemic, first confirmed in December 2019, is defined as the worldwide spread of a disease caused by a new coronavirus labelled SARS-CoV-2 [3]. In this review, pandemic refers to the worldwide spread of that disease which forced a sudden change and transition from physical assessment strategies to online or virtual strategies. The majority of higher education institutions including health profession educators (HPEs) across the world had to transition from physical teaching and learning strategies to online strategies for emergency remote learning [4]. Continued pandemic restrictions imposed on face-to-face learning resulted in a decision to permanently transition a graduate nursing education advanced assessment course from a hybrid one to online learning [5–9]. With online learning, learning takes place partially or entirely over the Internet, making it an ideal course delivery model for adult learners wishing to develop new skills and competencies [10]. It is noticeable that online learning has become one of the most popular educational alternatives to meet the demands of today's global knowledge economy [11].

## 1.1. Background

Online assessment is a system that involves assessments through the web or intranet [12]. Supporting the above-mentioned definition, [13] define online assessment as an e-system that involves assessment of students in an online context. The use of technology in assessment first began in the 1920s, and e-assessment enhances the measurement of learner outcomes, making it possible for them to obtain immediate and direct feedback [7]. With e-assessment, online or virtual assessment is witnessing significant changes to compliment the e-learning strategies established as a result of the pandemic. In this narrative review, the terms online assessment, virtual assessment and e-assessment are used interchangeably. Online assessment is used to assess applied knowledge and skills that can be assessed online [14].

Among their other roles and competencies, nurse educators are expected to execute professional teaching of knowledge and skills to facilitate teaching and learning, enable learner development, and supports learners' continuous life-long learning [15]. In this regard, the student nurse educators are assessed on their skills in preparation of their journey to becoming competent nurse educators. It has been suggested that there is a need for formal preparation for nurse educators who foster the ongoing development of nurses in clinical practice; therefore, nurse educators, regardless of the setting in which they work or are preparing to work, must receive formal instruction about online teaching [16].

## 1.2. Online or Virtual Practical Examination

There are several virtual or online practical examinations assessed in the literature including virtual streaming and screen activity recordings. These online practical examinations are conducted through the form of live streaming, video-conferencing style platforms that provide the opportunity to have several participants at a time. These platforms are mainly laptop and/or mobile phone app based, where an individual speaking directly to the camera on a mobile phone has the facility to invite several people to chat on-screen simultaneously.

Based on the literature, video conferencing seems to be the method utilised for medical and nursing students' virtual examinations. Several web-based video-conferencing platforms have emerged over the last decade that deliver audio, video, and screen-sharing experiences across various devices, enabling users to host webinars, virtual meetings, video demonstrations, video-conferences, and online training [17]. Video conferencing, as another method of virtual practical examination, offers assessors the potential for distance assessment of student skills. Online practical examinations such as webinars enhance students' knowledge and confidence, and have increasingly been adopted for continuing medical education [18]. It is suggested that due to their wide accessibility, webinars are a way of conferencing that can facilitate learning while ensuring high quality at low cost. Furthermore, webinars enable teachers to share information with students anywhere and at any time using different Internet-capable devices [19]. However, even though the use of video-conferencing has been utilised in the past by some HSE institutions, common barriers reported with this type of virtual assessment include instability of connection and lack of on-site technology and instructional design support. This narrative intends to provide an understanding of the synthesised opportunities and challenges presented by online practical examinations that emerged during the COVID-19 pandemic.

## 1.3. Health Sciences Education (HSE) Practical Examination for Student Nurse Educators

HSE is a specialised area that prepares students for a variety of careers related to medicine, dentistry and nursing. Assessment in HSE has become extremely critical, and learner assessment regimes need to have the capacity to accurately evaluate competences that include attitude, skills and the knowledge acquired during the training of healthcare professionals [20]. In South Africa, as in other countries, professional nurses who are intending to specialise in nursing education must undergo additional training at an accredited university in order to be registered as nurse educators with the South African Nursing Council (SANC) [21]. HSE is part of an undergraduate Bachelor of Arts in Nursing Science degree (BA CUR) qualification that consists of 10 modules including a one-year practical module with 12 credits [22]. The module aims "to enable students to practise the didactical skills of HSE in a simulated teaching environment" [22]. The training may take one to three years, depending on whether the intention is to acquire an advanced diploma only or a degree qualification that allows the graduates to practise as Nurse Educators post completion. The programme is offered via satellite transmission with limited face-to-face interaction with educators from an Open Distance e-Learning (ODeL) institution. In their study, [10] explored the effects of the length of online nurse educator courses and stated that online distance education is an effective strategy to increase nurses' access to nursing degrees and build program capacity.

Traditionally, the HSE practical examination involved face-to-face interactions conducted either in an actual or a simulated classroom, depending on the university requirements, and which take place through physical interaction between the student nurse educator, the students and the facilitator. It is common knowledge that the nursing education practical is primarily delivered through a traditional means of instruction, including face-to-face classroom instruction and clinical experiences in various practice settings [23]. Nursing education has been in alignment with the constructivist view, which believes that learning takes place via interaction with others [24], as cited by [25]. According to Summers (2017) [26], "teaching requires a skill set of its own". It is for that reason that learning how to teach and facilitate knowledge acquisition in nursing students requires preparation and additional formal education for nurse educators to be competent in their teaching role [26]. This preparation was previously conducted in face-to-face settings. However, as the need to maintain a safe physical distance during the pandemic rapidly increased, the online provision of health professions education accelerated technology adoption in academic settings [27]. The same method was adopted for the HSE practical examination.

The aim of this paper is to present a comprehensive narrative review synthesising the opportunities and challenges presented by e-assessment in the HSE practical examination for student nurse educators during the pandemic. Furthermore, we aim to make recommendations as to how to overcome identified challenges and to promote identified opportunities.

*1.4. Problem Statement*

A nurse educator plays an important role in promoting student learning and professional development, as well as in offering high-quality nursing education [28]. Keating, Berland, Capone et al. (2021) [29] suggest that the capacity of effective nurse educators is a significant constraint when addressing the global shortage of nurses. According to the WHO [30], the preparedness and expectations of nursing graduates will continue to evolve rapidly as a result of social and demographic changes, increasingly complex healthcare needs and chronic conditions, threats of emerging infectious diseases, and environmental and climate related illnesses. The core competencies of nurse educators include competence in nursing practice, pedagogical competence, communication, collaboration skills, monitoring and evaluating, management, and digital technology [31]. According to SANC, the competencies of a nurse educator are classified into seven domains, with facilitation of learning being the first competence which includes the use of information technologies to skilfully support the teaching-learning process [21]. For registration after qualification, each student nurse educator is required to obtain a minimum number of clinical practicum hours as part of their training that provides opportunities to develop the core competencies that align with course and program outcomes [32].

Prior to the COVID-19 pandemic, it was a SANC requirement that student nurse educators be assessed on theoretical lessons as well as clinical lessons. During the assessment, a real class scenario was simulated with fellow students or at an accredited nursing education institution with student nurses. Students would be assessed by a registered nurse educator on issues that included lesson plan preparation, class facilitation including material used for facilitation and class control to meet the nurse educators' core competencies as stipulated by WHO [31]. To conform to government-imposed physical distancing regulations for restricted infection transmission [33], the method of assessment was changed. This led to a shift from the face-to-face practical examination to an online practical examination assessment. To overcome pedagogical challenges posed by the COVID-19 pandemic, pre-recorded instructional videos, narrated PowerPoint presentations, and live practical classes with students practising at home are some examples of the digitally enhanced teaching approaches adopted by health science educators to teach practical skills remotely [34]. Naik, Deshpande, Shivananda et al. (2021) [35] reported that in efforts to combat this inevitable crisis, educational sectors began conducting online classes and this sudden changeover in the teaching and learning method raised new challenges and opportunities.

Given the background, it is noteworthy to report that much has been achieved with respect to online teaching and learning in HSE. However, none of the currently available studies have focused specifically on virtual practical examinations for student nurse educators. Therefore, this review aims to synthesise evidence that describes those challenges and opportunities presented by e-assessment in the HSE practical examination for student nurse educators during the COVID-19 pandemic. Furthermore, we aim to make recommendations that might help higher education institutions, particularly those offering nursing education, to enhance the use of e-assessment for practical examinations as an essential assessment tool rather than being one only to be used in such emergency situations as the COVID-19 pandemic.

*1.5. Definition of Key Concepts*

**Human Sciences:** This involves the study and understanding of human beings [36] and nursing as a human science focuses on the humaneness of the person and seeks to provide patient centred care which is directed towards improving the life of a unique individual [37].

**Higher Education**: Higher education is viewed as a vehicle for intellectual development, developing a flexible mind and, regardless of the field of study, helping students acquire knowledge and intellectual skills that can be applied in a variety of different contexts [38]. Higher nursing education is nursing education specifically offered in a university setting, with the aim of preparing nursing graduates with complex knowledge and skills [39].

**Nursing Education** refers to the professional education for the preparation of nurses to enable them to render professional nursing care to people of all ages, in all phases of health and illness, in a variety of settings. According to SANC, Nursing Education is a "specialist field that focuses on education and training students who are undertaking undergraduate and or postgraduate programme in nursing" [21].

**Nurse Educator** refers to a professional with an additional qualification in Nursing Education and is registered as such with the SANC [21]. In this review, the term student nurse educators refers to those professional nurses who are studying to obtain their basic degree qualification in Nursing Education, as explained in the definition above.

*1.6. Review Purpose*

The purpose of this narrative review was to synthesise the current evidence on opportunities and challenges presented by e-assessment in the HSE practical examination for student nurse educators during the COVID-19 pandemic.

*1.7. Review Question*

This narrative review aim to answer the following question:

What are the opportunities and challenges presented by e-assessment in the HSE practical examination for student nurse educators during the COVID-19 pandemic?

## 2. Materials and Methods

A comprehensive literature search was carried out on Google Scholar, PubMed/MEDLINE, Science direct, Directory of Open Access Journals, Complementary Index, SCOPUS, and Cumulative Index to Nursing and Allied Health Literature (CINAHL) with the intention of identifying opportunities and challenges presented by e-assessment in the HSE practical examination for student nurse educators during the COVID-19 pandemic. The search was conducted between August and November 2022.

*2.1. Data Collection*

Narrative reviews, also referred to as literature reviews, are a method used to identify and consolidate that which has been previously published on a specific topic; this consolidation prevents duplication and allows identification of any omissions or gaps for potential new studies [40,41]. This narrative review was conducted following the four steps as suggested [41]. The four proposed steps of narrative review are as follows: (1) a systematic search process and application of inclusion and exclusion criteria; (2) data extraction and synthesis of results; (3) the analysis of key findings by the narrative review; and (4) a quality appraisal procedure that included all studies. For the purpose of this narrative review, this method allowed a thorough search for extant literature, integration and interpretation of findings from varied study types which covered diverse online or virtual practical examinations or assessments in the fields of HSE and the quality appraisal of those studies.

*2.2. Inclusion and Exclusion Criteria*

The selection criteria included the following: (i) studies and reports written in English that reported on opportunities and challenges of e-assessment or online/virtual assessment in health science education or nursing education; (ii) articles and reports published in peer-reviewed journals; and (iii) published between 2020 and 2022. The search terms used were online practical assessment; virtual practical assessment; e-assessment practical tests; electronic assessment practical; digital practical assessment; virtual practical examination; student nurse educator; student nurse lecturer; student faculty nurse; student nurse teacher.

Articles and reports were excluded if they (i) focused only on e-learning and teaching; (ii) focused on virtual simulation assessment but were published before 2020; and/or (iii) were published in non-peer-reviewed journals. Thesis and dissertations outside health sciences institution repositories were also omitted.

*2.3. Selection Process*

The Preferred Reporting Items for Systematic Reviews and Meta-Analysis were applied in order to determine the most appropriate articles for review [42]. The search focused on full articles that included the key concepts. The thorough search generated 266 results, including reports and research articles; after duplicates were removed, the remaining 166 were reviewed at title, abstract and relevance level. This review resulted in the further removal of 129 articles. The remaining 37 were closely read to verify the methodology and the population, resulting in the further removal of 22 records. Fifteen articles then remained for critical review. The PRISMA diagram in Figure 1 illustrates the steps followed in selection of included articles.

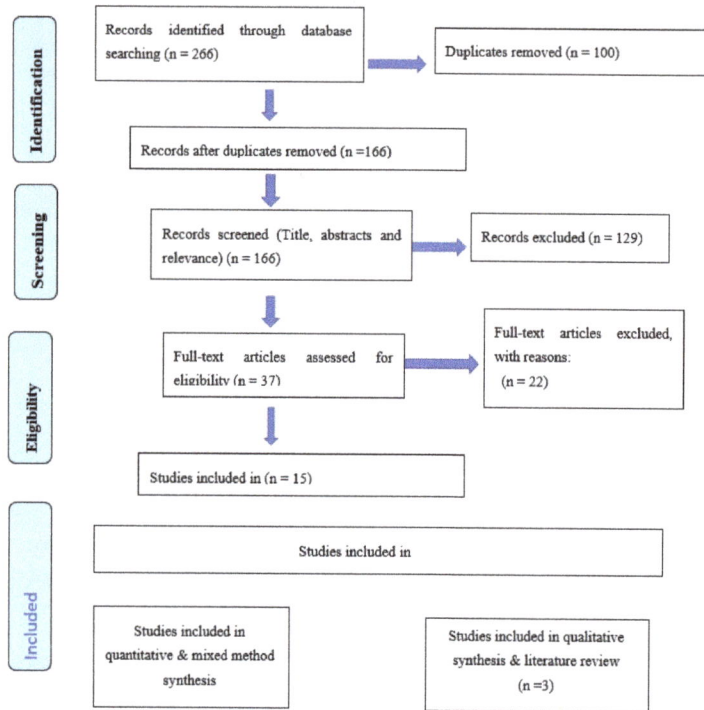

**Figure 1.** Flow diagram of the narrative review [42].

*2.4. Data Extraction, Analysis, Synthesis and Quality/Critical Appraisal*

Data were extracted on study details (author/s and country of study), methods (population, sample and sample size, collection and analysis methods), key results and conclusions. Studies were organised and tabulated into classifications by area of specialised fields. The data were analysed using inductive and descriptive synthesis [43]. The review question was used as the basis for searching the data for relevant expressions, which were then further tabulated. To synthesise the data, the author used tabulation to search the data for similarities and differences and further organise the data into categories named according to the content. The author critically evaluated the final articles using the Joanna Briggs Institute Critical Appraisal tools for qualitative and quantitative studies. The JBI tool with ten items was applied to rate the quality of qualitative studies [44], whereas another JBI tool with eight items was used to evaluate the quantitative (cross-sectional) studies [45]. Finally, 15 studies that met the quality appraisal criteria were retained (n = 15). Table 1 shows the JBI for quantitative and mixed method studies included (n = 12). The included qualitative articles, presented in Table 2, scored yes (n = 2), and the single literature review is presented in Table 3.

*2.5. Ethical Considerations*

The review was conducted ethically throughout the conceptualisation, planning, implementation and dissemination phases. No permission was needed to conduct this review; however, all sources used are duly acknowledged in the text and in the reference list.

**Table 1.** Critical appraisal checklist for the included quantitative and mixed method studies.

| Study/Criterion | [46] Alkhateeb, Ahmed, Al-Tawil et al. (2022) | [47] Donn, Scott, Binnie et al. (2021) | [48] Elzainy, El Sadik and Al Abdulmonem (2020) | [49] Fatima, Idrees, Jabeen et al. (2021) | [50] Ghaheri, Maghsoudi, Mobarak et al. (2022) Iran | [51] Fogg, Wilson, Trinka et al. (2020) | [52] Kuravi, Gogineni, Bhargav et al. (2021) | [53] Patra and Tekulapally (2021) | [54] Phillips, Munn and George (2020) | [55] Polancich, Steadman, Moneyham et al. (2021) | [56] Przymuszała, Zielińska-Tomczak, Kłos et al. (2022) | [57] Sadeesh, Prabavathy and Ganapathy (2021) India |
|---|---|---|---|---|---|---|---|---|---|---|---|---|
| 1. The criteria for inclusion in the sample was clearly defined | U | U | Y | Y | Y | U | Y | Y | Y | Y | Y | Y |
| 2. The study subjects and the setting were described in detail | Y | Y | Y | Y | Y | Y | Y | Y | Y | Y | Y | Y |
| 3. The exposure was measured in a valid and reliable way. | Y | Y | Y | Y | Y | Y | Y | Y | Y | Y | Y | Y |
| 4. Objective, standard criteria were used for measurement of the condition | Y | Y | Y | Y | Y | Y | Y | Y | Y | Y | Y | Y |
| 5. Confounding factors were identified? | Y | Y | Y | Y | Y | Y | Y | Y | Y | Y | Y | Y |
| 6. Strategies to deal with confounding factors were stated | Y | Y | Y | Y | Y | Y | Y | Y | Y | Y | Y | Y |
| 7. The outcomes were measured in a valid and reliable way | Y | Y | Y | Y | Y | Y | Y | Y | Y | Y | Y | Y |
| 8. Appropriate statistical analysis was used | Y | Y | Y | Y | Y | U | Y | Y | Y | Y | Y | Y |

Source: JBI Critical Appraisal Checklist for Analytical Cross-Sectional Studies (2017). Key: Yes = Y; No = N; Unclear = U; Not Applicable = N/A.

**Table 2.** Critical appraisal checklist for the included qualitative studies.

| Study/Criterion | [58]<br>Roman et al. (2022) | [59]<br>Thampy et al. (2022) |
|---|---|---|
| 1. Aim and objectives clearly described | Y | Y |
| 2. Research methods appropriate | Y | Y |
| 3. Research design appropriate to address the aim | Y | Y |
| 4. Recruitment of participants adequately described. | Y | Y |
| 5. Data collection addressed. | Y | Y |
| 6. Relationship between researcher and participants has been adequately considered | Y | Y |
| 7. Ethical issues adequately taken into consideration | Y | Y |
| 8. Data analysis sufficiently rigorous | Y | Y |
| 9. Findings clearly described | Y | Y |
| 10. Value of the research is adequately described | Y | Y |

Source: JBI Critical Appraisal Checklist for Systematic Reviews and Research Syntheses (2017). Key: Yes = Y; Cannot tell = CN; No = N.

**Table 3.** Critical appraisal checklist for the systematic reviews and research syntheses.

| Study/Criterion | [60]<br>Forde and Obrien (2022). Ireland |
|---|---|
| 1. Is the review question clearly and explicitly stated? | Y |
| 2. Were the inclusion criteria appropriate for the review question? | Y |
| 3. Was the search strategy appropriate? | Y |
| 4. Were the sources and resources used to search for studies adequate? | Y |
| 5. Were the criteria for appraising studies appropriate? | Y |
| 6. Was critical appraisal conducted by two or more reviewers independently? | Y |
| 7. Were there methods to minimise errors in data extraction? | Y |
| 8. Were the methods used to combine studies appropriate? | Y |
| 9. Was the likelihood of publication bias assessed? | Y |
| 10. Were recommendations for policy and/or practice supported by the reported data? | Y |
| 11. Were the specific directives for new research appropriate? | Y |

Source: JBI Critical Appraisal Checklist for Systematic Reviews and Research Syntheses (2017). Key: Yes = Y; No = N; Unclear=U; Not Applicable = N/A.

## 3. Results

On the basis of the studies included in this review, e-assessment was shown to be controversial among scholars due to the opportunities and challenges presented during the COVID-19 pandemic. Despite all the challenges, which include connectivity issues leading to frustration and stress and the unpreparedness and attitudes of students and facilitators, there are some opportunities that emerged from e-assessment that are believed to be beneficial to both the students and the facilitators, as well as the institution. Opportunities include reduced administrative burden, improved teaching and learning and immediate feedback from facilitators to students and from students to facilitators.

*Details of Empirical Studies*

Details of the 15 studies reviewed from the different fields of HSE are indicated in Table 4, below.

**Table 4.** Summary of included articles.

| Author/s/Country | Aim | Methods | Participants/Sample Size | Results |
|---|---|---|---|---|
| 1. Alkhateeb, Ahmed, Al-Tawil et al. (2022). Iraq [46] | To share the experience of conducting an online assessment with the academic community and to assess its effectiveness from both examiners' and students' perspectives. | A cross-sectional study | Examiners & medical students | The response rates among examiners and students were 69.4% and 88.5%, respectively. |
| 2. Donn, Scott, Binnie et al. (2021) UK [47] | A pilot of a Virtual Objective Structured Clinical Examination (VOSCE) in dental education. A response to COVID-19 | Quantitative | Undergraduate dental students | With careful planning, the VOSCE is a useful assessment method in difficult times. Feedback from staff and students was favourable. |
| 3. Elzainy, El Sadik and Al Abdulmonem (2020) Saudi Arabia [48] | Experience of e-learning and online assessment during the COVID-19 pandemic at the College of Medicine, Qassim University | Descriptive cross-sectional study | Undergraduate medical students and staff | The study observed higher student achievements and promising staff perceptions with obvious improvement in their technological skills. These findings support the shift towards future implementation of more online medical courses. |
| 4. Fatima, Idrees, Jabeen et al. (2021) Pakistan [49] | To evaluate online assessment in undergraduate medical education: Challenges and solutions from a LMIC university | Cross-sectional study | Medical students | The students reported that attempting the online exam on VLE with ZOOM support was user friendly. Ninety percent of the class was supportive of the continuing with the online assessments. |
| 5. Ghaheri, Maghsoudi, Mobarak et al. (2022) Iran [50] | Evaluation of Medical Students' Satisfaction with the Virtual Assessment of Cardiac Physiology Course | Quantitative | Medical students | The students preferred summative assessment questions to be multiple-choice due to the difficulty of the cardiac physiology course. More research should be conducted on this subject with a larger sample size in future studies. |
| 6. Fogg, Wilson, Trinka et al. (2020) USA [51] | To develop evidence-based recommendations for simulation hour equivalence ratios and compile a list of virtual activities and products faculty could use to complete clinical experiences. | Survey | Undergraduate and graduate nursing students | Tailoring learning opportunities such as continuing education courses, open-lab technology sessions, and appropriate reference materials can help to ensure faculty are prepared should the need for online transition be required again in the future. |
| 7. Kuravi, Gogineni, Bhargav et al. (2021) India [52] | Evaluation of experience with virtual conduction of semester practical exams for medical graduates. | A Prospective study | Medical students & Examiners | No problems occurred except a few short-duration (less than 5 min) interruptions due to internet connectivity issues. A total of 125/150 (83.5%) medical students and all examiners (2 internal and 2 external) expressed satisfaction with virtual medical evaluation. |
| 8. Patra and Tekulapally (2021) India [53] | Second-year dental students' perception of effectiveness of formative assessment in an online learning environment during COVID-19 pandemic | A cross-sectional study | Dental students | Immediate and faceless feedback in the form of a summary of overall performance was preferred by most of the students. |

**Table 4.** *Cont.*

| Author/s/Country | Aim | Methods | Participants/Sample Size | Results |
|---|---|---|---|---|
| 9. Phillips, Munn and George (2020) USA [54] | To evaluate the impact of incorporating telehealth simulation into objective structured clinical examinations (OSCEs) in the family nurse practitioner (FNP) and bachelor of science in nursing (BSN) programs. | Mixed-methods study | Nurse Practitioner students | Students' telehealth knowledge, skills, and confidence were improved after the telehealth OSCE experience. |
| 10. Polancich, Steadman, Moneyham et al. (2021) US [55] | Unexpected COVID-19 opportunity: applied experience for nurse educator students | Programmatic evaluation, using a 10-item Likert scale evaluation tool | Nurse Educator students | Aggregate mean evaluation scores ranged from 2.7 to 4.3. The nurse educator students attributed an aggregate mean of 4.3 to the possibility of spending additional clinical hours providing oversight to nursing students participating in this process. |
| 11. Przymuszała, Zielińska-Tomczak, Kłos et al. (2022) Poland [56] | Distance learning and assessment during the COVID-19 pandemic—pperspectives of Polish medical and healthcare students | Online questionnaire | Medical Students | Students noticed positive aspects of online learning. However, they also noticed its disadvantages. |
| 12. Sadeesh, Prabavathy and Ganapathy (2021). India [57] | Quantifying students' experience with virtual assessment. | Quantitative study | Medical students | Completed feedback forms were submitted by 228 students. More than 50% of students favoured online anatomy spotter examinations. |
| 13. Roman, Ruiz-Gonzalez, Rodriguez-Arrastia et al. (2022) Spain [58] | To explore nursing students' perceptions of the use of a serious game-like model in their final online objective structured clinical examination (OSCE). | Qualitative study | Nursing students | The two main themes were (i) generating emotions and feelings in times of virtuality; and (ii) online assessment: a potential alternative to educational barriers. |
| 14. Thampy, Collins, Baishnab et al. (2022) UK [59] | Virtual clinical assessment in medical education: an investigation of online conference technology | Qualitative study | Medical students | Four themes were identified, namely: optimising assessment design for online delivery, ensuring clinical authenticity, recognising and addressing feelings and apprehensions, and anticipating challenges through incident planning and risk mitigation. |
| 15. Forde and Obrien (2022) - [60] | To address this gap and to provide recommendations for overcoming identified challenges. | Literature Review | 29 articles | This literature review demonstrates the acceptability and usability of digitally enhanced practical teaching in health science education among students and educators. |

## 4. Discussion

The focus of this paper is primarily on the virtual practical examination of student nurse educators in HSE, although related experiences from other graduate nursing education and other multi-disciplinary fields during the COVID-19 pandemic are included where relevant. Assessment is considered an integral part of the learning process. Traditional assessment methods are often based on the student being treated as an isolated individual with limited access to resources and other people [61]. The evolution of technology together with the interruption from the COVID-19 pandemic, new opportunities for assessment are explored to acknowledge the increasingly important role e-assessment is playing in Higher Education. The discussion section will be based on the opportunities or advantages as well as challenges or disadvantages.

*4.1. Opportunities*

Virtual teaching and learning and assessment platforms in HSE, including nursing education, provide innovations and growth opportunities for both students and facilitators. Online practical assessments are innovative in a new reality for most student nurses and teachers and may empower students' nurses by helping them to remove perceived barriers in face-to-face assessments [58]. Technology assessments such as videos and web-based simulation for advance practice programs in the nursing education institutions were considered due to limited access to healthcare facilities during a period of social distancing [62]. Online practical examination such as telecommunication technology simulation can be an effective strategy to assess clinical skills competencies and provides personalised effective and immediate feedback to students [47,54]. Furthermore, it is suggested that online evaluation had benefits and expected impacts on student and teacher happiness and performance during the COVID-19 pandemic [63], and also improved the teaching and learning process both in managing distance education, increasing class size and staff workload [48,50]. Despite the concerns that included unfamiliarity and limited virtual assessment experience and the insufficient number of information technology technicians that interferes with proper digitalisation [48], the convenience of virtual clinical assessment including the removal of travelling to examination centres provides opportunity to partake at the comfort of both students and the examiners' homes [59]. As learning to teach and facilitate knowledge acquisition requires preparation and additional formal education to ensure competency in teaching [26], collaboration to ensure effective online assessment practical examination is critical [52,55,64].

*4.2. Challenges*

Virtual practical examination requires sufficient and effective logistics preparation including students' and facilitators' training on how to run and partake in the assessment, internet access and proper connections, availability of ICT structural support, as well as infrastructures. Moreover, conducting practical examinations is a challenging aspect during the COVID-19 pandemic; however, virtual-based practical assessment sessions can help teachers to conduct practical examinations effectively [65]. Practical examinations have a role in protecting patients [66] and it is important to continue their delivery via innovative methods of measuring the same knowledge, understanding, and capabilities with amended assessments such using video conferencing platforms to conduct vivas [66]. Additionally, problems with internet connection and other technical aspects, the attitudes of teachers, limited interpersonal relations, limited learning of practical skills, health concerns, students' engagement and distractions during assessment [49,56,67,68] were reported to be worrying factors. The use of virtual practical examination requires abundant preparation on the part of both student nurse educators and the facilitators. Therefore, these issues are undeniably contributory factors to high stress levels experienced by both students as well as the facilitators in HSE during online assessment [12,51]. Furthermore, financial costs and time consumption as the preparation requires more time than the traditional assessment method [69,70] remain part of the challenges. Teachers would require the acquisition of new skills to use digital tools and designing of significant evaluation activities to be used, whereas students are forced to acquire digitals skills that will enable them to use new forms of education [71]. To overcome challenges presented by virtual practical examination during the COVID-19 pandemic is to acknowledge and find ways to deal with those challenges which include collaboration among relevant stakeholders [60,72].

Another challenge presented by virtual practical examination was the question as to whether this method was relevant for some content in HSE. Instances where students could not feel the structure using their hands during virtual practical examination made it difficult for them to identify the structure, its relations and its vascular supply [57,60,73]. It can be argued that despite the positive perceptions, online examinations are not suitable for assessing the physical examination skills [46]. To overcome this challenge, academics in HSE have the responsibility to design and implement strategies that will ensure that the objectives of online practical examination are met which will lead to competent practitioners after completion.

*4.3. Limitations*

There may be some possible limitations in this study. Therefore, the author acknowledges several limitations related to the methods. Narrative reviews are known to be biased in nature [41]. Firstly, although the narrative reviews does not necessarily follow a systematic approach like other reviews [74], the author took steps to attempt to prevent bias by describing the methods followed during including literature search and selection, and discussion of results. However, despite the fact that there is no strict rule on the number of authors required to conduct a narrative review [74] being a single author, she may have been biased during the review process. Secondly, the review only included studies published between 2020 and 2022, which led to limited number of studies that met the set criteria, whereas there were other Pandemics prior to COVID-19. Finally, the majority of the studies used in this review focused on the perceptions and experiences of students and academics regarding virtual practical examination in other health sciences disciplines. This is an indication of a gap in the virtual assessment of practical examinations for student nurse educators. Therefore, the results cannot be generalised, but might provide a framework for future research.

*4.4. Recommendations*

Although educational technologies are increasingly being used in HSE, there is the question as to whether or not it is possible to completely substitute the traditional assessment method [75], particularly for HSE practical examinations. Khoshnevisan (2019) [76] suggests that the technological tools are predominantly far from achieving authentic interaction, and related literature has illustrated that many of these tools do not foster genuine interaction. For these reasons, the level of competence can still be explored. Therefore, because the objectives of the Nursing Education practical module is to prepare a fully competent nurse educator who is able to meet the teaching and learning needs of the students in an increasingly digital, networked world, it is paramount that the effects of virtual practical examinations as an assessment strategy on the competence of nursing educators is identified and explored in further research. Secondly, there is a need for further research into the perceptions and experiences of student nurse educators as well as those of the facilitators regarding online assessment during practical examination in the midst of the COVID-19 pandemic to fully understand the opportunities and challenges presented in HSE.

## 5. Conclusions

Based on the literature reviewed, the researcher concluded that the majority of HSE institutions adopted an online mode of assessment for their students. However, factors such as lack of infrastructure and computer literacy either from the students or from the facilitators can hinder the use of virtual assessment as an essential tool, especially with the HSE practical examination. The uncertainties brought about by the outbreak of the COVID-19 pandemic mandated that HSE facilitators propose durable distance assessment strategies that would minimise physical contact but still maintain the real class presentation skills for student nurse educators to complete the academic year. However, despite all the challenges outlined in this review, the author believes this study provides relevant insights into the opportunities brought by online assessment in the HSE practical examination. By eliminating these challenges, online assessment can be improved, causing it to be of great benefit to the student nurse educators as well as those student nurses who will be in the hands of these educators on completion of their speciality in order to meet the educational needs during and after the pandemic crisis. This is supported by the conclusion that suggested that transformative change in medical education using technology for assessment offers new opportunities for students and that the benefits of the pandemic need to be enhanced in a post-COVID era [53].

*Significance of This Study*

The shift from face-to-face practical examination to the virtual mode has gradually been adopted and implemented in HSE and its challenges and opportunities, implications and effects including the competence of graduates need to be thoroughly investigated. Even though this paper was based on the author's experiences of virtual practical examination, this study highlights the need for innovative ways to conduct and assess practical examination for student nurse educators in HSE during and beyond the Pandemic. The study also suggests that, despite the number of challenges presented by virtual practical examination in HSE, this pedagogical approach can still provide innovation and growth opportunities for both students and facilitators. This means that introduction and implementation of new modern pedagogical approaches such as online practical examination is of great significance and can be used post-pandemic. This study also suggests that since the majority of HSE institutions including nursing education has significantly adopted online teaching and learning, it is important to have future educators who are knowledgeable and comfortable with the use of technology in order to meet the learning needs of the future students. Therefore, virtual practical examination for student nurse educators is a better method to prepare for the task in nursing education.

**Funding:** This research received no external funding.

**Institutional Review Board Statement:** Not applicable.

**Informed Consent Statement:** Not applicable.

**Data Availability Statement:** Not applicable.

**Acknowledgments:** The author acknowledge all authors of the studies used.

**Conflicts of Interest:** The author declares no conflict of interest.

# References

1. Akimov, A.; Malin, M. When old becomes new: A case study of oral examination as an online assessment tool. *Assess. Eval. High. Educ.* **2020**, *45*, 1205–1221. [CrossRef]
2. Zhang, N.; He, X. A comparison of virtual and in-person instruction in a physical examination course during the COVID-19 pandemic. *J. Chiropr. Educ.* **2022**, *36*, 142–146. [CrossRef] [PubMed]
3. Matlhaba, K.L.; Khunou, S.H. Transition of graduate nurses from student to practice during the COVID-19 pandemic: Integrative review. *Int. J. Afr. Nurs. Sci.* **2022**, *17*, 100501. [CrossRef] [PubMed]
4. Crick, T.; Knight, C.; Watermeyer, R.; Goodall, J. The impact of COVID-19 and "Emergency Remote Teaching" on the UK computer science education community. In Proceedings of the United Kingdom & Ireland Computing Education Research Conference, Glasgow, UK, 3–4 September 2020; pp. 31–37.
5. Barnes, E.R.; Vance, B.S. Transitioning a Graduate Nursing Physical Examination Skills Lab to an Online Learning Modality. *Nurse Educ.* **2022**, *47*, 322–327. [CrossRef]
6. Gause, G.; Mokgaola, I.O.; Rakhudu, M.A. Information technology for teaching and learning in a multi-campus public nursing college. *Health SA Gesondheid* **2022**, *27*, 10. [CrossRef]
7. Alruwais, N.; Wills, G.; Wald, M. Advantages and challenges of using e-assessment. *Int. J. Inf. Educ. Technol.* **2018**, *8*, 34–37. [CrossRef]
8. Harerimana, A.; Mtshali, N.G. E-learning in nursing education in Rwanda: A middle-range theory. *J. Nurs. Educ. Pract.* **2021**, *11*, 78–88. [CrossRef]
9. Molato, B.J.; Sehularo, L.A. Recommendations for online learning challenges in nursing education during the COVID-19 pandemic. *Curationis* **2022**, *45*, 2360. [CrossRef]
10. Tiedt, J.A.; Owens, J.M.; Boysen, S. The effects of online course duration on graduate nurse educator student engagement in the community of inquiry. *Nurse Educ. Pract.* **2021**, *55*, 103164. [CrossRef]
11. Ferreira, D.; MacLean, G.; Center, G.E. Andragogy in the 21st century: Applying the assumptions of adult learning online. *Lang. Res. Bull.* **2018**, *32*, 10–19.
12. Ul Ain, N.; Jan, S.; Yasmeen, R.; Mumtaz, H. Perception of Undergraduate Medical and Health Sciences Students Regarding Online Formative Assessments During COVID-19. *Pak. Armed Forces Med. J.* **2022**, *72*, 882–886. [CrossRef]
13. Itani, M.; Itani, M.; Kaddoura, S.; Al Husseiny, F. The impact of the COVID-19 pandemic on on-line examination: Challenges and opportunities. *Glob. J. Eng. Educ.* **2022**, *24*, 105–120.

14. Moro, C.; Birt, J.; Stromberga, Z.; Phelps, C.; Clark, J.; Glasziou, P.; Scott, A.M. Virtual and augmented reality enhancements to medical and science student physiology and anatomy test performance: A systematic review and meta-analysis. *Anat. Sci. Educ.* **2021**, *14*, 368–376. [CrossRef]
15. Satoh, M.; Fujimura, A.; Sato, N. Competency of academic nurse educators. *SAGE Open Nurs.* **2020**, *6*, 2377960820969389. [CrossRef]
16. Matthias, A.D.; Gazza, E.A.; Triplett, A. Preparing future nurse educators to teach in the online environment. *J. Nurs. Educ.* **2019**, *58*, 488–491. [CrossRef]
17. Li, C.H.; Rajamohan, A.G.; Acharya, P.T.; Liu, C.S.J.; Patel, V.; Go, J.L.; Kim, P.E.; Acharya, J. Virtual read-out: Radiology education for the 21st century during the COVID-19 pandemic. *Acad. Radiol.* **2020**, *27*, 872–881. [CrossRef]
18. Nadama, H.U.H.; Tennyson, M.; Khajuria, A. Evaluating the usefulness and utility of a webinar as a platform to educate students on a UK clinical academic programme. *J. R. Coll. Physicians Edinb.* **2019**, *49*, 317–322. [CrossRef]
19. Wagner, F.; Knipfer, C.; Holzinger, D.; Ploder, O.; Nkenke, E. Webinars for continuing education in oral and maxillofacial surgery: The Austrian experience. *J. Cranio-Maxillofac. Surg.* **2019**, *47*, 537–541. [CrossRef]
20. Mugimu, C.B.; Mugisha, W.R. Assessment of Learning in Health Sciences Education: MLT Case Study. *J. Curric. Teach.* **2017**, *6*, 21–34. [CrossRef]
21. South African Nursing Council (SANC). *Competencies for a Nurse Educator*. 2005. Available online: https://www.sanc.co.za/wp-content/uploads/2020/06/SANC-Competencies-Nurse-Educator.pdf (accessed on 25 October 2022).
22. University of South Africa. Department of Health Studies. *Health Sciences Education: Practical. Only Study Guide for HSE2603*; Unisa: Pretoria, South Africa, 2018. Available online: https://www.unisa.ac.za/sites/corporate/default/Register-to-study-through-Unisa/Subjects-&-modules/All-subjects/HEALTH-SCIENCES-EDUCATION (accessed on 21 October 2022).
23. Vandenberg, S.; Magnuson, M. A comparison of student and faculty attitudes on the use of Zoom, a video conferencing platform: A mixed-methods study. *Nurse Educ. Pract.* **2021**, *54*, 103138. [CrossRef]
24. Vygotsky, L. *Mind in Society: The Development of Higher Psychological Processes*; Harvard University Press: Cambridge, MA, USA, 1980.
25. Erlam, G.D.; Smythe, L.; Clair, W.S. Simulation is not a pedagogy. *Open J. Nurs.* **2017**, *7*, 779–787. [CrossRef]
26. Summers, J.A. Developing competencies in the novice nurse educator: An integrative review. *Teach. Learn. Nurs.* **2017**, *12*, 263–276. [CrossRef]
27. Jeffries, P.R.; Bushardt, R.L.; DuBose-Morris, R.; Hood, C.; Kardong-Edgren, S.; Pintz, C.; Posey, L.; Sikka, N. The role of technology in health professions education during the COVID-19 pandemic. *Acad. Med.* **2022**, *97*, S104–S109. [CrossRef] [PubMed]
28. Salminen, L.; Tuukkanen, M.; Clever, K.; Fuster, P.; Kelly, M.; Kielé, V.; Koskinen, S.; Sveinsdóttir, H.; Löyttyniemi, E.; Leino-Kilpi, H. The competence of nurse educators and graduating nurse students. *Nurse Educ. Today* **2021**, *98*, 104769. [CrossRef] [PubMed]
29. Keating, S.A.; Berland, A.; Capone, K.; Chickering, M.J. Global nursing education: International resources meet the NLN core competencies for nurse educators. *OJIN: Online J. Issues Nurs.* **2021**, *26*, 1–9. [CrossRef]
30. World Health Organization. State of the World's Nursing 2020: Executive Summary. 2020. Available online: https://apps.who.int/iris/bitstream/handle/10665/331673/9789240003293-eng.pdf?sequence=1&isAllowed=y (accessed on 25 October 2022).
31. World Health Organization. Nurse Educator Core Competencies. 2016. Available online: https://apps.who.int/iris/bitstream/handle/10665/258713/9789241549622eng.pdf?sequence=1&isAllowed=y (accessed on 25 October 2022).
32. Hawkins, S.; Fogg, N.; Wilson, C.; Browne, J. Establishing a tutoring and academic support center: Collaborating with nurse educator students. *J. Prof. Nurs.* **2022**, *39*, 19–25. [CrossRef]
33. Pather, N.; Blyth, P.; Chapman, J.A.; Dayal, M.R.; Flack, N.A.; Fogg, Q.A.; Green, R.A.; Hulme, A.K.; Johnson, I.P.; Meyer, A.J.; et al. Forced disruption of anatomy education in Australia and New Zealand: An acute response to the COVID-19 pandemic. *Anat. Sci. Educ.* **2020**, *13*, 284–300. [CrossRef]
34. Ng, T.K.; Reynolds, R.; Chan, M.Y.H.; LI, X.; Chu, S.K.W. Business (teaching) as usual amid the COVID-19 pandemic: A case study of online teaching practice in Hong Kong. *J. Inf. Technol. Educ. Res.* **2020**, *19*, 775–802.
35. Naik, G.L.; Deshpande, M.; Shivananda, D.C.; Ajey, C.P.; Manjunath Patel, G.C. Online Teaching and Learning of Higher Education in India during COVID-19 Emergency Lockdown. *Pedagog. Res.* **2021**, *6*, em0090.
36. Pratt, M. The utility of human sciences in nursing inquiry. *Nurse Res.* **2012**, *19*, 12–15. [CrossRef]
37. Watson, J. *Human Caring Science*; Jones & Bartlett Publishers: Burlington, MA, USA, 2012.
38. Mtshali, N.G.; Zwane, Z.P. Positioning public nursing colleges in South African higher education: Stakeholders' perspectives. *Curationis* **2019**, *42*, 1–11.
39. Zhang, J.; Cui, Q. Collaborative learning in higher nursing education: A systematic review. *J. Prof. Nurs.* **2018**, *34*, 378–388. [CrossRef]
40. Grant, M.J.; Booth, A. A typology of reviews: An analysis of 14 review types and associated methodologies. *Health Inf. Libr. J.* **2009**, *26*, 91–108. [CrossRef]
41. Ferrari, R. Writing narrative style literature reviews. *Med. Writ.* **2015**, *24*, 230–235. [CrossRef]
42. The Joanna Briggs Institute (Producer). The Joanna Briggs Institute Critical Appraisal Tools for Use of in JBI Systematic Review. *Checklist for Qualitative Research*. 2017. Available online: https://jbi.global/sites/default/files/2019-06/JBI_Critical_Appraisal-Checklist_for_Qualitative_Research2017.docx (accessed on 22 November 2022).

43. The Joanna Briggs Institute (Producer). The Joanna Briggs Institute Critical Appraisal Tools for Use of in JBI Systematic Review. *Checklist for Cross-Sectional Studies.* 2017. Available online: https://jbi.global/sites/default/files/2019-05/JBI_Critical_Appraisal-Checklist_for_Analytical_Cross_Sectional_Studies2017_0.pdf (accessed on 22 November 2022).
44. Moher, D.; Liberati, A.; Tetzlaff, J.; Altman, D. Preferred reporting items for systematic reviews and meta-analyses: The PRISMA statement. *PLoS Med.* **2009**, *6*, e1000097. [CrossRef]
45. Polit, D.F.; Beck, C.T. *Nursing Research: Generating and Assessing Evidence for Nursing Practice*, 11th ed.; Wolters Kluwer: Alphen aan den Rijn, The Netherlands, 2021.
46. Alkhateeb, N.E.; Ahmed, B.S.; Al-Tawil, N.G.; Al-Dabbagh, A.A. Students and examiners perception on virtual medical graduation exam during the COVID-19 quarantine period: A cross-sectional study. *PLoS ONE* **2022**, *17*, e0272927. [CrossRef]
47. Donn, J.; Scott, J.A.; Binnie, V.; Bell, A. A pilot of a Virtual Objective Structured Clinical Examination in dental education. A response to COVID-19. *Eur. J. Dent. Educ.* **2021**, *25*, 488–494. [CrossRef]
48. Elzainy, A.; El Sadik, A.; Al Abdulmonem, W. Experience of e-learning and online assessment during the COVID-19 pandemic at the College of Medicine, Qassim University. *J. Taibah Univ. Med. Sci.* **2020**, *15*, 456–462. [CrossRef]
49. Fatima, S.S.; Idrees, R.; Jabeen, K.; Sabzwari, S.; Khan, S. Online assessment in undergraduate medical education: Challenges and solutions from a LMIC university. *Pak. J. Med. Sci.* **2021**, *37*, 945. [CrossRef]
50. Ghaheri, S.Z.; Maghsoudi, F.; Mobarak, S.; Radmanesh, E. Evaluation of Medical Students' Satisfaction with the Virtual Assessment of Cardiac Physiology Course. *Educ. Res. Med. Sci.* **2022**, *11*, e122572. [CrossRef]
51. Fogg, N.; Wilson, C.; Trinka, M.; Campbell, R.; Thomson, A.; Merritt, L.; Tietze, M.; Prior, M. Transitioning from direct care to virtual clinical experiences during the COVID-19 pandemic. *J. Prof. Nurs.* **2020**, *36*, 685–691. [CrossRef] [PubMed]
52. Kuravi, B.G.; Gogineni, S.; Bhargav, P.R.K.; Mayilvaganan, S.; Shanthi, V.; Ch, S. Utility of Virtual Platform for Conducting Practical Examination for Medical Students During Covid Times: A Prospective Study from Gynaecology Department. *J. Obstet. Gynecol. India* **2021**, *71*, 47–51. [CrossRef] [PubMed]
53. Patra, V.; Tekulapally, K. Second-year dental students' perception of effectiveness of formative assessment in an online learning environment during COVID-19 pandemic. *Natl. J. Physiol. Pharm. Pharmacol.* **2021**, *11*, 810–814. [CrossRef]
54. Phillips, T.A.; Munn, A.C.; George, T.P. Assessing the Impact of Telehealth Objective Structured Clinical Examinations in Graduate Nursing Education. *Nurse Educ.* **2020**, *45*, 169–172. [CrossRef] [PubMed]
55. Polancich, S.; Steadman, L.; Moneyham, L.; Poe, T. Unexpected COVID-19 Opportunity: Applied Experience for the Nurse Educator Student. *J. Nurs. Educ.* **2021**, *60*, 642–645. [CrossRef]
56. Przymuszała, P.; Zielińska-Tomczak, Ł.; Kłos, M.; Kowalska, A.; Birula, P.; Piszczek, M.; Cerbin-Koczorowska, M.; Marciniak, R. Distance Learning and Assessment During the COVID-19 pandemic—Perspectives of Polish Medical and Healthcare Students. *SAGE Open* **2022**, *12*, 21582440221085016. [CrossRef]
57. Sadeesh, T.; Prabavathy, G.; Ganapathy, A. Evaluation of undergraduate medical students' preference to human anatomy practical assessment methodology: A comparison between online and traditional methods. *Surg. Radiol. Anat.* **2021**, *43*, 531–535. [CrossRef]
58. Roman, P.; Ruiz-Gonzalez, C.; Rodriguez-Arrastia, M.; Granero-Molina, J.; Fernández-Sola, C.; Hernández-Padilla, J.M. A serious game for online-based objective structured clinical examination in nursing: A qualitative study. *Nurse Educ. Today* **2022**, *109*, 105246. [CrossRef]
59. Thampy, H.; Collins, S.; Baishnab, E.; Grundy, J.; Wilson, K.; Cappelli, T. Virtual clinical assessment in medical education: An investigation of online conference technology. *J. Comput. High. Educ.* **2022**, 1–22. [CrossRef]
60. Forde, C.; O'Brien, A. A Literature Review of Barriers and Opportunities Presented by Digitally Enhanced Practical Skill Teaching and Learning in Health Science Education. *Med. Educ. Online* **2022**, *27*, 2068210. [CrossRef]
61. Guàrdia, L.; Crisp, G.; Alsina, I.; Guàrdia, L.; Crisp, G.; Alsina, I. Trends and challenges of e-assessment to enhance student learning in Higher Education. *Innov. Pract. High. Educ. Assess. Meas.* 2017; 36–56.
62. De Tantillo, L.; Christopher, R. Transforming graduate nursing education during an era of social distancing: Tools from the field. *Nurse Educ. Today* **2020**, *92*, 104472. [CrossRef]
63. Fathurrochman, I. Online Evaluation System in the Pandemic Disruption in Madrasah: Opportunities and Challenges Based on Qualitative Report. *J. Iqra Kaji. Ilmu Pendidik.* **2021**, *6*, 184–197.
64. Foronda, C.L.; Alfes, C.M.; Dev, P.; Kleinheksel, A.J.; Nelson, D.A., Jr.; O'Donnell, J.M.; Samosky, J.T. Virtually nursing: Emerging technologies in nursing education. *Nurse Educ.* **2017**, *42*, 14–17. [CrossRef]
65. Vijayanarayanan, N.; Kondaguli, S.V. Lesson Learned During COVID-19 pandemic: Impact, Challenges and Opportunities in Nursing Education–A Review. *Int. J. Adv. Nurs. Manag.* **2021**, *9*, 417–422.
66. Sneyd, J.R.; Mathoulin, S.E.; O'Sullivan, E.P.; So, V.C.; Roberts, F.R.; Paul, A.A.; Cortinez, L.I.; Ampofo, R.S.; Miller, C.J.; Balkison, M.A. Impact of the COVID-19 pandemic on anaesthesia trainees and their training. *Br. J. Anaesth.* **2020**, *125*, 450–455. [CrossRef]
67. Joshi, A.; Vinay, M.; Bhaskar, P. Impact of coronavirus pandemic on the Indian education sector: Perspectives of teachers on online teaching and assessments. *Interact. Technol. Smart Educ.* **2020**, *18*, 205–226. [CrossRef]
68. O'Keefe, R.; Auffermann, K. Exploring the effect of COVID-19 on graduate nursing education. *Acad. Med.* **2022**, *97*, S61. [CrossRef]
69. Joshi, A.; Virk, A.; Saiyad, S.; Mahajan, R.; Singh, T. Online assessment: Concept and applications. *J. Res. Med. Educ. Ethics* **2020**, *10*, 49–59. [CrossRef]
70. Gurajala, S. Maximizing the utility of online assessment tools in the pandemic era-A narrative review. *J. Educ. Technol. Health Sci.* **2021**, *7*, 80–85. [CrossRef]

71. Torres-Madroñero, E.M.; Torres-Madroñero, M.C.; Ruiz Botero, L.D. Challenges and possibilities of ICT-mediated assessment in virtual teaching and learning processes. *Future Internet* **2020**, *12*, 232. [CrossRef]
72. Regmi, K.; Jones, L. A systematic review of the factors–enablers and barriers–affecting e-learning in health sciences education. *BMC Med. Educ.* **2020**, *20*, 91. [CrossRef] [PubMed]
73. Pettit, M.; Shukla, S.; Zhang, J.; Sunil Kumar, K.H.; Khanduja, V. Virtual exams: Has COVID-19 provided the impetus to change assessment methods in medicine? *Bone Jt. Open* **2021**, *2*, 111–118. [CrossRef] [PubMed]
74. Toronto, C.E.; Remington, R. (Eds.) *A Step-By-Step Guide to Conducting an Integrative Review*; Springer International Publishing: Cham, Switzerland, 2020.
75. Jin, J.; Bridges, S.M. Educational technologies in problem-based learning in health sciences education: A systematic review. *J. Med. Internet Res.* **2014**, *16*, e3240. [CrossRef] [PubMed]
76. Khoshnevisan, B. To integrate media and technology into language education: For and against. In *Errors. Advances in Global Education and Research Book Series Are not Copyrighted*; University of South Florida M3 Center Publishing: Sarasota, FL, USA, 2019; Volume 85, Available online: https://core.ac.uk/download/pdf/216961905.pdf#page=91 (accessed on 27 November 2022).

**Disclaimer/Publisher's Note:** The statements, opinions and data contained in all publications are solely those of the individual author(s) and contributor(s) and not of MDPI and/or the editor(s). MDPI and/or the editor(s) disclaim responsibility for any injury to people or property resulting from any ideas, methods, instructions or products referred to in the content.

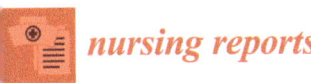 

*Case Report*

# A Novel Approach to Managing a COVID-19 Outbreak at a Farm in Outer Regional Victoria, Australia

Mwila Kabwe [1,2,*], Jennifer L. Dittmer [1], Jaimee Oxford [1], Catina Eyres [1], Ancara Thomas [1], Andrew Mahony [1] and Bruce Bolam [1]

1. The Loddon Mallee Public Health Unit, Bendigo Health, P.O. Box 126, Bendigo 3552, Australia
2. Department of Rural Clinical Sciences, La Trobe Rural Health School, La Trobe University, P.O. Box 199, Bendigo 3552, Australia
* Correspondence: m.kabwe@latrobe.edu.au

**Abstract:** The coronavirus disease (COVID-19) has been established as a major occupational health and safety issue that compounds pre-existing socioeconomic inequalities such as access to basic health services. This is exacerbated in migrant farmworkers who are an essential workforce in maintaining food supply across the country. An outbreak occurred in a remote part of Victoria with limited access to healthcare resources. Existing relationships allowed the Loddon Mallee Public Health Unit to quickly engage farm management and local pathology services and provide cultural and language support. After contact-tracing and comprehensive clinical review, rather than isolate positive cases, those who were asymptomatic and willing to work continued to do so whilst negative workers were in quarantine. Outbreak management and public health actions were quickly implemented even when the nationwide state-testing and contact-tracing systems were experiencing significant strain due to the rapid escalation in case numbers. Despite a large outbreak (68/74 workers), the management of the outbreak allowed asymptomatic cases to perform their work so farm productivity remained uninterrupted. Cases' health status was closely monitored, with no adverse outcomes in a high-risk population. COVID-19 negative workers safely quarantined away from positive cases until the closure of the outbreak.

**Keywords:** coronavirus disease (COVID-19); outbreak management; seasonal farmworkers; remote rural farms; culturally and linguistically diverse

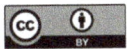

## 1. Introduction

Local farms are critical for maintaining food security in Australia and abroad [1,2]. In response to the global pandemic of the severe acute respiratory syndrome—2 (SARS-CoV-2) virus, the causative agent of the coronavirus disease (COVID-19), the Australian government and Department of Health (DH) highlighted guidelines for the management of COVID-19 across the country [3]. In farms specifically, the primary aim of these guidelines were to reduce or prevent the impact of COVID-19 on the health and productivity of farms through a COVIDSafe plan [4]. In Victoria, COVID-19 cases and outbreaks were ultimately managed by nine local public health units, including the Loddon Mallee Public Health Unit (LMPHU).

Not unique to Australia, seasonal farmworkers around the world are disproportionally affected by both communicable and non-communicable diseases [5]. In the COVID-19 pandemic, this was greatly exacerbated [6]. In Australia, foreign and temporary workers make up nearly 30% of the total workforce with a similar proportion among farmworkers [7]. When Australia shut its borders to international travel at the end of March 2020 [8], a shortage of farmworkers was quickly realised, emphasising the significance of imported labour from the Pacific Island nations through the Pacific Australia Labour Mobility (PALM) scheme, a partnership created in 2005 [9]. As COVID-19 vaccinations were mandated in

Victoria in October 2021 for all workers, only the PALM scheme provided a fully vaccinated farm workforce protected from the COVID-19 severe disease [10].

In late December 2021 and early January 2022, in Colignan, a small outer regional town in northern Victoria, there was a significant COVID-19 outbreak among seasonal farmworkers. This is a region where the economy depends on the agricultural production of citrus, grapes, garlic, melons, asparagus, and almonds [11]. This major outbreak provided insights into the vulnerabilities and challenges faced in the implementation of public health control measures in a culturally and linguistically diverse (CALD) population.

This report highlighted the epidemiological investigation and public health intervention approach aimed at limiting spread and morbidity whilst striving to maintain the productivity of the farm during a period where food security in Victoria was being impacted by rapidly rising numbers of COVID-19 cases.

## 2. Materials and Methods

### 2.1. Outbreak Investigation Team

This outbreak investigation and management was coordinated by the LMPHU, internally comprising a team of medical leads, communicable disease team leaders, public health officers, an epidemiologist, and an infection prevention control (IPC) consultant and support from the Department of Health Infection Prevention Control Advice and Response (IPCAR) team. To overcome hurdles in testing, PCR testing was outsourced to a local pathology provider and tertiary hospital, and linked into cultural support and language translation support services. Data collected were managed through the Victorian Government Department of Health Transmission and Response Epidemiology Victorian (TREVI) system [12].

### 2.2. Outbreak Detection and Case Finding

Notification of the outbreak was received by the LMPHU from the pathology provider with three confirmed cases identified; an assessment of the site was performed by public health officers in the LMPHU identifying an additional eleven symptomatic workers. Confirmed outbreak cases were epidemiologically linked workers with a positive COVID-19 test through either polymerase chain reaction (PCR; confirmed cases) or rapid antigen test (RAT; probable cases). Epidemiologically linked cases were cases who had contact with other previously confirmed cases for at least 15 min or 2 h cumulatively, within 48 h of either symptom onset or date of sample collection in asymptomatic cases [13]. Cultural and language translation services were employed to ensure speedy case confirmation and accurate information collection to facilitate contact-tracing. Infections were considered active within seven days of testing positive, as per DH case-definition guidelines [13].

### 2.3. Analysis

Case, contact, and site assessments were conducted over the telephone and via Microsoft Teams application. Data collected were securely stored and managed through the Victorian Department of Health TREVI system. Descriptive analysis of cases was performed in Microsoft® Office Excel and R Studio using the EpiCurve package.

### 2.4. Public Health Interventions

Before the outbreak was identified, routine targeted vaccination programs run by the LMPHU vaccination outreach team meant that by the time the outbreak was declared on the 8 January 2022, all workers had received at least 2 doses of the Pfizer-BioNTech (COMIRNATY) vaccine. None of the workers were reported to have had their last dose of COVID-19 vaccination more than 6 months or less than 10 days before outbreak declaration (considered for vaccine protection efficacy) or had COVID-19 infection 6 weeks prior (considered re-infection window at the time of the outbreak) [13]. Immediately after receiving the outbreak notification, which occurred late on a Saturday afternoon, the farm was contacted by one of the LMPHU public health officers to undertake a risk assessment;

this assessment identified that the seasonal workers lived onsite in accommodation that consisted of a single or double room, with shared facilities and communal spaces. The pathology provider was then contacted and requested to assist in performing onsite-testing for all workers; they delivered seventy rapid-antigen-testing kits the next day. Further testing was subsequently undertaken on the fourth and sixth days on all workers who had previously tested negative to COVID-19 to ensure that any late onset infections were ruled out. The cultural and language support services assisted in providing instructions for performing a RAT to all workers and also provided pastoral care support to all onsite. The IPCAR and IPC consultant liaised with the farm management to ensure that appropriate infection control measures were in place to limit infection transmission among workers. An outbreak management team (OMT) was established to discuss with all stakeholders and workers the optimal measures to manage the outbreak. During this meeting after consulting with the LMPHU medical leads, it was determined that all symptomatic workers would be treated as COVID-19-positive due to the delays in obtaining the results of COVID-19 PCRs that were occurring at the time. The local tertiary public hospital supported the outbreak by performing a clinical assessment on cases as they were identified; they then met with the site daily during the outbreak to monitor the clinical status of all cases.

## 3. Results

### 3.1. Epidemiological Investigation and Case Identification

The LMPHU was notified of farmworkers who were symptomatic and presented to the pathology centre for SARS-CoV-2 viral PCR testing, which subsequently identified nine cases. Through contact tracing, further PCR testing, and rapid antigen testing, a cumulative total of 68 cases of the 74 farmworkers were identified, including 9 (13.8%) PCR-confirmed and 59 (86.8%) probable (Table 1). There were 42 staff contacts of which 3 later tested positive using a RAT and were able to isolate from their homes.

**Table 1.** Characteristics of COVID-19 cases in the outbreak ($n = 68$).

| Characteristics of COVID-19 Cases | Number of Cases | Percent of Total |
|---|---|---|
| **Cases** | | |
| Confirmed | 9 | 13.8% |
| Probable | 59 | 86.8% |
| **Clinical Assessment** | | |
| No symptoms | 58 | 85.3% |
| Symptomatic | 10 | 14.7% |
| Hospitalisations | 0 | 0.0% |
| Deaths | 0 | 0.0% |
| **Sex** | | |
| Men | 57 | 83.8% |
| Women | 11 | 16.2% |
| **Age Groups** | | |
| 18–29 | 24 | 35.3% |
| 30–39 | 35 | 51.5% |
| 40–49 | 9 | 13.2% |

Initially, three confirmed cases were notified to the LMPHU on 8 January 2022 with their samples collected on 7 January 2022. This result turnaround was considerably quick considering the national overload all pathology services were experiencing due to the peaking of the Omicron variant of concern (VoC) in Australia. All cases in this cohort were cleared by 19 January 2022 (Figure 1). Figure 1 shows this as a point source outbreak with the epi curve flattening after 9 January 2022 and the last three probable cases diagnosed on 12 January 2022. The SARS-CoV-2 virus VoC agent for this outbreak was not determined. All cases that were initially symptomatic on testing or during the infection period were assessed as asymptomatic at least 24 h before clearance date and released from isolation. COVID-19-negative contacts were tested on 9, 12, and 14 January 2022 and continued to quarantine until 19 January 2022 when the last positive cases were considered to be no longer infectious.

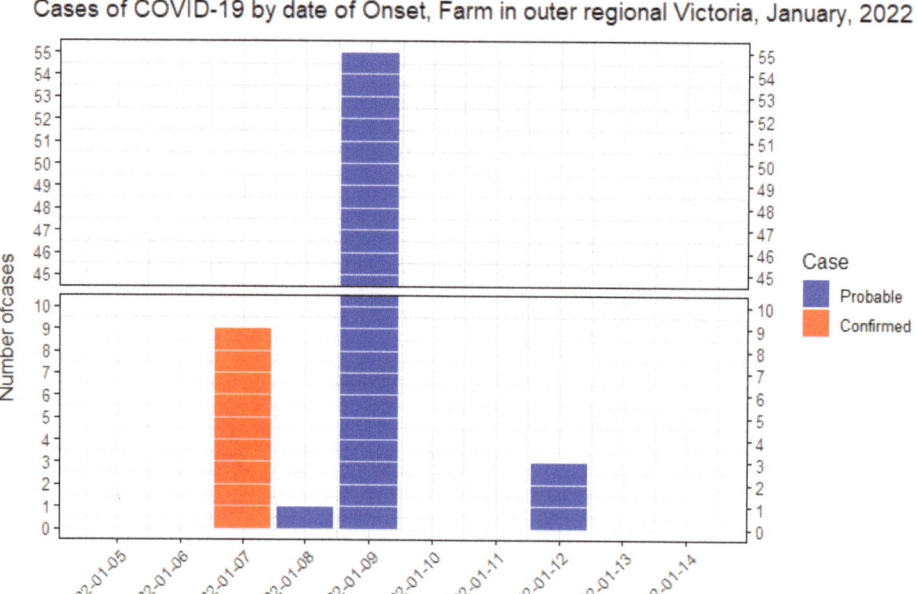

**Figure 1.** Epidemic curve of confirmed and probable cases. Nine cases were initially identified by PCR on 7 January 2022; then a further 56 showed positive RAT tests on 8 and 9 January, and the last 3 were identified on 12 January 2022.

During the outbreak period, there were no deaths or requirements for hospitalisations among all workers; however, 10 (14.7%) cases had had minor COVID-19-related symptoms. Due to the few cases with minor symptoms, risk factors associated with the severity of infections could not be analysed. This cohort was mostly composed of male workers [57 (83.8%)]. The age group was mostly 30–39 years old [35 (51.5%)] followed by the 18–29 years old age group [24 (35.3%)]. All workers were younger than 50 years old (Table 1). Six workers that remained COVID-19-negative throughout the outbreak were all men with a median age of 28 years, whereas the case cohort had a median age of 32 years.

*3.2. Outbreak Management and Implementation of Cohorting*

After the notification of initial cases on the 8 January 2022, the LMPHU declared the farm an outbreak site and initiated public health actions as per the public health and wellbeing act of 2008. An outbreak was defined as five or more cases in a high-risk residential setting in accordance with the DH COVID-19 control strategy. Identification of close contacts was completed, and requests for further testing and quarantine of all farmworkers were initiated, cohorting the positive cases after clinical assessment.

On the second day of the outbreak, an IPCAR referral was made, and a site visit occurred on the third day (Figure 2). The visit highlighted the need for all staff to undergo training regarding the recommended infection control measures to prevent further spread of the SARS-CoV-2 virus. This visit also reinforced a two-step cleaning approach with a detergent to clean before using a disinfectant, the use of facemasks, and physical distancing.

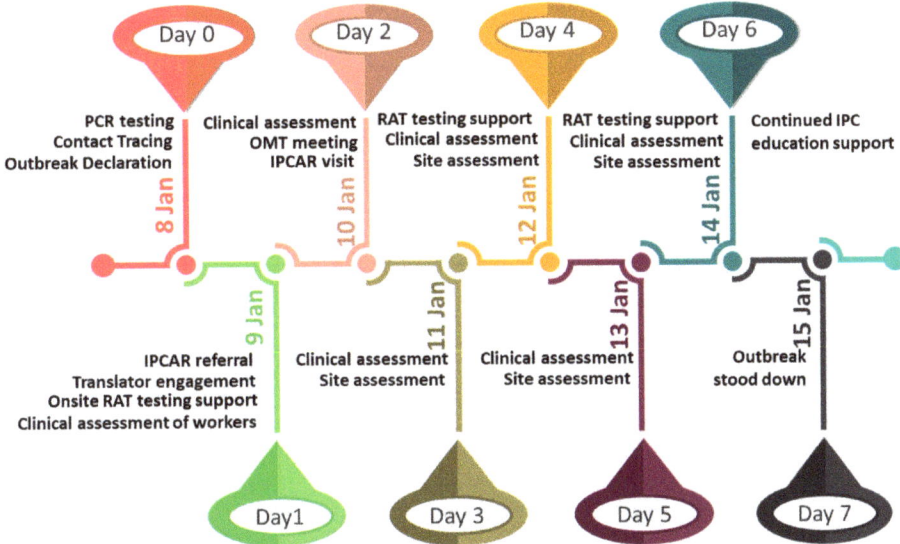

**Figure 2.** Timeline for key outbreak management interventions from date the outbreak was declared to date of stand-down.

Cultural support and translation services were engaged on the second day as well and complimented the efforts for contact tracing, testing, and quarantine compliance as all workers had indicated Samoan as the preferred language. Further onsite RA testing and daily clinical assessment of all workers were performed before the outbreak was stood down on 15 January 2022 (Figure 2), noting that this was no longer a transmission site, i.e., all workers that did not test positive had completed their quarantine period.

All outbreaks managed by the LMPHU have an OMT. In this outbreak, an OMT was organised with farm management, the workers, and other stakeholders including pathology services, cultural and support services, an IPC consultant, medical leads, a local tertiary public hospital, and the local rural city council—emergency management. This OMT ensured that the farm was adequately supported to manage the outbreak; this was achieved through the provision of personal protective equipment, rapid antigen tests, and food for workers onsite. At the time of the OMT, more than 80% of the farmworkers were identified as either confirmed or probable cases. Considering the risks due to COVID-19 disease epidemiology, the LMPHU in liaison with the farm management provided an exemption for all asymptomatic individuals with positive RAT to be able to return to work with appropriate introduction of personal protective equipment (PPE). This was authorised by the deputy chief health officer and aided in ensuring that food distribution was not impacted.

COVID-19 cases globally were mandated to stay at home and isolate. In workplaces, this minimised the spread of COVID-19 to workers who remained asymptomatic and tested negative, facilitating industry productivity and minimising impact on the economy as we transitioned to the "new normal" [14]. However, asymptomatic cases were able to choose to work from home whilst completing mandatory isolation, depending on their work requirements [15]. In this case study, after the initial screening, all cases were isolated, and, when more were identified, it was no longer possible to effectively isolate them but was much easier to quarantine their contacts. For this reason, all who remained negative could not return to work. The LMPHU recognised that it was important to ensure that asymptomatic RAT positive staff members were not coerced to attend work. As such, a cultural support officer external to the business regularly visited the site. This worker was able to communicate with cases in their preferred language and discussed with the cases their rights to ensure that they were not being coerced to attend work. The LPMHU director and medical lead advised that only cases who were asymptomatic and consenting were able to attend work. A further stipulation to this arrangement was that the farm health supervisor would be required to monitor staff to ensure that they were not presenting to work with symptoms. All cases received daily health monitoring through the local health service, and food relief was provided by the local multicultural support service. Both the farm health supervisor and cultural support worker provided language support to the cases; this was to ensure that instructions were communicated in preferred language for donning and doffing of personal protective equipment and for the use of rapid antigen tests. Overall, this public health response ensured improved health and social welfare of both cases and contacts throughout the outbreak period.

The positive farmworkers were cohorted in the accommodation onsite, whereas the negative workers were provided with single-room accommodation so that they could safely quarantine. All negative residents had to quarantine until all positive cases had completed their infection period, and effective cleaning of communal areas had been performed. This was ideal as there were challenges with fewer areas for appropriate quarantine, and only 6/74 (8.1%) workers had remained negative during the outbreak. Furthermore, the LMPHU engaged the IPCAR team to offer COVIDSafe training for workers in liaison with farm management on how to safely work with COVID-19-positive cases, PPE, isolation and quarantine requirements, and their implications.

## 4. Discussion

With support from the LMPHU vaccination outreach team, many farms across the region were prepared for this pandemic and ensured that cases did not have severe outcomes. The outer regional and remote areas of Australia had virtually no COVID-19 in 2020 and the first half of 2021 due to government-imposed lockdowns. The rapid response teams involving the local pathology service, cultural and language support services, and farm management enabled adequate risk assessment and allowed for farm work to continue in the face of the outbreak. Even though the initiative to allow asymptomatic workers to continue working was not the norm for all outbreaks, it has also been reported elsewhere with favourable outcomes [16].

Although the viral genomics were not performed to identify the VoC in this outbreak, confirmation with PCR was important to understand the severity of the outbreak and negate the low sensitivity for the RAT as per DH guidelines [3]. Once established, follow-up tests for contacts were performed by RAT, and all who tested positive were considered probable cases. Although the outbreak coincided with the peaking of the Omicron VoC in the country, in this rural town, it is difficult to ascertain whether the causative agent was Delta or Omicron as infections have historically shown a delay compared with the more populated metropolitan regions. The high infectivity and low symptom severity may point towards a possible Omicron VoC as the causative agent [17–19].

In this case report, the farmworkers were managed by contractors and initially worked across different farms. Yet, they lived together in the farm's accommodation camps where they shared facilities. This added another layer of complexity in contact-tracing and efficient communication between the farm management and contractors in identifying close contacts between different farms. However, after multiple site contact-tracing and testing, all contacts that lived elsewhere were able to quarantine in their homes, further reducing the risk of spread. No new cases or exposures were generated from these contacts. Other risks in this outbreak were mainly due to the timing coinciding with the peak of the Omicron COVID-19 VoC and the collapse of the pathology PCR testing capacity across the country. The RATs were introduced; however, the reporting system was not yet live online until the outbreak was well underway. Another challenge in managing this outbreak was that it occurred in a CALD group with low levels of written and spoken English. This proved a barrier to reading the provided instructions for responding to the outbreak, such as testing; reporting of RAT results; and compliance with isolation, quarantine, and appropriate facemask requirements. Furthermore, migrant populations have significantly higher proportions of undiagnosed co-morbidities and do not have access to many government support initiatives, such as Medicare, that promote equitable access to healthcare [20,21], which was reinforced during the COVID-19 pandemic [22].

Colignan is an outer regional town on the banks of the Murray River located at least 40 min from the rural city of Mildura where the main public hospital, testing, and vaccination clinics are located. Its remote location provides excessive challenges with access to healthcare. This cohort experienced barriers including the limited provision of appropriate local health options, limited transport, and fear of accessing services in many instances. The migrant farmworkers did not have Medicare cards, and whilst they did have private insurance, there were concerns expressed about the out-of-pocket costs they would incur should they need to access healthcare. Further communication barriers made it difficult to ensure that public health orders were complied with and testing requirements with RATs were correctly performed. As the case numbers were increasing during the outbreak, organising food and accommodation for effective isolation and quarantine became challenging.

Engagement with the farm management and cultural support for overcoming communication barriers was important for gaining trust between the LMPHU and workers who were living through a COVID-19 outbreak. The introduction and delivery of RAT kits further helped alleviate the challenges with PCR testing, which, at this point, had turnaround times not ideal to make useful public health actions. Although RATs are generally considered to have lower sensitivity to detect infections [23,24], they are regarded as a vital public health tool for the management of outbreaks [3]. The LMPHU has now engaged the services of an outer regional coordinator who will work hand-in-hand with key stakeholders such as community health services to specifically target more farms in the Mildura region for coordinated vaccination programs.

*Lessons Learned*

Outreach targeted testing and vaccination have allowed for the communities in the remote locations of the Loddon Mallee region to have access to vaccines, and this has subsequently reduced the burden of adverse events associated with COVID-19 infection. In our report, even though we had a large outbreak, the outcome of infection was excellent, the cases were still able to perform their work, and the productivity of the industry continued.

The trust between the LMPHU, farm management, pathology service, and cultural support made all the difference with the rapid response in screening, contact tracing, and innovative thinking and outbreak management to reduce spread and maintain workforce in this critical sector. The stakeholder engagement and cultural support including translation services for reporting test results were critical in evaluating the risk and extent of the outbreak. This provided the opportunity for the industry to continue to operate with a workforce that was asymptomatic yet RAT positive, and the few negative workers were able to safely quarantine, reducing the spread of infection whilst maintaining the workforce. The farm management and its workers readily embraced the COVIDSafe training for donning and doffing PPE allowing for public health actions to be implemented and complied with. Fostering existing relationships and building new ones with key stakeholders across the Loddon Mallee region was key to managing outbreaks. The collaborations have remained critical in gathering information, providing on-the-ground support, and achieving better outcomes for those impacted.

## 5. Conclusions

This farm outbreak in outer regional Victoria was the first major outbreak in the Loddon Mallee region during the time when the highly infectious Omicron VoC was spreading throughout Victoria. The pathology testing service was under unprecedented demand, and testing with RATs had just been introduced. The reporting system came online when this outbreak was underway. Furthermore, the outbreak occurred in a vulnerable population with limited English literacy, limited access to healthcare, and higher comorbidity per age compared with the rest of the country. This was a community of seasonal farmworkers who provide essential support to the agriculture industry, the mainstay of the economy in this part of the state. The LMPHU quickly acted to engage the farm management, local pathology service, and local health service and provided cultural and language support. This efficient collaboration enabled the continued productivity of the farm and provided extra training through the IPC consultant, which is and will be an invaluable asset for any future disease exposures and/or outbreaks.

**Author Contributions:** Conceptualization, B.B. and J.O.; methodology, A.M., A.T., B.B., C.E., J.L.D., J.O. and M.K.; formal analysis, M.K. and J.L.D.; investigation, all authors; writing—original draft preparation, M.K.; writing—review and editing, all authors; supervision, B.B.; project administration, J.O.; funding acquisition, B.B. All authors have read and agreed to the published version of the manuscript.

**Funding:** This work was supported by the Victorian Government Department of Health.

**Institutional Review Board Statement:** Not applicable.

**Informed Consent Statement:** Informed consent was obtained from all participants.

**Data Availability Statement:** Data available at reasonable request with permission from the Victorian Government Department of Health.

**Acknowledgments:** We would like to acknowledge all individuals at the LMPHU who support this outbreak investigation and management. We would also like to thank all the stakeholders who efficiently worked to support the case identifications and cultural and language support.

**Conflicts of Interest:** The authors declare no conflict of interest.

## References

1. Lawrence, G.; Richards, C.; Lyons, K. Food security in Australia in an era of neoliberalism, productivism and climate change. *J. Rural Stud.* **2013**, *29*, 30–39. [CrossRef]
2. Millar, J.; Roots, J. Changes in Australian agriculture and land use: Implications for future food security. *Int. J. Agric. Sustain.* **2011**, *10*, 25–39. [CrossRef]
3. Holley, A.; Coatsworth, N.; Lipman, J. The Australian response to the COVID-19 pandemic: A co-ordinated and effective strategy. *Anaesth. Crit. Care Pain Med.* **2021**, *40*, 100859. [CrossRef] [PubMed]
4. Department of Health—Victorian Government. COVIDSafe Plan. 2022. Available online: https://www.coronavirus.vic.gov.au/covidsafe-plan#creating-a-covidsafe-plan (accessed on 23 June 2022).
5. Murray, L.R. Sick and Tired of Being Sick and Tired: Scientific Evidence, Methods, and Research Implications for Racial and Ethnic Disparities in Occupational Health. *Am. J. Public Health* **2003**, *93*, 221–226. [CrossRef] [PubMed]
6. Etienne, C.F. COVID-19 has revealed a pandemic of inequality. *Nat. Med.* **2022**, *28*, 17. [CrossRef] [PubMed]
7. Australian Beureau of Statistics. Characteristics of Employment, Australia. 2021. Available online: https://www.abs.gov.au/statistics/labour/earnings-and-working-conditions/characteristics-employment-australia/latest-release#data-download (accessed on 23 June 2022).
8. Parliament of Australia. COVID-19: A Chronology of State and Territory Government Announcements (up until 30 June 2020). 2020. Available online: https://www.aph.gov.au/About_Parliament/Parliamentary_Departments/Parliamentary_Library/pubs/rp/rp2021/Chronologies/COVID-19StateTerritoryGovernmentAnnouncements#_Toc52275792 (accessed on 23 June 2022).
9. MacLellan, N.; Mares, P. Labour Mobility in the Pacific: Creating seasonal work programs in Australia. In *Globalization and Governance in the Pacific Islands*; ANU E Press: Canberra, Australia, 2006; pp. 137–171. ISBN 192094298X.
10. Pacific Australia Labour Mobility. Supporting Workers While They Are in Australia. 2022. Available online: https://www.palmscheme.gov.au/ (accessed on 23 June 2022).
11. Nangiloc; Colignan; Iraak. Nangiloc, Colignan and Iraak. 2022. Available online: https://nangiloc.vic.au/ (accessed on 23 June 2022).
12. Department of Health—Victorian Government. *Transmission and Response Epidemiology Victorian (TREVI) System*; Department of Health—Victorian Government: Melbourne, Australia.
13. Victorian Department of Health. Coronavirus (COVID-19) Victoria. Available online: https://www.coronavirus.vic.gov.au/ (accessed on 23 June 2022).
14. Jamaludin, S.; Azmir, N.A.; Ayob, A.F.M.; Zainal, N. COVID-19 exit strategy: Transitioning towards a new normal. *Ann. Med. Surg.* **2020**, *59*, 165–170. [CrossRef] [PubMed]

15. Department of Health—Victorian Government. Coronavirus (COVID-19) Guidance Note for the Victorian Public Service and Sector. 16 August 2021. Available online: https://www.vic.gov.au/coronavirus-covid-19-guidance-note-victorian-public-service-and-sector (accessed on 23 June 2022).
16. Mema, S.; Frosst, G.; Hanson, K.; Yates, C.; Anderson, A.; Jacobsen, J.; Guinar, C.; Lima, A.; Andersen, T.; Roe, M. COVID-19 outbreak among temporary foreign workers in British Columbia, March to May 2020. *Can. Commun. Dis. Rep. = Relev. des Mal. Transm. au Can.* **2021**, *47*, 5–10. [CrossRef] [PubMed]
17. Maslo, C.; Friedland, R.; Toubkin, M.; Laubscher, A.; Akaloo, T.; Kama, B. Characteristics and outcomes of hospitalized patients in South Africa during the COVID-19 Omicron wave compared with previous waves. *JAMA* **2022**, *327*, 583–584. [CrossRef] [PubMed]
18. Veneti, L.; Bøås, H.; Kristoffersen, A.B.; Stålcrantz, J.; Bragstad, K.; Hungnes, O.; Storm, N.L.; Aasand, N.; Rø, G.; Starrfelt, J.; et al. Reduced risk of hospitalisation among reported COVID-19 cases infected with the SARS-CoV-2 Omicron BA. 1 variant compared with the Delta variant, Norway, December 2021 to January 2022. *Eurosurveillance* **2022**, *27*, 2200077. [CrossRef]
19. Ward, I.L.; Bermingham, C.; Ayoubkhani, D.; Gethings, O.J.; Pouwels, K.; Yates, T.; Khunti, K.; Hippisley-Cox, J.; Banerjee, A.; Walker, A.S.; et al. Risk of COVID-19 related deaths for SARS-CoV-2 omicron (B.1.1.529) compared with delta (B.1.617.2): Retrospective cohort study. *BMJ* **2022**, *378*, e070695. [CrossRef] [PubMed]
20. Castañeda, H.; Carrion, I.V.; Kline, N.; Tyson, D.M. False hope: Effects of social class and health policy on oral health inequalities for migrant farmworker families. *Soc. Sci. Med.* **2010**, *71*, 2028–2037. [CrossRef] [PubMed]
21. McElfish, P.A.; Hallgren, E.; Yamada, S. Effect of US Health Policies on Health Care Access for Marshallese Migrants. *Am. J. Public Health* **2015**, *105*, 637–643. [CrossRef] [PubMed]
22. Okonkwo, N.E.; Aguwa, U.T.; Jang, M.; Barré, I.A.; Page, K.R.; Sullivan, P.S.; Beyrer, C.; Baral, S. COVID-19 and the US response: Accelerating health inequities. *BMJ Evid.-Based Med.* **2020**, *26*, 176–179. [CrossRef] [PubMed]
23. Jeewandara, C.; Guruge, D.; Pushpakumara, P.D.; Madhusanka, D.; Jayadas, T.T.; Chaturanga, I.P.; Aberathna, I.S.; Danasekara, S.; Pathmanathan, T.; Jayathilaka, D.; et al. Sensitivity and specificity of two WHO approved SARS-CoV2 antigen assays in detecting patients with SARS-CoV2 infection. *BMC Infect. Dis.* **2022**, *22*, 276. [CrossRef]
24. Peña, M.; Ampuero, M.; Garcés, C.; Gaggero, A.; García, P.; Velasquez, M.S.; Luza, R.; Alvarez, P.; Paredes, F.; Acevedo, J.; et al. Performance of SARS-CoV-2 rapid antigen test compared with real-time RT-PCR in asymptomatic individuals. *Int. J. Infect. Dis.* **2021**, *107*, 201–204. [CrossRef] [PubMed]

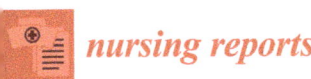 

*Article*

# COVID-19 Infection among Nursing Students in Spain: The Risk Perception, Perceived Risk Factors, Coping Style, Preventive Knowledge of the Disease and Sense of Coherence as Psychological Predictor Variables: A Cross Sectional Survey

Diego Serrano-Gómez [1], Verónica Velasco-González [2,*], Ana Rosa Alconero-Camarero [3], José Rafael González-López [4], Montserrat Antonín-Martín [5], Alicia Borras-Santos [5], Montserrat Edo-Gual [5], Vicente Gea-Caballero [6], José L. Gómez-Urquiza [7], Alfonso Meneses-Monroy [8], Montserrat Montaña-Peironcely [9] and Carmen Sarabia-Cobo [3]

1. Faculty of Health Sciences, Universidad de Burgos, 09001 Burgos, Spain
2. Nursing Care Research Group (GICE), Department of Nursing, Faculty of Nursing, Universidad de Valladolid, 47005 Valladolid, Spain
3. Faculty of Nursing, Universidad de Cantabria, IDIVAL Nursing Research Group, 39008 Santander, Spain
4. Department of Nursing, Faculty of Nursing, Physiotherapy and Podiatry, Universidad de Sevilla, 41009 Sevilla, Spain
5. Escola Universitària d'Infermeria, Escoles Universitàries Gimbernat, Universitat Autònoma de Barcelona, 08174 Barcelona, Spain
6. Faculty of Health, Universidad Internacional de Valencia, 46002 Valencia, Spain
7. Faculty of Health Sciences, Universidad de Granada, 18071 Granada, Spain
8. Faculty of Nursing, Physiotherapy and Podiatry, Universidad Complutense de University of Madrid, 28040 Madrid, Spain
9. Parc Taulí Hospital Universitari, Grup Recerca d'Infermeria, Institut d'Investigació i Innovació Parc Taulí (I3PT), Universitat Autònoma de Barcelona, 08208 Sabadell, Spain
* Correspondence: veronica.velasco.gonzalez@uva.es; Tel.: +34-983184165

**Abstract:** The exploration of patterns of health beliefs about COVID-19 among nursing students may be beneficial to identify behaviors, attitudes and knowledge about contagion risk. We sought to analyze the variables of risk perception, perceived risk factors, coping style, sense of coherence and knowledge of preventive measures as possible predictors of having suffered from COVID-19. Participants were nursing students from 13 universities in Spain. Sociodemographic and health variables were collected. To test the independent variables, the Perception Risk Coping Knowledge (PRCK-COVID-19) scale was created and validated because there was no specific survey for young people adapted to the pandemic situation of COVID-19. It was validated with adequate psychometric properties. A total of 1562 students (87.5% female, mean age 21.5 ± 5.7 years) responded. The high perception of the risk of contagion, the high level of knowledge and a coping style focused on the situation were notable. Significant differences by gender were found in the coping styles, problem-focused, avoidance and knowledge scales, with women scoring higher in all categories. The multiple regression analysis was significant (F = 3.68; $p < 0.001$). The predictor variables were the coping styles subscale search for support and the intrinsic and extrinsic perceived risk factors. Our model predicts that nursing students with a social support-based coping style are at a higher risk of becoming infected with COVID-19, based on their own health belief model.

**Keywords:** nursing students; coping behaviors; COVID-19; salutogenesis; risk factors; nurses

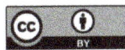

## 1. Introduction

It is evident that the recommendations to the population for the adoption of safety measures against COVID-19 have failed [1]. Classified as a worldwide pandemic, COVID-19 has affected more than 83 million people worldwide (1,893,502 in Spain) and caused more than 1.8 million deaths (50,000 in Spain) [2,3]. Recent research shows that health systems have allocated more resources to hospital and clinical care than to community care [4]. Experts warn that the key is to prevent the onset of the disease and not just treat it when its spread cannot be contained [5]. Hence, community and public health strategies are keys in prevention efforts.

These strategies are in line with the Health Belief Model [6,7] (Rosenstock, 1966, 1976), by which people, in general, present greater illusory optimism and a lower perception of risk, which are well-studied facts in processes such as adherence to treatment or prevention of risky behaviors (drugs, sexual practices, etc.) [8]. Rosenstock's Health Belief Model (HBM) is "a theoretical model concerned with health decision-making. The model attempts to explain the conditions under which a person will engage in individual health behaviors, such as preventative screenings or seeking treatment for a health condition" [6,7]. The model is based on the assumption that people's willingness to change their health behaviors primarily comes from their health perceptions. Individual beliefs about health and health conditions play a role in determining health-related behaviors. The psychological and cognitive processes underlying the Health Belief Models indicate that psychological constructs such as risk perception, coping style and knowledge perception are keys in the adoption of preventive measures against certain communicable diseases [9]. Thus, recent studies on COVID-19 focus on these psychological constructs [10]. Among the health models, one model that stands out in the field of public health and health promotion is the salutogenic model [11], which relates one's approach to stressful situations (such as the COVID-19 pandemic) to the individual's capacity for self-management of such situations [12]. This model develops concepts such as sense of coherence (SOC), which is directly related to the ability to employ cognitive, affective and instrumental strategies to better cope with stress [11].

Studies relating other psychological constructs besides SOC to the risk of acquisition of COVID-19 are unknown. Our study focused on nursing students (NS). Their lack of clinical experience, combined with their knowledge of preventive measures, may be valuable indicators for developing a predictive model relating psychological constructs such as SOC and coping styles to the likelihood of contracting the virus. This study constitutes an important aid in designing health education strategies in two manners: one, to inform the teachers of NS who perform their clinical placements, and two, based on general policies, since young people under 30 years of age seem to have a lower perception of risk in relation to the transmission of COVID-19 [13]. Our hypothesis considers that it is possible to predict the risk of contagion in nursing students, based on knowledge of psychological variables that, according to the literature, can act as mediators in this sense. These variables would have to relate to knowledge and coping strategies in the face of contagion, such as those we have described.

The main objective was to analyze the variables of risk perception, perceived risk factors, coping styles, SOC and knowledge of preventive measures among NS as possible mediating and predictor variables for contracting COVID-19.

## 2. Materials and Methods

*2.1. Design*

An observational single-group cross-sectional study was conducted. The participants were nursing students of 13 Spanish universities in all years of the degree. In Spain, the degree in nursing has a duration of four years and the students carry out clinical placements in health institutions from the second year onwards. Data collection was anonymous and did not entail any academic benefit for the students. Students were informed that participation was voluntary and that their involvement in the study would not affect their grade. We followed the Strengthening the Reporting of Observational Studies in Epidemiology (STROBE) [14]. All students received the instructions about the study by email with an information sheet and informed consent agreement. It was explained to them that their participation was anonymous, confidential and had no repercussions for the results.

### 2.2. Sample Size

Purposeful sampling methods were used. The study universe comprised a total of 7479 students. The sample size was calculated taking into account the statistical formula for prevalence of a known universe using the Grammo program (https://www.imim.es/ofertadeserveis/software-public/granmo/, accessed on 1 September 2020). It was increased by 20% to account for possible losses. Obtaining a minimum sample size of 366 students was thus sufficient to estimate a representative population mean, with 95% confidence and a margin of error of 5.

### 2.3. Variables and Instruments

Sociodemographic variables were collected, including age, gender, place of residence (rural/urban), course, chronic diseases, number of cohabitants during confinement and smoking habits.

A series of COVID-19 variables were also considered (questions with yes/no responses): Have you had COVID-19? Has anyone in your close environment suffered from the virus? Has anyone in your close environment died from COVID-19?

Having suffered from the disease was considered the dependent variable (DV).

The following independent variables were collected:

- Sense of coherence was evaluated using the Orientation to Life Questionnaire—13 Items (OLQ-13 or SOC-13) [15]. This instrument measures a global personality orientation that facilitates adaptive problem solving in stressful situations. The 13-item questionnaire also measures the dimensions of understandability (5 items), manageability (4 items) and meaningfulness (4 items). The scores express the strength of the person's SOC; the higher the score, the greater the strength. The answers offer a continuum of degree from minus to plus in 7 response options on a Likert scale from 1 to 7 ("never" "rarely" to "very often" or "always"), both in the positive and negative dimensions of the question. The OLQ-13 scale presents suitable internal consistency, with a Cronbach's alpha between 0.70 and 0.92 [16,17], and retains the same psychometric qualities as the original 29-item version. In this study, the internal consistency of the items was analyzed using Cronbach's alpha for the total scale (0.71) and for the comprehensibility (0.81), manageability (0.79) and significance (0.71) subscales.

For the assessment of risk perception, perceived risk factors and coping styles in the face of COVID-19, an ad hoc survey was designed by a panel of 6 experts based on the literature [18–20]. This survey, called the Perception. Risk. Coping. Knowledge (PRCK-COVID-19) scale, was created and validated because there was no specific survey for young people adapted to the pandemic situation of COVID-19. It was validated on a sample of 30 students, with adequate psychometric properties. The scales have been validated, piloted and created for the Spanish population. This survey consists of four scales:

- Perceived risk scale (3 items). The degree of agreement was shown on an LS (0, none and 10, maximum risk). The maximum score is 30 points, indicating that the higher the score, the higher the perceived risk of COVID-19 infection. Factor analysis identified a one-factor structure (Cronbach's alpha = 0.735).

- Perceived risk factors scale (16 items). The degree of agreement according to an LS was shown (from 1, strongly disagree to 5, strongly agree). The factor analysis identified a two-factor structure (total Cronbach's alpha = 0.781; FR1 alpha = 0.721; FR2 alpha = 0.841). The two factors identified correspond to risk factors perceived as external or dependent on the environment (9 items, extrinsic factor or FR1) or as personal factors that depend on their own behavior (7 items, intrinsic factor or FR2). The higher the score, the greater the weight of one risk factor over the other. The intrinsic factors are desirable because they refer to "the things I can do to protect myself", whereas the extrinsic factors refer to the inevitability of the disease and "factors that are beyond my control and for which I can do nothing" [21].
- Coping styles scale in the face of contagion (19 items). This scale gathered the degree of agreement according to an LS (from 1, strongly disagree to 5, strongly agree). Eight items are reversed. Factor analysis identified a three-factor structure (total Cronbach's alpha = 0.889). The three factors identified correspond to three coping styles when faced with COVID-19: EA1, reality-focused (7 items); EA2, avoidance (7 items); and EA3, support-seeking (5 items). The higher the score, the greater the weight of one risk factor over the other. Of the coping styles that coincide with the literature, reality-focused (greater self-efficacy) and support-seeking (5 items) are preferred [22].
- Preventive knowledge of COVID-19 scale (19 items). The degree of agreement was shown (from 1, strongly disagree to 5, strongly agree). The factor analysis identified a single factor structure called knowledge (Cronbach's alpha = 0.57). Reverse items are included in this scale. The maximum score is 60 points; a score range from 50 to 60 points indicates high knowledge, and lower scores indicate less knowledge.

### 2.4. Procedure

All variables were integrated into an online survey using Google Forms that was sent to all participating universities for dissemination, for convenience, through mailing lists, between November 2020 and January 2021. Multiple responses were avoided with the response identification protocol. Completing the questionnaire took an average of 6 min. The students only completed the questionnaires indicated in this work.

### 2.5. Statistical Analysis

IBM SPSS Statistics 22 was used for the statistical analysis. A bilateral contrast and a confidence level of 95% were adopted. To analyze possible missing values, we used the EM method (expected maximization). A descriptive analysis was performed for all the variables studied (means and SD for quantitative variables and percentages for qualitative variables). Comparisons were made between the categories defined by the independent variables for all the scales evaluated (SOC, coping styles, risk factors and knowledge) by means of Student's $t$-test for independent samples. A bivariate correlation analysis was performed between all the variables using Pearson's r test. A forward stepwise multiple regression analysis was calculated using the dependent variable of having suffered from COVID-19 and the predictor variables of different SOC scales, risk perception, risk factors, coping styles and knowledge.

### 2.6. Ethics

The researchers had no conflicts of interest. Ethical approval was obtained from the Research Ethics Committee of the University of Cantabria, Spain (CE Proyectos 13/2020). The treatment of the data guaranteed their confidentiality and their exclusive use for this project, respecting the legislation in force. At the beginning of the questionnaire, there was a specific box for giving consent to participate.

## 3. Results

### 3.1. Descriptive Analysis of the Sample

A total of 1562 people responded (response rate = 20.88%). Women accounted for 87.5% of the sample. The mean age was 21.5 ± 5.7 years. Up to 76.8% resided in urban areas. Participation of NS was equal for all four academic years. Overall, 67.9% did not suffer from any chronic disease, and 86.3% were non-smokers. In relation to COVID-19, only 9% had suffered from the virus, confirmed with a PCR test. For 52.8%, someone in their environment had suffered from the disease and of these, 6.9% died from it (Table 1).

**Table 1.** Sociodemographic variables of the sample and questions related to COVID-19.

|  |  | N | % |
|---|---|---|---|
| Gender [†] | Female | 1366 | 87.5% |
|  | Male | 193 | 12.4% |
| Age [†] |  | M 21.5 | DE 5.7 |
| Place of residence [†] | Rural | 351 | 22.5% |
|  | Urban | 1200 | 76.8% |
| Academic year [†] | 1st | 432 | 27.7% |
|  | 2nd | 413 | 26.4% |
|  | 3rd | 346 | 22.2% |
|  | 4th | 355 | 22.7% |
| Do you have any of the following chronic diseases? | No | 1060 | 67.9% |
|  | Allergy | 224 | 14.3% |
|  | Asthma | 109 | 7.0% |
|  | Diabetes | 11 | 0.7% |
|  | Hypertension | 7 | 0.4% |
|  | Obesity | 22 | 1.4% |
|  | Others * | 129 | 8.3% |
| Do you currently smoke? [†] | No | 1348 | 86.3% |
|  | Yes | 204 | 13.1% |
| Have you had COVID-19 (confirmed by PCR and/or serology)? [†] | No | 1406 | 90.0% |
|  | Yes | 140 | 9.0% |
| Has anyone in your close environment suffered from the virus? [†] | No | 726 | 46.5% |
|  | Yes | 824 | 52.8% |
| Has anyone close to you died from COVID-19? [†] | No | 1443 | 92.4% |
|  | Yes | 108 | 6.9% |

[†] Variable not answered by the totality of the sample. * Other diseases such as asthma, hypertension, hypothyroidism, diabetes, hyperlipidemia, cancer, bronchitis, etc.

## 3.2. Perceived Risk, Risk Factors and Preventive Knowledge about COVID-19

The students analyzed showed a medium-high perception of risk of COVID-19 infection (67.2%), with a greater weight of extrinsic factors (FR1, 75.6%) than intrinsic factors (FR2, 56.9%). Those who stated that someone in their close environment had suffered from COVID-19 scored significantly higher. Those who had experienced COVID-19 scored significantly higher on FR1 (extrinsic), and those who had not suffered COVID-19 scored higher on FR2 (intrinsic). Intrinsic factors scored differently depending on the academic year. The score obtained on the knowledge scale, which reached a high level in the general population (54.25 +/− 4.95 out of 60), was significantly higher in women and in those in more senior years (Table 2).

**Table 2.** Gender variables, academic year and having suffered COVID-19 by risk perception, risk factors and knowledge subscales (descriptive and differential analysis).

| Variable | N | Total Perceived Risk (Range 0–30) M/SD | FR1 (Range 9–45) M/SD | FR2 (Range 7–35) M/SD | Knowledge (Range 50–60) M/SD |
|---|---|---|---|---|---|
| Total | 1559 | 20.15 (4.27) | 34.00 (4.04) | 19.93 (2.88) | 54.25 (4.95) |
| Gender | | | | | |
| Female | 1366 | 20.17 (4.25) | 34.05 (4.06) | 19.97 (2.88) | 54.44 ** (4.88) |
| Male | 193 | 20.03 (4.45) | 33.63 (3.94) | 19.58 (2.86) | 52.91 (5.23) |
| Academic year | | | | | |
| 1st | 432 | 20 (4.32) | 33.71 (4.25) | 19.89 (2.92) * | 53.62 ** (5.38) |
| 2nd | 413 | 20.2 (4.20) | 33.98 (3.85) | 20.25 (2.80) * | 54.15 (4.70) |
| 3rd | 346 | 20.05 (4.29) | 33.88 (3.99) | 19.49 (2.89) * | 54.08 (5.28) |
| 4th | 355 | 20.34 (4.30) | 34.49 (4.06) | 19.89 (2.86) * | 55.25 (4.16) |
| Have you had COVID-19 (confirmed by PCR and/or serology)? | | | | | |
| Yes | 140 | 19.99 (4.92) | 34.07 (3.95) * | 19.43 (3.18) * | 54.55 (4.78) |
| No | 1406 | 20.16 (4.21) | 33.20 (4.82) | 19.97 (2.84) | 54.24 (4.97) |
| Has anyone close to you died from COVID-19? | | | | | |
| Yes | 108 | 20.15 (3.98) | 33.78 (3.83) | 20.02 (2.39) | 54.68 (4.24) |
| No | 1443 | 20.14 (4.30) | 34.01 (4.05) | 19.92 (2.91) | 54.21 (5.00) |
| Has anyone in your close environment suffered from COVID-19? | | | | | |
| Yes | 726 | 20.58 (4.25) ** | 34.11 (4.03) | 19.93 (2.74) | 54.29 (4.77) |
| No | 824 | 19.65 (4.26) | 33.88 (4.06) | 19.92 (3.02) | 54.19 (5.15) |

* $p$ value < 0.05. ** $p$ value < 0.001. FR1 = extrinsic risk factors. FR2 = intrinsic risk factors.

### 3.3. Coping Styles in the Face of COVID-19

EA1 (reality-focused) coping styles, which acquired greater weight in the sample of students analyzed, scored significantly higher among females. AE2 (avoidance), which ranked last when analyzing the entire sample, scored significantly higher among females, first-year students and those who reported that someone in their close environment had suffered or died from COVID-19. AE3 (seeking support) scored significantly higher among fourth-year students and those who reported that they or someone close to them had suffered from COVID-19 (Table 3). Of the three styles, only for EA3 did those who had experienced COVID-19 score significantly higher.

### 3.4. Sense of Coherence towards COVID-19

The mean total SOC for the entire sample was 52.77 ± 6.71 points (out of 91), with the relative order of the dimensions, according to their percentage of each total, being understandability, manageability and meaningfulness. Females and first-year students scored significantly higher for the total SOC and in the understandability and meaningfulness dimensions. Males scored significantly higher in the manageability dimension. Those who stated that someone in their environment had died from COVID-19 scored significantly higher in the total SOC and the manageability dimension (Table 4).

**Table 3.** COVID-19 coping styles. EA1 (situation-focused coping style); EA2 (avoidance coping style); EA3 (support-seeking coping style).

| Variable | N | EA1 (Range 7–35) M/SD | EA2 (Range 7–35) M/SD | EA3 (Range 5–25) M/SD |
|---|---|---|---|---|
| Total | 1532 | 27.79 (4.15) | 18.27 (5.48) | 17.16 (3.96) |
| Gender | | | | |
| Female | 1366 | 27.92 (4.12) ** | 18.51 (5.44) ** | 17.18 (3.97) |
| Male | 193 | 26.8 (4.25) | 16.69 (5.46) | 17.04 (3.89) |
| Academic year | | | | |
| 1st | 432 | 27.53 (4.47) | 19.16 (5.69) ** | 16.62 (4.15) |
| 2nd | 413 | 27.63 (3.97) | 18.58 (5.47) | 17.24 (3.68) |
| 3rd | 346 | 27.73 (4.27) | 17.65 (5.27) | 16.96 (4.12) |
| 4th | 355 | 28.32 (3.81) * | 17.47 (5.31) | 17.93 (3.78) ** |
| Have you had COVID-19 yourself (confirmed by PCR and/or serology)? | | | | |
| Yes | 140 | 28.22 (4.02) | 18.60 (5.60) | 18.24 (3.9) ** |
| No | 1406 | 27.74 (4.16) | 18.23 (5.46) | 17.06 (3.95) |
| Has anyone close to you died from COVID-19? | | | | |
| Yes | 106 | 28.05 (3.75) | 19.58 (5.92) * | 17.74 (4.40) |
| No | 1423 | 27.76 (4.18) | 18.17 (5.43) | 17.11 (3.92) |
| Has anyone in your close environment suffered from COVID-19? | | | | |
| Yes | 814 | 27.70 (4.13) | 18.64 (5.57) ** | 17.41 (3.93) * |
| No | 718 | 27.88 (4.17) | 17.86 (5.35) | 16.90 (3.97) |

\* $p$ value < 0.05. ** $p$ value < 0.001. EA1 = situation-focused; EA2 = avoidance; EA3 = support-seeking.

**Table 4.** Sense of coherence (SOC) versus COVID-19.

| Variable | N | SOC Total (Range 13–91) M/SD | SOC1 (Range 5–35) M/SD | SOC2 (Range 4–28) M/SD | SOC3 (Range 4–28) M/SD |
|---|---|---|---|---|---|
| Total | 1520 | 52.77 (6.71) | 16.58 (3.63) | 14.39 (2.67) | 17.55 (2.62) |
| Gender | | | | | |
| Female | 1366 | 52.94 (6.67) * | 16.67 (3.58) * | 14.34 (2.65) | 17.64 (2.59) ** |
| Male | 193 | 51.60 (6.91) | 16.04 (3.97) | 14.78 (2.76) * | 16.90 (2.71) |
| Academic year | | | | | |
| 1st | 432 | 54.09 (6.4) ** | 17.24 (3.36) ** | 14.64 (2.71) | 17.82 (2.62) * |
| 2nd | 413 | 52.84 (7) | 16.72 (3.71) | 14.25 (2.77) | 17.64 (2.64) |
| 3rd | 346 | 52.37 (6.37) | 16.37 (3.66) | 14.35 (2.44) | 17.42 (2.44) |
| 4th | 355 | 51.56 (6.8) | 15.89 (3.67) | 14.31 (2.69) | 17.23 (2.72) |
| Have you had it (confirmed by PCR and/or serology)? | | | | | |
| Yes | 140 | 52.8 (6.69) | 16.59 (3.06) | 14.54 (2.9) | 17.48 (2.66) |
| No | 1406 | 52.76 (6.68) | 16.57 (3.69) | 14.38 (2.64) | 17.56 (2.6) |
| Has anyone close to you died from COVID-19? | | | | | |
| Yes | 105 | 54.66 (6.44) * | 17.12 (3.42) | 14.96 (2.84) * | 17.92 (2.33) |
| No | 1412 | 52.62 (6.72) | 16.53 (3.65) | 14.35 (2.65) | 17.52 (2.64) |
| Has anyone in your close environment suffered from COVID-19? | | | | | |
| Yes | 802 | 52.95 (6.76) | 16.72 (3.59) | 14.39 (2.62) | 17.59 (2.56) |
| No | 714 | 52.54 (6.66) | 16.42 (3.67) | 14.39 (2.69) | 17.50 (2.68) |

\* $p$ value < 0.05. ** $p$ value < 0.001. SOC1 (comprehensibility); SOC2 (manageability); SOC3 (significance).

### 3.5. Predictive Factors of Having Suffered from COVID-19

The correlational analysis indicated a significant association between the variable of having suffered from COVID-19 and all the SOC subscales (total $r = -0.23$, $p < 0.001$; comprehensibility $r = -0.58$, $p < 0.001$; manageability $r = -0.21$, $p < 0.001$; significance $r = -0.22$, $p < 0.001$), the risk perception scale ($r = -0.47$, $p < 0.001$), the risk factor subscales (FR1 $r = -0.84$, $p < 0.001$; FR2 $r = -0.41$, $p < 0.001$), the coping style subscales (EA1 $r = -0.57$, $p < 0.001$; EA2 $r = -0.61$, $p < 0.001$; EA3 $r = -0.84$, $p < 0.001$) and knowledge ($r = -0.25$, $p < 0.001$).

A forward stepwise multiple regression analysis was performed using having suffered from COVID-19 as the dependent variable and the different SOC scales, risk perception, risk factors, coping style and knowledge as predictor variables. The model was significant (F = 3.68; $p < 0.001$) and managed to explain 15% of the variance in the criterion variable (suffering from COVID-19) by means of the predictor variables EA3, FR1 and FR2. The subscale EA3 (support-seeking) is the most relevant predictor (beta = $-0.12$; $p < 0.001$), explaining 8% of the variance of the criterion variable, followed by FR1 (extrinsic factors) (beta = 0.07; $p = 0.008$) and FR2 (intrinsic factors) (beta = 0.06; $p < 0.001$) (Table 5).

**Table 5.** Multiple regression analysis.

| Predictors | Increase in $R^2$ | Increase in Adjusted $R^2$ | B | Standard Error | Beta | t | Sig. |
|---|---|---|---|---|---|---|---|
| EA3 | 0.8 | 0.8 | −0.68 | 0.10 | −0.12 | −6.64 | 0.000 |
| FR1 | 0.04 | 0.04 | −0.22 | 0.08 | 0.07 | −2.63 | 0.008 |
| FR2 | 0.03 | 0.04 | 0.06 | 0.28 | 0.06 | 2.65 | 0.000 |

Dependent variable: having suffered from COVID-19. EA3 = support-seeking; FR1= extrinsic risk factors; FR2 = intrinsic risk factors. $R^2$ total for the model = 0.15; $R^2$ total model adjustment = 0.15 (F = 3.68; $p < 0.001$).

## 4. Discussion

*Geographical context of the pandemic in the country of study.*

Spain is a country that has stood out throughout the pandemic considering two aspects in the management executed by the authorities. First, control has been exercised from the central government, but each region of the country has its own competencies in health legislation. This means that although a state of alarm was decreed throughout the national territory (with the mandatory confinement of the entire population between March and June 2020, limitation of mobility, control of capacity in premises, mandatory use of a mask indoors, etc.), each region, as of September 2020, has implemented its own measures, which could not contradict State regulations, but which sometimes differed from one area of the country to another. This situation, similar to other countries such as Italy and Portugal, led to an unequal approach to the control of the pandemic, with large differences in contagion and control. Shelling the comparative aspects of the sample by country zone exceeds the objectives of this study, but that is why it is representative of most regions of the country. It is usual in this type of study to carry out an extensive data collection (longitudinal and cross-sectional study design) and with a sample that is as geographically heterogeneous as possible. The second important milestone in Spain was the premature vaccination campaign (December 2020) compared to other European countries, with a high vaccination rate throughout the national territory. However, this fact comes after the data collection of this study, so even in spite of its relevance (in terms of the explanation of risk perception, coping styles and sense of coherence in the face of health behaviors such as getting vaccinated), it is not worth discussing here.

### 4.1. Descriptive Analysis of the Sample

Risk perception makes it possible to assess why people do or do not take measures to protect themselves from external threats [23]; therefore, it would be desirable for the scores to be proportionally higher in the intrinsic subscale ("I can control my behavior to avoid risk factors"). In our study, we found that the extrinsic risk factor (FR1) was the highest in the sample. This variable is related to the disease as a risk (linked to the inevitability of the disease and "factors that are alien to me and over which I have no influence"). Our results could be justified in part by the "inevitability" of the disease, transmitted through the media and the lack of reliable data in the face of an unknown disease that generates fear, stress and uncertainty [24].

Both subscales of risk perception factors revealed medium-high values, in agreement with those obtained by other authors in Belgian NS populations [25], Saudi populations [26], German populations [20], Pakistani populations [23] and Spanish populations [27]. As in other professions, being in higher years of study [26] is associated with an increased perception of risk. Surprisingly, in contrast to the results obtained by others [20,23,26,27], gender does not seem to influence risk perception, which may be due to the low male representation in our sample. Having close experiences with COVID-19 reduces the perception of risk, in contrast with previous findings [25,27], although in these former studies, the "experiences" involve professional patient care, and in our study, the experiences are more related to the family or social environment.

The population analyzed showed high knowledge of prevention, which coincides with other studies conducted among nursing students [25,28] and medical students [29]. This is probably due to the fact that in the latter, data collection was carried out at the beginning of the pandemic, when numerous studies were being conducted [24,27]. In line with other authors, women [26,28] and students in higher years [26] who carried out their clinical practices during the pandemic showed greater knowledge. Unlike what was observed for risk factors, in our sample, knowledge was not affected by experiences related to COVID-19.

In relation to the coping styles scale, several papers have been published that use different scales to study the coping strategies used by the general population [20,23,30] or NS in particular [29,30] in the face of the pandemic. In line with our findings, other studies [31,32] have also found that situation-focused coping strategies are the most employed by students to face COVID-19, and they are more employed by females [20,23,31]. In our study, significant differences were found between men and women for the situation-centered and avoidance coping styles, with higher scores among women in both. It is also noteworthy that EA3 (support-seeking) yielded statistically significant differences between people who have suffered from the disease and those who have not, with higher scores in the former [33].

The most significant findings in SOC values revealed medium values on the total scale and on the three subscales, which is in line with similar studies [34,35]. Women scored significantly higher on the comprehensibility and meaningfulness subscales, while men scored significantly higher on the manageability subscales, consistent with a former study [36]. Men present more practical and applied coping values than women, who find more meaning and understanding in what is happening, finding a meaning that allows them to deal better with stressful situations [37]. However, despite the significant values in the SOC variable, this has not played any relevant role in the predictive model, unlike other studies [38,39]. It is likely that this may be due to the fact that the variables of the coping styles and risk perception scales have displaced this other scale when it comes to coping with the situation, a fact that is corroborated by studies on prevention and health promotion [40,41].

*4.2. Predictive Model*

From the perspective of psychological variables related to prevention and a model of health beliefs, we found three variables to predict having suffered from the disease: the coping styles subscale, *search for support*, and the intrinsic and extrinsic perceived risk factors, which explain 15% of the variance. These results seem to indicate that people who, according to our support-seeking subscale, seek support in the opinion of experts, the media, third parties or government measures, contracted COVID-19. Relying on changing and contradictory information from authorities could justify this coping style, as has been partially suggested by other studies [13,42]. Those with an extrinsic risk factor present passive behaviors and attitudes, focused on the inevitability of the situation versus those with an intrinsic style focused on their own ability to protect themselves and take action. Both styles could be related to internal and external locus of control, as suggested by previous authors [43]. Interestingly, both are predictor variables, although to a lesser extent. Whereas the extrinsic factor is contemplated in other studies, as it favors adopting a passive and non-preventive attitude towards contagion [44], the intrinsic factor is not so easy to explain, suggesting the need for further research.

This study has several limitations. It is important to note that a sampling selection was used, and although it was intended to be a representative sample, generalization of the findings should be considered with caution. It should also be noted that although the questionnaire used was validated with adequate psychometric properties, it is necessary to confirm these findings on a larger sample. Analysis of long-term maintenance of acquired knowledge and reinforced attitudes may be a future line of research. It would be interesting to extend the sample to the same universities as well as to other students of health sciences, such as medicine. We must also be cautious with the generalization of the results in these types of studies due to the design (cross-sectional study). Another important limitation is that all the measures were self-report questionnaires so that the subjective value of responding is conditioned by the circumstances surrounding the person.

## 5. Conclusions

Our predictive model allows us to predict that NS with a coping style based on social support and a perception of high intrinsic and extrinsic risk factors present a greater risk of contracting COVID-19, according to their own model of health beliefs. Women presented greater knowledge of preventive measures and a more situation-focused coping style than men.

Female students in their final years, with more knowledge and experience in clinical practice, also presented more knowledge, a more extrinsic risk perception and a more situation-focused and less avoidant coping style than younger students. In terms of SOC, females scored significantly higher in total SOC and in the comprehensibility and meaningfulness dimensions, whereas males scored significantly higher in the manageability dimension.

Our study provides a model of health beliefs that can be considered when focusing on the preventive measures to be implemented among NS who must undertake their clinical practices.

Investing in training and educating in a health belief model that addresses psychological variables such as risk perception, coping styles and sense of coherence may have important benefits for career and internship curriculum design.

**Author Contributions:** Conceptualization, C.S.-C.; Data curation, C.S.-C.; Formal analysis, C.S.-C.; Investigation, D.S.-G., V.V.-G., A.R.A.-C., J.R.G.-L., M.A.-M., A.B.-S., M.E.-G., V.G.-C., J.L.G.-U., A.M.-M. and M.M.-P.; Methodology, C.S.-C.; Project administration, C.S.-C.; Writing—original draft, D.S.-G., V.V.-G., A.R.A.-C. and C.S.-C.; Writing—review and editing, D.S.-G., V.V.-G., A.R.A.-C. and C.S.-C. All authors have read and agreed to the published version of the manuscript.

**Funding:** This research did not receive any specific grant from funding agencies in the public, commercial, or not-for-profit sectors.

**Institutional Review Board Statement:** The study was conducted according to the guidelines of the Declaration of Helsinki and approved by the Research Ethics Committee of the University of Cantabria, Spain (CE Proyectos 13/2020).

**Informed Consent Statement:** Informed consent was obtained from all subjects involved in the study.

**Data Availability Statement:** The data presented in this study are available on request from the corresponding author.

**Acknowledgments:** We are grateful to all participating institutions and students.

**Conflicts of Interest:** The authors declare no potential conflict of interest with respect to the research, authorship and/or publication of this article.

# References

1. Broucke, S.V.D. Why health promotion matters to the COVID-19 pandemic, and vice versa. *Health Promot. Int.* **2020**, *35*, 181–186. [CrossRef] [PubMed]
2. World Health Organization, 2021. COVID-19 Weekly Epidemiological Update 22–12 January 2021. World Health Organ. 1–3. Available online: https://apps.who.int/iris/handle/10665/339547 (accessed on 11 January 2022).
3. World Health Organization. Infection Prevention and Control during Health Care When COVID-19 Is Suspected, Interim Guidance. 2021. Available online: https://apps.who.int/iris/handle/10665/331495 (accessed on 11 January 2022).
4. Smith, J.A.; Judd, J. COVID-19: Vulnerability and the power of privilege in a pandemic. *Health Promot. J. Aust.* **2020**, *31*, 158–160. [CrossRef] [PubMed]
5. Carson, A. Deadly Choices: The importance of health promotion and prevention during the COVID-19 pandemic. *Health Voices* **2020**, *9*, 26.
6. Rosenstock, I.M. Why people use health services. *Milbank Meml. Fund Q.* **1966**, *44*, 94–127. [CrossRef]
7. Rosenstock, I.M. Historical Origins of the Health Belief Model. *Health Educ. Monogr.* **1974**, *2*, 328–335. [CrossRef]
8. Anderson, R.M.; Heesterbeek, H.; Klinkenberg, D.; Hollingsworth, T.D. How will country-based mitigation measures influence the course of the COVID-19 epidemic? *Lancet* **2020**, *395*, 931–934. [CrossRef]
9. Tagini, S.; Brugnera, A.; Ferrucci, R.; Mazzocco, K.; Compare, A.; Silani, V.; Pravettoni, G.; Poletti, B. It won't happen to me! Psychosocial factors influencing risk perception for respiratory infectious diseases: A scoping review. *Appl. Psychol. Health Well-Being* **2021**, *13*, 835–852. [CrossRef]
10. Kebede, Y.; Yitayih, Y.; Birhanu, Z.; Mekonen, S.; Ambelu, A. Knowledge, perceptions and preventive practices towards COVID-19 early in the outbreak among Jimma university medical center visitors, Southwest Ethiopia. *PLoS ONE* **2020**, *15*, e0233744. [CrossRef]
11. Mittelmark, M.B.; Sagy, S.; Eriksson, M.; Bauer, G.F.; Pelikan, J.M.; Lindström, B.; Espnes, G.A. *The Handbook of Salutogenesis*; Springer International Publishing: Cham, Switzerland, 2016. [CrossRef]

12. Becker, C.M.; Glascoff, M.A.; Felts, W.M. Salutogenesis 30 Years Later: Where Do We Go from here? *Int. Electron. J. Health Educ.* **2010**, *13*, 25–32.
13. Andrews, J.L.; Foulkes, L.; Blakemore, S.-J. Peer Influence in Adolescence: Public-Health Implications for COVID-19. *Trends Cogn. Sci.* **2020**, *24*, 585–587. [CrossRef]
14. Von Elm, E.; Altman, D.G.; Egger, M.; Pocock, S.J.; Gøtzsche, P.C.; Vandenbroucke, J.P.; STROBE Initiative. The Strengthening the Reporting of Observational Studies in Epidemiology (STROBE)statement: Guidelines for reporting observational studies. *J Clin Epidemiol.* **2008**, *61*, 344–349. [CrossRef] [PubMed]
15. Antonovsky, A. The structure and properties of the sense of coherence scale. *Soc. Sci. Med.* **1993**, *36*, 725–733. [CrossRef]
16. Antonovsky, A. The salutogenic model as a theory to guide health promotion. *Health Promot. Int.* **1996**, *11*, 11–18. [CrossRef]
17. Eriksson, M.; Lindström, B. Validity of Antonovsky's sense of coherence scale: A systematic review. *J. Epidemiol. Community Health* **2005**, *59*, 460–466. [CrossRef]
18. Brug, J.; Aro, A.R.; Oenema, A.; De Zwart, O.; Richardus, J.H.; Bishop, G.D. SARS Risk Perception, Knowledge, Precautions, and Information Sources, the Netherlands. *Emerg. Infect. Dis.* **2004**, *10*, 1486–1489. [CrossRef]
19. de Zwart, O.; Veldhuijzen, I.K.; Elam, G.; Aro, A.R.; Abraham, T.; Bishop, G.D.; Voeten, H.A.C.M.; Richardus, J.H.; Brug, J. Perceived Threat, Risk Perception, and Efficacy Beliefs Related to SARS and Other (Emerging) Infectious Diseases: Results of an International Survey. *Int. J. Behav. Med.* **2009**, *16*, 30–40. [CrossRef]
20. Gerhold, L. COVID-19: Risk perception and Coping strategies. *PsyArXiv* **2020**. preprint. [CrossRef]
21. Zhong, Y.; Liu, W.; Lee, T.-Y.; Zhao, H.; Ji, J. Risk perception, knowledge, information sources and emotional states among COVID-19 patients in Wuhan, China. *Nurs. Outlook* **2020**, *69*, 13–21. [CrossRef]
22. Greenaway, K.H.; Louis, W.R.; Parker, S.L.; Kalokerinos, E.K.; Smith, J.R.; Terry, D.J. Measures of coping for psychological well-being. In *Measures of Personality and Social Psychological Constructs*; Academic Press: Cambridge, MA, USA, 2015; pp. 322–351.
23. Rana, I.A.; Bhatti, S.S.; Aslam, A.B.; Jamshed, A.; Ahmad, J.; Shah, A.A. COVID-19 risk perception and coping mechanisms: Does gender make a difference? *Int. J. Disaster Risk Reduct.* **2021**, *55*, 102096. [CrossRef]
24. Hunter, P. The spread of the COVID-19 coronavirus. *EMBO Rep.* **2020**, *21*, e50334. [CrossRef]
25. Ulenaers, D.; Grosemans, J.; Schrooten, W.; Bergs, J. Clinical placement experience of nursing students during the COVID-19 pandemic: A cross-sectional study. *Nurse Educ. Today* **2021**, *99*, 104746. [CrossRef]
26. Albaqawi, H.M.; Alquwez, N.; Balay-Odao, E.; Bajet, J.B.; Alabdulaziz, H.; Alsolami, F.; Tumala, R.B.; Alsharari, A.F.; Tork, H.M.M.; Felemban, E.M.; et al. Nursing Students' Perceptions, Knowledge, and Preventive Behaviors Toward COVID-19: A Multi-University Study. *Front. Public Health* **2020**, *8*, 573390. [CrossRef]
27. Domínguez, J.M.M.; Jiménez, I.F.; Eraso, A.B.; Otero, D.P.; Pérez, D.D.; Vivas, A.M.R. Risk Perception of COVID–19 Community Transmission among the Spanish Population. *Int. J. Environ. Res. Public Health* **2020**, *17*, 8967. [CrossRef]
28. Gao, Z.; Ying, S.; Liu, J.; Zhang, H.; Li, J.; Ma, C. A cross-sectional study: Comparing the attitude and knowledge of medical and non-medical students toward 2019 novel coronavirus. *J. Infect. Public Health* **2020**, *13*, 1419–1423. [CrossRef]
29. Pandit, S.B.; Pandit, R.B. Knowledge, Attitude and Practices of Nursing Students towards COVID-19: A Cross Sectional Study. *Int. J. Health Sci. Res.* **2021**. Available online: www.ijhsr.org (accessed on 11 January 2020).
30. Li, D.-J.; Ko, N.-Y.; Chang, Y.-P.; Yen, C.-F.; Chen, Y.-L. Mediating Effects of Risk Perception on Association between Social Support and Coping with COVID-19: An Online Survey. *Int. J. Environ. Res. Public Health* **2021**, *18*, 1550. [CrossRef]
31. Huang, L.; Lei, W.; Xu, F.; Liu, H.; Yu, L. Emotional responses and coping strategies in nurses and nursing students during COVID-19 outbreak: A comparative study. *PLoS ONE* **2020**, *15*, e0237303. [CrossRef]
32. Savitsky, B.; Findling, Y.; Ereli, A.; Hendel, T. Anxiety and coping strategies among nursing students during the COVID-19 pandemic. *Nurse Educ. Pract.* **2020**, *46*, 102809. [CrossRef]
33. Ferdous, M.Z.; Islam, S.; Sikder, T.; Mosaddek, A.S.; Zegarra-Valdivia, J.A.; Gozal, D. Knowledge, attitude, and practice regarding COVID-19 outbreak in Bangladesh: An online-based cross-sectional study. *PLoS ONE* **2020**, *15*, e0239254. [CrossRef]
34. Salamonson, Y.; Ramjan, L.M.; Nieuwenhuizen, S.V.D.; Metcalfe, L.; Chang, S.; Everett, B. Sense of coherence, self-regulated learning and academic performance in first year nursing students: A cluster analysis approach. *Nurse Educ. Pract.* **2016**, *17*, 208–213. [CrossRef]
35. van der Riet, P.; Levett-Jones, T.; Aquino-Russell, C. The effectiveness of mindfulness meditation for nurses and nursing students: An integrated literature review. *Nurse Educ. Today* **2018**, *65*, 201–211. [CrossRef]
36. Länsimies, H.; Pietilä, A.-M.; Hietasola-Husu, S.; Kangasniemi, M. A systematic review of adolescents' sense of coherence and health. *Scand. J. Caring Sci.* **2017**, *31*, 651–661. [CrossRef]
37. Ribeiro, Í.J.S.; Pereira, R.; Freire, I.V.; de Oliveira, B.G.; Casotti, C.A.; Boery, E.N. Stress and Quality of Life Among University Students: A Systematic Literature Review. *Health Prof. Educ.* **2018**, *4*, 70–77. [CrossRef]
38. Chu, J.J.; Khan, M.H.; Jahn, H.J.; Kraemer, A. Sense of coherence and associated factors among university students in China: Cross-sectional evidence. *BMC Public Health* **2016**, *16*, 336. [CrossRef]
39. Barni, D.; Danioni, F.; Canzi, E.; Ferrari, L.; Ranieri, S.; Lanz, M.; Iafrate, R.; Regalia, C.; Rosnati, R. Facing the COVID-19 Pandemic: The Role of Sense of Coherence. *Front. Psychol.* **2020**, *11*, 578440. [CrossRef]
40. Commódari, E.; La Rosa, V.L. Adolescents in Quarantine During COVID-19 Pandemic in Italy: Perceived Health Risk, Beliefs, Psychological Experiences and Expectations for the Future. *Front. Psychol.* **2020**, *11*, 559951. [CrossRef]

41. Dymecka, J.; Gerymski, R.; Machnik-Czerwik, A. How does stress affect life satisfaction during the COVID-19 pandemic? Moderated mediation analysis of sense of coherence and fear of coronavirus. *Psychol. Health Med.* **2021**, *27*, 280–288. [CrossRef]
42. Hyland-Wood, B.; Gardner, J.; Leask, J.; Ecker, U.K.H. Toward effective government communication strategies in the era of COVID-19. *Humanit. Soc. Sci. Commun.* **2021**, *8*, 30. [CrossRef]
43. Armaş, I.; Cretu, R.Z.; Ionescu, R. Self-efficacy, stress, and locus of control: The psychology of earthquake risk perception in Bucharest, Romania. *Int. J. Disaster Risk Reduct.* **2017**, *22*, 71–76. [CrossRef]
44. Heydari, S.T.; Zarei, L.; Sadati, A.K.; Moradi, N.; Akbari, M.; Mehralian, G.; Lankarani, K.B. The effect of risk communication on preventive and protective Behaviours during the COVID-19 outbreak: Mediating role of risk perception. *BMC Public Health* **2021**, *21*, 54. [CrossRef]

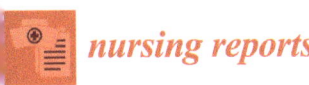 

*Article*

# Examining Healthcare Professionals' Telehealth Usability before and during COVID-19 in Saudi Arabia: A Cross-Sectional Study

Mohammed Gh. Alzahrani [1], Nazik M. A. Zakari [2], Dina I. Abuabah [2], Mona S. Ousman [2], Jing Xu [3] and Hanadi Y. Hamadi [3,*]

[1] Department of Respiratory Care, College of Applied Sciences, AlMaarefa University, Diriyah, Riyadh 13713, Saudi Arabia
[2] College of Applied Sciences, AlMaarefa University, Riyadh 11597, Saudi Arabia
[3] Department of Health Administration, Brooks College of Health, University of North Florida, Jacksonville, FL 32224, USA
* Correspondence: h.hamadi@unf.edu

**Abstract:** COVID-19 has placed substantial stress on healthcare providers in Saudi Arabia as they struggle to avoid contracting the virus, provide continued care for their patients, and protect their own families at home from possible exposure. The demand for care has increased due to the need to treat COVID-19. This pandemic has created a surge in the need for care in select healthcare delivery specialties, forcing other nonurgent or elective care to halt or transition to telehealth. This study provides a timely description of how COVID-19 affected employment, telehealth usage, and interprofessional collaboration. The STROBE checklist was used. We developed a cross-sectional online survey design that is rooted and grounded in the Technology Acceptance Model (TAM). The TAM model allows us to identify characteristics that affect the use of telehealth technologies. The survey was deployed in November 2021 to local healthcare providers in Saudi Arabia. There were 66 individuals in the final sample. Both interprofessional satisfaction on frequency and quality were positively correlated with the frequency of interactions. The odds for satisfaction of frequency and quality were about 12 times (OR = 12.27) and 8 times 110 (OR = 8.24) more, respectively, for the participants with more than three times of interaction than the participants with no interaction at all. We also found that change in telehealth usage during the pandemic was positively associated with the Telehealth Usability Questionnaire (TUQ) scores. The estimated score for the participants who reported an increase in telehealth usage was 5.37, while the scores were lower for the participants reporting 'no change' and 'decreased usage'. Additional training on telehealth use and integration to improve interprofessionalism is needed.

**Keywords:** COVID-19; telehealth; Saudi Arabia; interprofessionalism; usability

## 1. Introduction

COVID-19 and related precautions have affected various healthcare services that have been either temporarily closed or transitioned to virtual care delivery and have placed substantial stress on healthcare providers. Therefore, using telehealth technologies and its policy incentivizing is an emergent need now more than ever. While work demands have varied, it is very important to examine the usability of telehealth implementation and services in Saudi Arabia during COVID-19. The combination of higher costs for the acquisition of personal protective equipment and an increased number of health providers testing positive has created a strain on the healthcare workforce [1]. Frontline healthcare providers have been reporting increased symptoms of anxiety and depression related to burnout, and fatigue and chronic concern for lack of personal protective equipment (PPE) [2]. The demand for care is relatively consistent; however, this pandemic has created

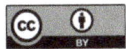

a surge in the need for care in select healthcare delivery specialties, forcing other nonurgent or elective care to halt or transition to telehealth [3]. Even with the slowdown or in some cases halting of elective surgeries [4–6], millions of individuals with chronic diseases or non-COVID-19 illnesses still required access to care [4,7]. COVID-19 has created the need for 'social distancing' [8,9] to slow the spread of the virus, thus reducing the ability to provide in-person healthcare services. This forced distancing made telehealth an ideal modality to deliver necessary care [10]. Telehealth technologies group synchronous (phone and video) and asynchronous (store and forward such as patient portals) communication and virtual agents (telemonitoring through wearable devices); all of these activities allow the delivery of care and the interaction of provider-to-patient or provider-to-provider [11]. During these strenuous times, the need for telehealth services has pushed many organizations to expand their telehealth capabilities to serve patients while maintaining their safety at home [12].

However, most organizations and professions were not telehealth ready before the pandemic, causing staff resistance and lack of utilization of this technology within the interprofessional setting when it was needed most [13]. The lack of prior utilization of this technology is not the only challenge, but also several challenges are encountered in the usage and uptake of telehealth. These include digital illiteracy, technology, and internet access, gender, age, rural location, and low-income patients [14,15]. For telehealth to be effective during a healthcare crisis, we must rapidly understand how such technologies are being utilized and integrated into models of care. Therefore, this study aims to understand how healthcare providers, telehealth utilization, and interprofessional interactions were affected during COVID-19.

## 2. Materials and Methods

*Study and Instrument Design*

We used a cross-sectional online survey design that is rooted and grounded in the Technology Acceptance Model (TAM). The TAM model allows us to identify characteristics that affect the use of telehealth technologies. Survey questions for this study were extracted from validated health surveys such as the Telehealth Usability Questionnaire (TUQ) [16–18]. This study expands on a previous study conducted in the United States and has been modified specifically for healthcare professionals in Saudi Arabia. The research team reviewed the survey instrument and ensured face validity. The study was submitted to the University Institutional Review Board (IRB), and received approval under 'expedited review'. The final web-based survey consisted of demographic questions, provider practice questions, patient engagement questions, and the TUQ. We included questions on telehealth use before the start of the pandemic and during the third wave of the COVID-19 pandemic. This survey was created and disseminated using the web-tool Qualtrics™. Informed consent was at the beginning of the survey. Participants acknowledge a statement of consent to participate in the anonymous survey.

Setting

This study was conducted in hospitals in Saudi Arabia. Healthcare professionals employed and providing care to patients in Saudi Arabia were recruited for the study. The findings from this study will inform the factors impacting telehealth utilization and interprofessional interactions.

Participants

The inclusion criteria were for the healthcare professional to be employed and licensed. The survey was emailed to physicians, nurses, respiratory therapists, EMS specialists, social workers, physical therapists, and occupational therapists. Professions were identified based on the most common health providers for multidisciplinary healthcare work and involvement in COVID-19 treatment. Professionals were identified through snowballing sampling. The healthcare team's local healthcare professional network was used to initiate the first responses and asked that the survey be shared with those individual colleagues from November 2021 until March 2022. Of those who opened the survey link, 63% completed the survey; there were 127 surveys started and 80 completed. Among the 66 individuals in the final sample, 50% were female, and 43.9% were citizens of Saudi Arabia. Regarding the primary profession, 66.7% were nurses, followed by physicians (18.2%), respiratory therapists (10.6%), and EMS specialists (4.6%). The majority of the participants (66.7%) had been licensed for less than 10 years, with each of the other categories (11–15 years, 16–20 years, and more than 21 years) representing about 33.3% of the sample (Table 1).

**Table 1.** Participants' demographic characteristics, $n$ = 66.

|  | n | % |
|---|---|---|
| Gender |  |  |
| Male | 33 | 50 |
| Female | 33 | 50 |
| Expatriate |  |  |
| No (Saudi citizen) | 29 | 43.94 |
| Yes (non-Saudi citizen) | 35 | 50.03 |
| No Response | 2 | 3.03 |
| Primary profession |  |  |
| Physician | 12 | 18.18 |
| Nurse | 44 | 66.67 |
| Respiratory Therapist | 7 | 10.61 |
| Emergency Medical Services Specialist | 3 | 4.55 |
| Level of engagement in direct patient care |  |  |
| <1 day per week | 3 | 4.55 |
| 1–2 days per week | 6 | 9.09 |
| >2 days per week | 57 | 86.36 |
| Experience as a licensed provider |  |  |
| 0–5 years | 27 | 40.91 |
| 6–10 years | 17 | 25.76 |
| 11–15 years | 13 | 19.7 |
| 16–20 years | 6 | 9.09 |
| 21 or more years | 3 | 4.55 |

Data Analysis

Descriptive statistics were performed using SAS software Version 9.4.36. Descriptive statistics including means and frequencies were generated for participants ($n$ = 66) who provided direct patient care during the COVID-19 pandemic. For the telehealth and interprofessional components of the survey, the summary was provided at both the overall level and expatriate status. To ensure homogeneity of the results, a sensitivity analysis was performed on a subset of the sample ($n$ = 44) who were nurses and physicians.

## 3. Results

### 3.1. Satisfaction of Interprofessional Care Interactions

Of the 66 health professionals who participated in our survey 7.6% strongly agreed, 40.9% agreed, and 22.7% somewhat agreed that they were satisfied with the frequency of interprofessional care interaction 6 months before the pandemic (Table 2). In addition, 9.1% strongly agreed, 37.9% agreed, and 21.2% somewhat agreed that they were satisfied with the quality of interprofessional care interaction 6 months before the pandemic. When examining the time during the pandemic, 13.6% strongly agreed, 33.3% agreed, and 19.7% somewhat agreed that they were satisfied with the frequency of interprofessional care interaction. In addition, 15.2% strongly agreed, 31.8% agreed, and 16.7% somewhat agreed that they were satisfied with the quality of interprofessional care interaction. When we asked participants about telehealth usage for interprofessional collaboration during the COVID-19 pandemic compared to before the pandemic, 7 (10.6%) stated that their telehealth use decreased, 28 (42.4%) stated that their use did not change, and 31 (47%) stated that their telehealth use increased.

Table 2. Satisfaction on interprofessional care interaction and telehealth usage, $n = 66$.

|  | 6 Months before the Pandemic | | During the Pandemic | |
| --- | --- | --- | --- | --- |
|  | Satisfied with Frequency | Satisfied with Quality | Satisfied with Frequency | Satisfied with Quality |
| Strongly disagree | 6 (9.1%) | 7 (10.6%) | 7 (10.6%) | 6 (9.1%) |
| Disagree | 1 (1.5%) | 1 (1.5%) | 1 (1.5%) | 2 (3.0%) |
| Somewhat disagree | 5 (7.6%) | 3 (4.6%) | 7 (10.6%) | 4 (6.1%) |
| Neither agree nor disagree | 7 (10.6%) | 9 (13.6%) | 7 (10.6%) | 11 (16.7%) |
| Somewhat agree | 15 (22.7%) | 14 (21.2%) | 13 (19.7%) | 11 (16.7%) |
| Agree | 27 (40.9%) | 25 (37.9%) | 22 (33.3%) | 21 (31.8%) |
| Strongly agree | 5 (7.6%) | 6 (9.1%) | 9 (13.6%) | 10 (15.2%) |
| No Response | 0 | 1 (1.5%) | 0 | 1 (1.5%) |

Statistical analysis was conducted to explore the satisfaction data further (Table 3). Both interprofessional satisfaction on frequency and quality showed no significant difference between 6 months before and during the pandemic. However, both satisfactions were positively correlated with the frequency of interactions. For example, the odds of satisfaction of frequency and quality were about 12 times (OR = 12.27) and 8 times (OR = 8.24) more, respectively, for the participants with more than three times of interaction than the participants with no interaction at all. The change in telehealth usage was the other significant factor.

Table 3. Impact of COVID-19 on interprofessional satisfaction, $n = 66$.

|  | Odds Ratio | Lower Confidence Level | Upper Confidence Level |
| --- | --- | --- | --- |
| Satisfaction on Frequency of Interprofessional Interaction | | | |
| >3 per day vs. no interaction | 12.27 | 2.73 | 55.23 |
| >3 per day vs. <1 per week | 7.54 | 1.28 | 44.27 |
| >3 per day vs. >1 per week | 1.58 | 0.19 | 13.51 |
| >3 per day vs. 1–2 per day | 2.04 | 0.40 | 10.32 |
| Satisfaction on Quality of Interprofessional Interaction | | | |
| >3 per day vs. no interaction | 8.24 | 2.06 | 32.96 |
| >3 per day vs. <1 per week | 5.80 | 1.11 | 30.44 |
| >3 per day vs. >1 per week | 3.33 | 0.55 | 20.33 |
| >3 per day vs. 1–2 per day | 1.96 | 0.44 | 8.71 |

*3.2. Telehealth Usability*

The only significant factor that impacted the overall Telehealth Usability Questionnaire (TUQ) scores was the change in telehealth usage during the pandemic (Figure 1). The estimated score for the participants who reported an increase in telehealth usage was 5.37, while the scores were 4.60 and 4.29 for the participants reporting 'no change' and 'decreased usage', respectively. The profession, age, gender, and participants from Saudi Arabia did not impact the overall TUQ score.

*3.3. Subgroup Analysis*

A subgroup analysis was also conducted to focus on the subgroup of nurses and physicians (44 in total). The results (not shown) for the satisfaction analysis were similar except that the change in telehealth usage was no longer significant. The results for the overall TUQ score showed there were no significant predictors. Both were possibly due to the reduction in sample size.

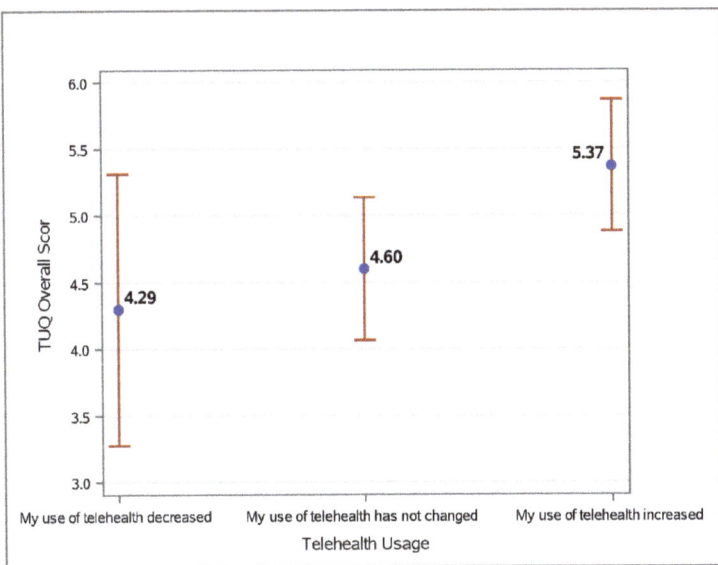

**Figure 1.** Least square mean estimates and 95% confidence interval for Telehealth Usability Questionnaire (TUQ) scores.

## 4. Discussion

To answer our research question, which is to understand how healthcare providers, telehealth utilization, and interprofessional interactions were impacted during COIVD-19, we found that both interprofessional satisfaction on frequency and quality were positively correlated with the frequency of interactions. Research has shown that incorporating interprofessional education can help improve both telehealth utilization and satisfy the need for and increase interprofessional interactions [19]. We also found that healthcare professionals in Saudi Arabia were more likely to use telehealth during the COVID-19 pandemic, according to our study's findings. For telehealth to be effective during the current COVID-19 pandemic and future healthcare crises, we must understand how it is being utilized and integrated into evolving models of care, and examine the ability of health providers to use these technologies to improve the care delivery framework. This change not only creates an excellent opportunity for providers to demonstrate the value of telehealth, but also points to considerable education gaps that must be rapidly filled to take full advantage of the opportunity [20].

An array of free and commercial telemedicine applications (apps) has been created in Saudi Arabia in response to the COVID-19 outbreak. To ensure long-term viability of these services after the pandemic, it is vital to conduct usability testing of these apps. The healthcare organizations that provide telemedicine services in Saudi Arabia must be aware of the existing governing legislation and the accrediting authorities when developing telemedicine apps. During the pandemic, these organizations made several efforts to build and update their regulations to serve as a reference for healthcare providers and developers. Additionally, the Saudi Commission for Health Specialties has just launched a national online training course for healthcare providers to ensure a uniform approach to delivering telemedicine care. By making use of these tools, we can guarantee a high level of quality in telemedicine care as well as a satisfying user experience.

From a public health and health capacity standpoint, in Saudi Arabia, health authorities have been prepared to tackle any potential spread of infectious diseases associated with mass gatherings (e.g., the Hajj season). Currently, they implement the Ministry of Health (MOH) strategy for handling the disease. This strategy follows the Saudi Vision 2030 plan that stresses the importance of adopting and developing a national telehealth network to improve healthcare services accessibility across the kingdom. To screen suspected cases, provide long-distance care, and track COVID-19 patients, the Saudi MOH provided many telehealth mobile applications (e.g., Seha, Mawid, Tawakklna, Tabaud, and Tetamman) to be used instead of visiting primary care clinics. These telehealth tools were found effective in facilitating healthcare delivery, control the spread of COVID-19, and flatten the growth curve [21].

*Limitations*

This study has several limitations that need to be recognized. First, this study was limited to a small sample of providers who are licensed in Riyadh, Saudi Arabia, so the results may not be generalizable to other care providers in other cities in Saudi Arabia or countries. Second, professionals' main practice area was asked on the survey without a follow-up question on subspecialty or multispecialty; furthermore, only two main professions answered the survey.

## 5. Conclusions

This study sheds light on the utilization of telehealth and access to healthcare services. The result of the present study confirms the outcome of the previous studies [14,22,23]. There will be an increasing demand for initiatives to improve telehealth benefits or use among patients as more information about the benefits and consequences of using telehealth becomes available. Policymakers appeared to be reacting to the impending pandemic's uncertainty as COVID-19 spread. Considering our findings, policymakers should think about making these temporary telehealth policies permanent in the event of another epidemic. To better prepare patients for future and unanticipated hurdles to in-person healthcare, authorities should consider adopting rules that favor the growth of telehealth services, such as specialized care. Owing to the potential benefits of telehealth services, policymakers should conduct additional analyses before devising strategies for managing future and unexpected obstacles that prevent patients from receiving in-person treatment.

**Author Contributions:** Study design: H.Y.H., N.M.A.Z. and J.X.; funding acquisition N.M.A.Z.; data collection and analysis: D.I.A., M.S.O. and M.G.A.; manuscript writing: H.Y.H., N.M.A.Z., J.X., D.I.A., M.S.O. and M.G.A.; agrees to be accountable for all aspects of work: H.Y.H., N.M.A.Z., J.X., D.I.A., M.S.O. and M.G.A. All authors have read and agreed to the published version of the manuscript.

**Funding:** This research was funded by AlMaarefa University, grant number TUMA-2021-25.

**Institutional Review Board Statement:** Institutional Review Board Statement: The study was conducted according to the guidelines of the Declaration of Helsinki and approved by the Institutional Review Board (or Ethics Committee) of AlMaarefa University (protocol code 2021-25).

**Informed Consent Statement:** Informed consent was obtained from all subjects involved in the study.

**Data Availability Statement:** The data that support the findings of this study are available on request from the corresponding author. The data are not publicly available due to privacy or ethical restrictions.

**Acknowledgments:** The authors would like to express their gratitude to AlMaarefa University, Riyadh, Saudi Arabia, for providing funding to this work under TUMA project grant number (TUMA-2021-25).

**Conflicts of Interest:** The authors declare no conflict of interest.

## References

1. Forsythe, E.; Kahn, L.B.; Lange, F.; Wiczer, D. Labor demand in the time of COVID-19: Evidence from vacancy postings and UI claims. *J. Public Econ.* **2020**, *189*, 104238. [CrossRef] [PubMed]
2. Shaukat, N.; Ali, D.M.; Razzak, J. Physical and mental health impacts of COVID-19 on healthcare workers: A scoping review. *Int. J. Emerg. Med.* **2020**, *13*, 40. [CrossRef] [PubMed]
3. Oh, H.; Reis, R. Targeted transfers and the fiscal response to the great recession. *J. Monet. Econ.* **2012**, *59*, S50–S64. [CrossRef]

4. Bloem, B.R.; Dorsey, E.R.; Okun, M.S. The coronavirus disease 2019 crisis as catalyst for telemedicine for chronic neurological disorders. *JAMA Neurol.* **2020**, *77*, 927–928. [CrossRef] [PubMed]
5. Donley, G.; Chen, B.A.; Borrero, S. The legal and medical necessity of abortion care amid the COVID-19 pandemic. *J. Law Biosci.* **2020**, *7*, lsaa013. [CrossRef]
6. Fu, S.J.; George, E.L.; Maggio, P.M.; Hawn, M.; Nazerali, R. The consequences of delaying elective surgery: Surgical perspective. *Ann. Surg.* **2020**, *272*, e79. [CrossRef]
7. Lu, J.F.; Chi, M.J.; Chen, C.M. Advocacy of home telehealth care among consumers with chronic conditions. *J. Clin. Nurs.* **2014**, *23*, 811–819. [CrossRef]
8. Ferguson, N.; Laydon, D.; Nedjati Gilani, G.; Imai, N.; Ainslie, K.; Baguelin, M.; Bhatia, S.; Boonyasiri, A.; Cucunuba Perez, Z.; Cuomo-Dannenburg, G.; et al. Report 9: Impact of non-pharmaceutical interventions (NPIs) to reduce COVID19 mortality and healthcare demand. *Imp. Coll. Lond.* **2020**, *10*, 491–497.
9. Lewnard, J.A.; Lo, N.C. Scientific and ethical basis for social-distancing interventions against COVID-19. *Lancet Infect. Dis.* **2020**, *20*, 631–633. [CrossRef]
10. Calton, B.; Abedini, N.; Fratkin, M. Telemedicine in the time of coronavirus. *J. Pain Symptom Manag.* **2020**, *60*, e12–e14. [CrossRef]
11. Mehrotra, A.; Jena, A.B.; Busch, A.B.; Souza, J.; Uscher-Pines, L.; Landon, B.E. Utilization of telemedicine among rural Medicare beneficiaries. *JAMA* **2016**, *315*, 2015–2016. [CrossRef] [PubMed]
12. Nouri, S.; Khoong, E.C.; Lyles, C.R.; Karliner, L. Addressing equity in telemedicine for chronic disease management during the COVID-19 pandemic. *NEJM Catal. Innov. Care Deliv.* **2020**, *1*, 1–13.
13. Smith, A.C.; Thomas, E.; Snoswell, C.L.; Haydon, H.; Mehrotra, A.; Clemensen, J.; Caffery, L.J. Telehealth for global emergencies: Implications for coronavirus disease 2019 (COVID-19). *J. Telemed. Telecare* **2020**, *26*, 309–313. [CrossRef]
14. Hamadi, H.Y.; Zhao, M.; Haley, D.R.; Dunn, A.; Paryani, S.; Spaulding, A. Medicare and telehealth: The impact of COVID-19 pandemic. *J. Eval. Clin. Pract.* **2022**, *28*, 43–48. [CrossRef] [PubMed]
15. Sizer, M.A.; Bhatta, D.; Acharya, B.; Paudel, K.P. Determinants of Telehealth Service Use among Mental Health Patients: A Case of Rural Louisiana. *Int. J. Environ. Res. Public Health* **2022**, *19*, 6930. [CrossRef]
16. Langbecker, D.; Caffery, L.J.; Gillespie, N.; Smith, A.C. Using survey methods in telehealth research: A practical guide. *J. Telemed. Telecare* **2017**, *23*, 770–779. [CrossRef]
17. Parmanto, B.; Lewis, A.N., Jr.; Graham, K.M.; Bertolet, M.H. Development of the telehealth usability questionnaire (TUQ). *Int. J. Telerehabil.* **2016**, *8*, 3. [CrossRef] [PubMed]
18. Hicks-Roof, K.K.; Xu, J.; Zeglin, R.J.; Bailey, C.E.; Hamadi, H.Y.; Osborne, R. COVID-19 impacts on Florida's healthcare professionals. *Hosp. Top.* **2022**, *100*, 112–122. [CrossRef]
19. World Health Organization (WHO). *Coronavirus Disease 2019 (COVID-19): Situation Report*; World Health Organization (WHO): Geneva, Switzerland, 2020; Volume 80.
20. Lee, A.C. COVID-19 and the advancement of digital physical therapist practice and telehealth. *Phys. Ther.* **2020**, *100*, 1054–1057. [CrossRef]
21. Alghamdi, S.M.; Alqahtani, J.S.; Aldhahir, A.M. Current status of telehealth in Saudi Arabia during COVID-19. *J. Fam. Community Med.* **2020**, *27*, 208. [CrossRef]
22. Xu, J.; Hamadi, H.Y.; Hicks-Roof, K.K.; Zeglin, R.J.; Bailey, C.E.; Zhao, M. Healthcare Professionals and Telehealth Usability during COVID-19. *Telehealth Med. Today* **2021**, *6*. [CrossRef]
23. Zhao, M.; Hamadi, H.; Xu, J.; Haley, D.R.; Park, S.; White-Williams, C. Telehealth and hospital performance: Does it matter? *J. Telemed. Telecare* **2022**, *28*, 360–370. [CrossRef] [PubMed]

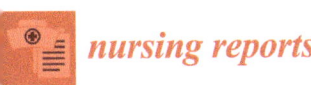 

*Protocol*

# Changes in Clinical Training for Nursing Students during the COVID-19 Pandemic: A Scoping Review Protocol

Catarina Lobão [1,*], Adriana Coelho [1,2], Rui Gonçalves [1], Vitor Parola [1,2], Hugo Neves [1,2] and Joana Pereira Sousa [2,3]

1. Health Sciences Research Unit: Nursing (UICISA: E), Nursing School of Coimbra (ESEnfC), 3000-232 Coimbra, Portugal; adriananevescoelho@esenfc.pt (A.C.); rgoncalves@esenfc.pt (R.G.); vitorparola@esenfc.pt (V.P.); hugoneves@esenfc.pt (H.N.)
2. Portugal Centre for Evidence-Based Practice: A Joanna Briggs Institute Centre of Excellence, 3000-232 Coimbra, Portugal; joana.sousa@ipleiria.pt
3. Center for Innovative Care and Health Technology—ciTechCare, School of Health Sciences-Polytechnic of Leiria, 2411-091 Leiria, Portugal
* Correspondence: catarinalobao@esenfc.pt

**Abstract: Backgrounds**: The COVID-19 pandemic has had consequences for social, economic, cultural and educational life, affecting nursing training and practice. To date, no previous scoping reviews addressing this objective have been found. This study aims to map the literature related to changes in clinical training for nursing students during the COVID-19 pandemic. **Methods**: A scoping review will be carried out according to the Joanna Briggs Institute's latest guidance regarding methodology. A set of relevant electronic databases and grey literature will be searched using terms such as clinical practice, nursing students, COVID-19. **Results**: This scoping review will consider any type of quantitative, qualitative, and mixed-methods study and systematic review designs for inclusion, focusing on changes in clinical training for nursing students during the COVID-19 pandemic. **Conclusion**: Pedagogical criteria had to be changed due to the COVID-19 pandemic, especially face-to-face clinical training for nursing students. Identifying the changes in clinical training for nursing students during the COVID-19 pandemic will help educators to understand the potential impact of this specific context and trace possible gaps. This protocol is registered at Open Science Framework.

**Keywords:** changes; clinical training; COVID-19; nursing students; review

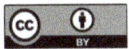

## 1. Introduction

The emergence of the SARS-CoV-2 coronavirus and its rapid spread worldwide prompted the World Health Organization to declare a pandemic state on 11 March 2020. Changes were required in world dynamics and society in general to combat the spread of the new coronavirus [1].

There was a need to reinvent strategies and readapt the teaching, learning, and assessment processes in nursing education [2,3], through digital training programs or tools such as simulation and telehealth [4,5].

The nursing discipline focuses on human responses to health-disease phenomena and life processes, with face-to-face nursing care being essential [6]. Thus, the training of health professionals to take care of people requires developing skills resulting from the action and articulation of various actors, encouraging debate, exchanging experiences, interaction, reflection, and critical thinking [6].

The impact of the new coronavirus has created unusual learning methods for nursing students. The clinical placement can be experienced as a challenging part of training, even discounting from the pandemic situation. Students already struggle to be part of a care team, where professional self is not yet defined, leading to feelings of insecurity about their competence [7].

The pandemic has raised several challenges in teaching nursing students, namely in the clinical context. Uncertainty about the reception of students in healthcare teams or even the interruption of clinical training enhanced the need for a solution to promote clinical training by means of a simulation interface [7,8].

Additionally, students could not develop their practical activities in the clinical context at pre-licensing and advanced practice levels. This phenomenon required ingenious solutions to promote students' training, allowing them to complete their training programs at the usual schedule [8].

Training nursing students in a pandemic context is an urgent need. However, many clinical settings have interrupted or postponed the nursing students' clinical training due to lockdown policies, scarcity of material (specifically, individual protection equipment (IPE)), workload-related burnout, and the obligation to reduce the movement of people in clinical practice care settings [4,9]. Nevertheless, final year undergraduates have contributed to the fight against the pandemic in many contexts. This reality allowed for continuing the learning processes in clinical education by integrating the health teams created to respond to the pandemic [4,9]. However, while some students participating in this catastrophic scenario saw this as an extremely attractive challenge, which allowed knowledge consolidation in a historical era, the challenge has been seen as demanding and painful by others [9].

Despite recognizing the challenges that the pandemic has created, in clinical internships, nursing students revealed understanding and acceptance of the needed change. On the other hand, students mentioned that it was difficult to find an inbound clinical setting [7,8], which influenced their ability to adapt to this new reality, personally and academically. The need for an adjustment is reflected in students' achievements and expectations [3], based on their wellbeing [10–12], stress levels [13] and perception of their quality of life [14].

In all graduation levels, students will play a crucial role in future pandemics. When students are not adequately prepared in the art of care, simulation training improves anxiety and stress levels, especially in the simulation on managing critical patients and ventilatory support [15].

This scoping review is guided by the Joanna Briggs Institute's (J.B.I.) methodology to conduct scoping reviews, and aims to map the changes in clinical training for nursing students during the COVID-19 pandemic. An initial search of MEDLINE (PubMed), the J.B.I. Evidence Synthesis, the Cochrane Database of Systematic Reviews, PROSPERO, and Open Science Framework (O.S.F.) revealed that currently, there are no scoping reviews or systematic reviews (published or in progress) about this subject [16–18].

The main goal of this scoping review is to map the changes in clinical training for nursing students during the COVID-19 pandemic. It can significantly contribute to understanding this phenomenon to aid nursing educators in developing programs and proposals to target clinical teaching, learning, and assessment strategies for nursing students in similar contexts. This map will identify relevant topics to assist in advancing evidence-based nursing education, develop knowledge, and identify potential gaps.

This scoping review seeks to answer the following questions:
- What are the changes in clinical training for nursing students during the COVID-19 pandemic? (e.g., contamination risk; IPE);
- What is the context of clinical practice training for nursing students where the changes are described? (e.g., clinical training services);
- What are the educational implications of nursing students' learning processes reported? (e.g., postponement, withdrawal, interruption).

## 2. Materials and Methods

The protocol for this scoping review will be guided following the J.B.I.'s latest guidance regarding methodology [16–18]. The final review will be reported following the Preferred Reporting Items for Systematic Reviews and Meta-Analyses extension for Scoping Reviews

(PRISMA-ScR) guidelines [19]. This review protocol was registered in the Open Science Framework (https://osf.io/mduve/ (accessed on 21 April 2021)).

## 2.1. Inclusion Criteria

Based on the J.B.I. recommendations regarding the mnemonic "P.C.C." for scoping reviews, the inclusion criteria will include: participants—this review will consider studies that include undergraduate nursing students; concept—this review will consider studies exploring nursing students' clinical training changes during the COVID-19 pandemic; context—this review will consider studies, independently of the country of the study, conducted in any clinical practice setting; and types of sources—this scoping review will consider any quantitative, qualitative, mixed methods study designs, editor letters and guidelines for inclusion. Additionally, all types of systematic reviews will be considered for inclusion in the proposed scoping review.

## 2.2. Search Strategy

The search strategy will locate both published and unpublished primary studies and reviews.

Two reviewers developed the search strategy, which was peer-reviewed by the expert third reviewer considering the Peer Review of Electronic Search Strategies (PRESS) checklist [20]. The J.B.I.'s recommended three-step search strategy will be applied [16,18]. A limited preliminary search was undertaken on MEDLINE (via PubMed) and CINAHL Complete (EBSCOhost) to find articles on the topic. Thus, the text words in the titles and abstracts of pertinent articles and the index terms used to describe the articles were used to create a full search strategy for MEDLINE (via PubMed), as seen in Table 1. The search was conducted on 17 January 2022. The search strategy will be adapted to the specificities of each information source. Lastly, the reference lists of the articles included in the review will be screened for supplementary papers.

**Table 1.** Search strategy for MEDLINE (via Pubmed).

| Search | Query | Record Retrieved |
|---|---|---|
| #1 | "nursing students"[Title/Abstract] OR "nursing student"[Title/Abstract] OR "nurse students"[Title/Abstract] OR "nurse student" [Title/Abstract] OR "students, nursing"[MeSH Terms] | 34,097 |
| #2 | "clinical training"[Title/Abstract] OR "clinical learning"[Title/Abstract] OR "clinical practice"[Title/Abstract] OR "preceptorship"[MeSH Terms] OR "Preceptorship"[Title/Abstract] | 228,818 |
| #3 | "COVID-19"[MeSH Terms] OR "COVID-19"[Title/Abstract] OR "Sars-CoV-2"[Title/Abstract] OR "Sars-CoV-2"[MeSH Terms] | 212,741 |
| #4 | (("nursing students"[Title/Abstract] OR "nursing student"[Title/Abstract] OR "nurse students"[Title/Abstract] OR "nurse student"[Title/Abstract] OR "students, nursing"[MeSH Terms]) AND ("clinical training"[Title/Abstract] OR "clinical learning"[Title/Abstract] OR "clinical practice"[Title/Abstract] OR "preceptorship"[MeSH Terms] OR "Preceptorship"[Title/Abstract])) AND ("COVID-19"[MeSH Terms] OR "COVID-19"[Title/Abstract] OR "Sars-CoV-2"[Title/Abstract] OR "Sars-coV-2"[MeSH Terms]) | 67 |

Study languages will be restricted to those mastered by the authors—English, Spanish and Portuguese—in order to ensure a good-quality selection procedure and data extraction. Document studies in other languages, excluded based on language, will be stated for transparency in the scoping review report.

The databases to be searched will include MEDLINE (via PubMed), CINAHL complete (EBSCOhost), Cochrane Central Register of Controlled Trials, Cochrane Database of Systematic Reviews, LILACS, Scopus, and scientific libraries, such as SciELO. The search for unpublished studies will include DART-Europe; OpenGrey or other grey literature (e.g., Editor letters or guidelines).

2.3. Study Selection

All of the records identified during the database search will be retrieved and stored in the Mendeley® V1.19.4 (Mendeley Ltd., Elsevier, Amsterdam, The Netherlands), and duplicates removed. Two reviewers will independently screen the titles and abstracts. A pilot test will be undertaken to verify whether inclusion criteria are met. Potentially eligible studies will be assessed according to whether the full text is available, whether they meet the inclusion criteria, whether the abstract is unclear, and whether the study's relevance is uncertain, while their citation details will be imported into the J.B.I. System for the Unified Management, Assessment and Review of Information (JBI SUMARI; J.B.I., Adelaide, Australia) [21]. Secondly, the full text of selected citations will be assessed in detail, against the inclusion criteria, by the two independent reviewers. Full-text studies will be excluded if they do not meet the inclusion criteria. In addition, the reasons for exclusion will be provided in an appendix in the final report of the scoping review. Finally, the references of all the included studies in the review will be hand-searched. Disagreements between the two reviewers will be resolved through discussion or with a third reviewer at each stage of the selection process. In the case of an inaccessible full article, the author will be contacted.

The search results will be detailed in the final scoping review and presented in a Preferred Reporting Items for Systematic Reviews and Meta-analyses for Scoping Reviews (PRISMA-ScR) flow diagram [19].

2.4. Data Extraction

Extracted data from included articles will be charted according to the J.B.I.-proposed template by the two independent reviewers [16,18] and aligned with the goals and research questions. A draft extraction tool is presented in Table 2. The draft data extraction tool could be revised as necessary during data extraction from each included paper. Levac, Colquhoun and O'Brien [22] suggested that to ensure consistency of data extraction, a priori pilot charting of the first five to ten studies should be made by two reviewers, independent of each other. The decision of a third reviewer will solve any disagreements in data extraction.

Study authors will be contacted for further data information in the case of missing data. Because review studies will be included, reviewers will choose to report the preliminary study in the case of data duplication.

**Table 2.** Data extraction tool.

| Scoping Review Details | |
|---|---|
| Scoping review title | Changes in clinical training for nursing students during the COVID-19 pandemic: a scoping review protocol |
| Review objective(s) | Map the changes in clinical training for nursing students during the COVID-19 pandemic situation. |
| Review question(s) | 1. What are the changes seen in clinical training for nursing students during the COVID-19 pandemic.<br>2. What are the nursing students' perceptions about the changes in clinical training during the COVID-19 pandemic (exploring causal factors);<br>3. What are the contexts of nursing students' clinical training where the changes are observed (context of learning/clinical training services);<br>4. What are the implications of the changes to nursing students' learning processes (academic and personal; postponement, withdrawal, interruption). |

**Table 2.** *Cont.*

| | |
|---|---|
| Inclusion/Exclusion Criteria | |
| Population | This review will consider studies that include undergraduate nursing students. |
| Context | This review will consider studies conducted in any clinical practice setting. |
| Concept | This review will consider studies that explore changes and challenges in clinical training for nursing students during the COVID-19 pandemic. |
| Types of evidence source | This scoping review will consider any quantitative, qualitative, and mixed methods study designs for inclusion. Additionally, systematic reviews will be considered for inclusion in the proposed scoping review. |
| Evidence Source Details and Characteristics | |
| Author(s) | |
| Year of publication | |
| Origin/country of origin (where the source was published or conducted) | |
| Aims/purpose | |
| Population and sample size | |
| Details/Results Extracted from the Source of Evidence (concerning the concept of the scoping review) | |
| Changes and challenges in clinical training | |
| Perception of nursing students | |
| Context of in clinical training | |
| Academic implications | |
| Personal implications | |

*2.5. Data Analysis and Presentation*

The data collected will be shown in tabular form (Table 3), depending on which is more appropriate to this review's objective. A descriptive summary will be provided regarding the charted result aligned with this scoping review's purpose [16,18] and a qualitative coding might emerge from the data analysis.

**Table 3.** Data collection in tabular form.

| | Study 1 | Study 2 | ... | ... |
|---|---|---|---|---|
| Changes in clinical training | | | | |
| Context of clinical training | | | | |
| Academic implications | | | | |
| Personal implications | | | | |

## 3. Discussion

This scoping review will only consider English, Portuguese, and Spanish studies, which can be registered as a potential study limitation. To overcome this limitation, abstracts of articles published in other languages, which could also be important to include in this review, will be translated through Google Translator and Linguee to prevent restricting ourselves to programs specific to certain cultures.

## 4. Conclusions

We believe that the academic community has reflected on the changes driven by the COVID-19 pandemic. Thus, this scoping review will allow pedagogical structures to embrace the strategies arising from these findings to establish programs that support clinical training for undergraduate nursing students. This scope will also identify possible gaps in future research work.

**Author Contributions:** Conceptualization: C.L., A.C., R.G., V.P., H.N. and J.P.S. Validation: V.P. and H.N. Writing—initial draft preparation: C.L., A.C., R.G., V.P., H.N. and J.P.S. Writing—review and editing: C.L., A.C., R.G., V.P., H.N. and J.P.S. All authors have read and agreed to the published version of the manuscript.

**Funding:** This research received no external funding.

**Institutional Review Board Statement:** Not applicable.

**Informed Consent Statement:** Not applicable.

**Data Availability Statement:** Not applicable.

**Acknowledgments:** The authors wish to acknowledge the Health Sciences Research Unit: Nursing, Nursing School of Coimbra, Portugal and the Portugal Centre for Evidence-Based Practice: a Joanna Briggs Institute Centre of Excellence, Portugal.

**Conflicts of Interest:** The authors declare no conflict of interest.

# References

1. World Health Organization. *Operational Planning Guidelines to Support Country Preparedness and Response*; World Health Organization: Geneva, Switzerland, 2020.
2. Agu, C.F.; Stewart, J.; McFarlane-Stewart, N.; Rae, T. COVID-19 Pandemic Effects on Nursing Education: Looking through the Lens of a Developing Country. *Int. Nurs. Rev.* **2021**, *68*, 153–158. [CrossRef] [PubMed]
3. dos Santos Ferreira, A.M.; Principe, F.; Pereira, H.; Oliveira, I.; Mota, L. COVimpact: Pandemia COVID-19 Nos Estudantes Do Ensino Superior Da Saúde. *Rev. Investig. Inovação Em Saúde* **2020**, *3*, 7–16. [CrossRef]
4. Intinarelli, G.; Wagner, L.M.; Burgel, B.; Andersen, R.; Gilliss, C.L. Nurse Practitioner Students as an Essential Workforce: The Lessons of Coronavirus Disease 2019. *Nurs. Outlook* **2021**, *69*, 333–339. [CrossRef] [PubMed]
5. Son, H.K. Effects of S-Pbl in Maternity Nursing Clinical Practicum on Learning Attitude, Metacognition, and Critical Thinking in Nursing Students: A Quasi-Experimental Design. *Int. J. Environ. Res. Public Health* **2020**, *17*, 7866. [CrossRef] [PubMed]
6. de Lira, A.L.B.C.; Adamy, E.K.; Teixeira, E.; da Silva, F.V. Educação Em Enfermagem: Desafios e Perspectivas Em Tempos Da Pandemia COVID-19. *Rev. Bras. Enferm.* **2020**, *73*, e20200683.
7. Ulenaers, D.; Grosemans, J.; Schrooten, W.; Bergs, J. Clinical Placement Experience of Nursing Students during the COVID-19 Pandemic: A Cross-Sectional Study. *Nurse Educ. Today* **2021**, *99*, 104746. [CrossRef] [PubMed]
8. Emerson, M.R.; Buchanan, L.; Golden, A. Telehealth Simulation with Graduate Nurse Practitioner Students. *Nurse Educ.* **2021**, *46*, 126–129. [CrossRef] [PubMed]
9. Swift, A.; Banks, L.; Baleswaran, A.; Cooke, N.; Little, C.; McGrath, L.; Meechan-Rogers, R.; Neve, A.; Rees, H.; Tomlinson, A.; et al. COVID-19 and Student Nurses: A View from England. *J. Clin. Nurs.* **2020**, *29*, 3111–3114. [CrossRef] [PubMed]
10. Xavier, B.; Camarneiro, A.; Loureiro, L.; Menino, E.; Cunha-Oliveira, A.; Monteiro, A. Impact of COVID-19 on the family, social, and academic dynamics of nursing students in Portugal. *Rev. Enferm. Ref.* **2020**, *4*, 1–10. [CrossRef]
11. Kochuvilayil, T.; Fernandez, R.S.; Moxham, L.J.; Lord, H.; Alomari, A.; Hunt, L.; Middleton, R.; Halcomb, E.J. COVID-19: Knowledge, Anxiety, Academic Concerns and Preventative Behaviours among Australian and Indian Undergraduate Nursing Students: A Cross Sectional Study. *J. Clin. Nurs.* **2021**, *30*, 882–891. [CrossRef] [PubMed]
12. Eweida, R.S.; Rashwan, Z.I.; Desoky, G.M.; Khonji, L.M. Mental Strain and Changes in Psychological Health Hub among Intern-Nursing Students at Pediatric and Medical-Surgical Units amid Ambience of COVID-19 Pandemic: A Comprehensive Survey. *Nurse Educ. Pract.* **2020**, *49*, 102915. [CrossRef] [PubMed]
13. Aslan, H.; Pekince, H. Nursing Students' Views on the COVID-19 Pandemic and Their Percieved Stress Levels. *Perspect. Psychiatr. Care* **2020**, *57*, 695–701. [CrossRef] [PubMed]
14. Ramos, T.H.; Pedrolo, E.; Santana, L.D.L.; Ziesemer, N.D.B.S.; Haeffner, R.; de Carvalho, T.P. O Impacto Da Pandemia Do Novo Coronavírus Na Qualidade de Vida de Estudantes de Enfermagem. *Rev. Enferm. Centro-Oeste Min.* **2020**, *10*, 1–11. [CrossRef]
15. Hernández-Martínez, A.; Rodríguez-Almagro, J.; Martínez-Arce, A.; Romero-Blanco, C.; García-Iglesias, J.J.; Gómez-Salgado, J. Nursing Students' Experience and Training in Healthcare Aid during the COVID-19 Pandemic in Spain. *J. Clin. Nurs.* **2021**, 1–8. [CrossRef] [PubMed]
16. Peters, M.D.J.; Godfrey, C.; Mcinerney, P.; Munn, Z.; Tricco, A.C.; Khalil, H. Chapter 11: Scoping Reviews. In *J.B.I. Manual for Evidence Synthesis*; Aromataris, E., Munn, Z., Eds.; 2020; Available online: https://synthesismanual.jbi.global (accessed on 8 March 2022).
17. Khalil, H.; Peters, M.; Godfrey, C.M.; McInerney, P.; Soares, C.B.; Parker, D. An Evidence-Based Approach to Scoping Reviews. *Worldviews Evid.-Based Nurs.* **2016**, *13*, 118–123. [CrossRef] [PubMed]

18. Peters, M.D.J.; Marnie, C.; Tricco, A.C.; Pollock, D.; Munn, Z.; Alexander, L.; McInerney, P.; Godfrey, C.M.; Khalil, H. Updated Methodological Guidance for the Conduct of Scoping Reviews. *JBI Evid. Synth.* **2020**, *18*, 2119–2126. [CrossRef] [PubMed]
19. Tricco, A.C.; Lillie, E.; Zarin, W.; Brien, K.K.O.; Colquhoun, H.; Levac, D.; Moher, D.; Peters, M.D.J.; Ma, Q.; Horsley, T.; et al. PRISMA Extension for Scoping Reviews (PRISMA-ScR): Checklist and Explanation. *Ann. Intern. Med.* **2018**, *169*, 467–473. [CrossRef] [PubMed]
20. McGowan, J.; Sampson, M.; Salzwedel, D.M.; Cogo, E.; Foerster, V.; Lefebvre, C. PRESS Peer Review of Electronic Search Strategies: 2015 Guideline Statement. *J. Clin. Epidemiol.* **2016**, *75*, 40–46. [CrossRef] [PubMed]
21. Munn, Z.; Aromataris, E.; Tufanaru, C.; Stern, C.; Porritt, K.; Farrow, J.; Lockwood, C.; Stephenson, M.; Moola, S.; Lizarondo, L.; et al. The Development of Software to Support Multiple Systematic Review Types. *Int. J. Evid. Based. Healthc.* **2019**, *17*, 36–43. [CrossRef] [PubMed]
22. Levac, D.; Colquhoun, H.; O'Brien, K. Scoping Studies: Advancing the Methodology. *Implement. Sci.* **2012**, *5*, 69. [CrossRef] [PubMed]

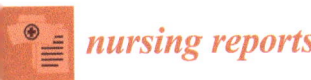 

*Article*

# Perceptions of COVID-19 Mitigation Strategies between Rural and Non-Rural Adults in the US: How Public Health Nurses Can Fill the Gap

Alan M. Beck [1,*], Amy J. Piontek [2], Eric M. Wiedenman [1,3] and Amanda Gilbert [1]

[1] Prevention Research Center, Washington University in St. Louis, St. Louis, MO 63130, USA; ericw@wustl.edu (E.M.W.); a.s.gilbert@wustl.edu (A.G.)
[2] Goldfarb School of Nursing, Barnes-Jewish College, St. Louis, MO 63110, USA; amy.piontek@barnesjewishcollege.edu
[3] Department of Surgery, Division of Public Health Sciences, Washington University in St. Louis, St. Louis, MO 63130, USA
* Correspondence: alan.beck@wustl.edu; Tel.: +1-314-935-0125

**Abstract:** The purpose of this study was to capture the perceptions of COVID-19 mitigations' efficacy of rural and non-rural participants, using the health belief model (HBM), as well as to describe where public health nursing may be able to fill behavior gaps in rural communities. Rural and non-rural participants completed electronic surveys. Surveys collected demographic information and perceptions of various mitigation strategies' effectiveness. Rurality was significantly associated with perceptions of the effectiveness of public health mitigation strategies including wearing facemasks, limiting time indoors, avoiding gatherings, non-essential business closure, and staying home. Our findings suggest people in rural areas perceive mitigations to be effective. Other researchers have consistently shown rural residents are least likely to partake in the same mitigations. Rural public health nurses on the front line serve as the key to closing the aforementioned gap. Understanding where their community's perceptions lie is pivotal in creating educational programs to continue mitigation efforts as we embark on the second year of this pandemic.

**Keywords:** rural; COVID-19; public health nursing

## 1. Introduction

At the onset of the SARS-CoV-2 (COVID-19) pandemic in the United States (US), metropolitan areas were the most highly impacted by the infection [1]. Rural areas were thought to have some protection from the virus inherently due to their sparse nature. Over time, however, this perceived protection of rural areas dwindled, thereby becoming the US's newest hot spot [1,2]. Unfortunately, as has been the normal trajectory with COVID-19, by September 2020 death rates in rural areas surpassed those in urban areas [1,3]. In fact, rural areas have been hit harder; roughly 1 in 434 rural Americans have died of COVID, compared to 1 in 513 urban Americans [4].

Rural local health departments (LHD) are key resources in their respective communities. Unfortunately, LHDs in rural areas are among the most understaffed and underfunded health departments in the nation [5,6]. While LHDs in rural areas serve smaller populations, these communities tend to have limited access to medical care [7,8], poor health outcomes [7–9], and experience health disparities related to risky health behaviors [7,10,11]. Leadership at most LHDs in metropolitan areas tends to be someone with a formal degree in public health [6]; in contrast, rural LHDs are three times as likely to be led by someone with a nursing degree [12–14]. Nurses are the linchpin that holds rural health departments together, especially considering rural LHDs frequently offer more direct clinical services [15,16]. Unfortunately, prior to the COVID-19 pandemic, there was an estimated

36% decrease in staffing of public health nurses [17]. Therefore, rural area LHDs were likely the most impacted given much of their staff are nurses. This amalgamation of the need for public health nurses in rural areas, services provided by rural LHDs, and a global pandemic, left rural LHDs at risk of being overwhelmed—their communities would need to do their part to protect themselves.

Practices such as avoiding contact with others who are ill, social distancing, covering the nose and mouth when coughing or sneezing, washing hands or using approved hand sanitizer, and using face coverings when in public places are all recommendations established by the Centers for Disease Control and Prevention (CDC) to reduce the spread of COVID-19 [18]. It is also recommended that when a person falls ill with COVID-19-like symptoms that they remain quarantined and away from others [19]. It has been well documented that mitigation strategies decrease the spread of COVID-19 in community and healthcare settings [20–22]. However, these strategies are only effective if consistently followed.

Overall, Americans report agreement with public health mitigations; though, few of the respondents in these studies were from rural areas [23–25]. There is hope now with the approval of vaccines; however, there is still a concern for variants coupled with vaccine hesitancy. Rural areas, and states with large rural populations, are demonstrating some of the lowest vaccine rates in the nation [26]. The coalescing of low vaccination rates, rural populations' increased vulnerability to serious infection, increased vaccine hesitancy, and the concern for variants, means public health mitigation strategies will likely continue to be warranted [3,27]. Due to the likely need for ongoing mitigation strategies, the present study was designed to capture the perceptions of mitigation strategies among a sample of rural residents as compared to non-rural residents.

## 2. Materials and Methods

Participants were recruited from social media posts (e.g., Facebook, Twitter) and email list serves from 26 August to 17 September 2020. An image, with a link imbedded, describing the study was posted to social media. (Example post, "If you live in a rural area, please take our survey for a chance to win an Amazon gift card!") Various local, regional, and national advocacy groups distributed social media posts and emails. Emails contained a brief description of the study with a link to the survey's consent form. Social media posts contained a link embedded in an image describing the study—when the potential participant clicked the image, they were routed to the consent form. If potential participants agreed, they were then taken to the survey. All responses were anonymous unless they wanted to be entered into the raffle for a gift card in which the participant would provide contact information. Inclusion criteria for participation were ≥18 years of age and the ability to read English. All data were collected in Qualtrics software [28]. The Washington University in St. Louis Institutional Review Board approved the study with an exempt status.

### 2.1. Theoretical Framework

The health belief model (HBM) first developed by Godfrey H. Hochbaum in the late 1950s is the theoretical framework supporting this study. Hochbaum developed the HBM to understand peoples' behaviors associated with their perceived susceptibility in contracting disease, perceived severity of the disease, perceived benefits to reducing the threat of disease, and perceived barriers to action in decreasing the risk of disease [29]. The first three constructs of perceived susceptibility, perceived severity, and perceived benefits were measured in this study.

### 2.2. Measures

2.2.1. Demographics

Participants were asked to provide their gender (male, female), age, education level (less than high school, some college/associates degree, college, more than college), race (black or African American, white, American Indian or Alaska Native, Asian, Native

Hawaiian, or Pacific Islander), ethnicity (Hispanic), marital status (married, widowed, divorced, separated, never married, unmarried couple), household income (less than 20,000, 20,000–49,999, 50,000–79,999, 80,000 or more), and zip code. In order to minimize the number of variables, educational level was used as a surrogate to income as they were highly correlated. To define rurality, each participant's zip code was compared to the Rural-Urban Continuum Codes (RUCC) [30]—a code of four or higher was operationally defined as rural [31,32].

#### 2.2.2. Impact of COVID-19

Participants were asked how COVID-19 influenced one's personal daily life for each of the following five domains (work, school, finances, physical health, and mental health). Five response options were provided ranging from not at all, a little, a moderate amount, a lot, to a great deal. Responses were collapsed into three categories, not at all (not at all), somewhat (a little, a moderate amount), and a lot (a lot, a great deal) for analysis.

#### 2.2.3. COVID-19 Worries

Participants were asked about their worries regarding the pandemic (e.g., contracting COVID-19, transmitting COVID-19 to someone else, family/friends contracting COVID-19, having enough food, and loss of income). Five response options were provided ranging from not at all, a little, a moderate amount, a lot, to a great deal. Responses were collapsed into three categories, not at all (not at all), somewhat (a little, a moderate amount), and a lot (a lot, a great deal) for analyses.

#### 2.2.4. Mitigation Strategies

Participants were asked about COVID-19 mitigation strategies for both individual behaviors (wearing of a facemask, consulting a health care provider if you feel sick, avoiding/limiting indoor public spaces, avoiding outdoor spaces, avoiding large gatherings, avoiding contact with people at high risk, and limiting errands requiring public places), and public health measures (closure of schools, closures of all shops not considered essential, non-essential workers stay home, and people over the age of 70 stay home). Five response options were provided ranging from not at all effective, slightly effective, moderately effective, very effective, to extremely effective. Responses were collapsed into three categories, not at all effective (not effective at all), moderately effective (slightly effective, moderately effective), and highly effective (very effective, extremely effective) for analysis.

### 2.3. Analysis

Quantitative data analysis was conducted using SPSS (version 26) (IBM Corporation. Armonk, NY, USA). The dependent variables were participant perceptions of the impact of COVID-19, COVID-19 worry, and perceptions of the effectiveness of COVID-19 mitigation strategies. The independent variable was rurality based on the RUCC and dichotomized into rural and urban. Descriptive statistics, frequency tables, and chi-squared analyses were conducted. Assumptions of sample size were met for chi-squared analyses.

## 3. Results

In total, 278 respondents completed the survey (Table 1). Fifty percent of participants were classified as rural and 50% as non-rural. Most participants were female (88%), white (96.7%), married (71%), and between the ages of thirty-six to sixty years old (61%). About half of the participants reported a household income of USD 80,000 or greater and around 60% had a college degree or higher. Among rural participants, 79% were female, 99% white, and 62% were between the ages of thirty-six and sixty. In regard to household income and marital status, 46% of rural participants reported an annual household income equal to or greater than USD 80,000 and 70% reported being married. Around 11% of rural participants had a high school degree or GED, with most (43%) completing some college or associates degree. Compared to rural participants, there were a higher percentage of non-rural participants who reported being female (87%), earning USD 80,000 or more (58%), having more than a college degree (41%) and being married (73%) and a lower percentage of non-rural participants reporting being white (94%), and aged between thirty-six and sixty years old (60%).

**Table 1.** Demographic characteristics of rural and non-rural respondents.

|  | Total ($n$ = 278) | Rural ($n$ = 139) | Non-Rural ($n$ = 139) |
|---|---|---|---|
| Female, $n$ (%) | 245 (88.1) | 125 (78.51) | 120 (87.0) |
| Race, $n$ (%) |  |  |  |
|   White | 265 (96.7) | 135 (99.3) | 130 (94.2) |
|   Black | 6 (2.2) | 1 (0.7) | 5 (3.6) |
|   Asian | 2 (0.7) | 0 (0.0) | 2 (1.4) |
|   American Indian or Alaska Native | 1 (0.4) | 0 (0.0) | 1 (0.7) |
| Hispanic/Latino, $n$ (%) | 1 (0.4) | 1 (0.7) | 0 (0.0) |
| Age, $n$ (%) |  |  |  |
|   35 and younger | 60 (22.5) | 27 (20.3) | 33 (24.6) |
|   36–60 years | 163 (61.0) | 83 (62.4) | 80 (59.7) |
|   61 and older | 44 (16.5) | 23 (17.3) | 21 (15.7) |
| Income, $n$ (%) |  |  |  |
|   Less than USD 20,000 | 13 (4.8) | 9 (6.6) | 4 (3.0) |
|   USD 20,000–49,999 | 52 (19.3) | 33 (24.3) | 19 (14.3) |
|   USD 50,000–79,999 | 64 (23.8) | 31 (22.8) | 33 (24.8) |
|   USD 80,000 or more | 140 (52.0) | 63 (46.3) | 77 (57.9) |
| Education, $n$ (%) |  |  |  |
|   High school/GED | 20 (7.2) | 15 (10.8) | 5 (3.6) |
|   Some college/associates degree | 87 (31.4) | 60 (43.2) | 27 (19.6) |
|   College | 91 (32.9) | 41 (29.5) | 50 (36.2) |
|   More than college | 79 (28.5) | 23 (16.5) | 56 (40.6) |
| Marital Status, $n$ (%) |  |  |  |
|   Married | 197 (71.4) | 97 (69.8) | 100 (73.0) |
|   Widowed | 5 (1.8) | 4 (2.9) | 1 (0.7) |
|   Divorced | 31 (11.2) | 21 (15.1) | 10 (7.3) |
|   Separated | 4 (1.4) | 2 (1.4) | 2 (1.5) |
|   Never married | 17 (6.2) | 6 (4.3) | 11 (8.0) |
|   Unmarried couple | 22 (8.0) | 9 (6.5) | 13 (9.5) |

*3.1. Perceptions on the Impact of COVID-19 on Daily Life*

Regarding the impact of the COVID-19 pandemic on work, 87% of the total sample reported the COVID-19 pandemic negatively impacted work some (53%) or a lot (34%), and 14% reported no impact at all. When asked about the financial impact of COVID-19, 66% reported being negatively impacted some (52%) or a lot (14%), and 87% reported being worried some (24%) or a lot (63%), about the potential for income loss. In terms of the negative impact of COVID-19 on health, 65% reported their physical health was negatively impacted some (53%) or a lot (12%) by the COVID-19 pandemic and 87% reported their mental health was negatively impacted some (53%) or a lot (34%). No significant correlations were found between rurality and COVID-19 impact.

*3.2. Participant Worries Regarding COVID-19*

Overall, 85% of participants worried some (48%) or a lot (37%) about getting COVID-19 and 78% worried some (39%) or a lot (39%) about giving COVID-19 to others. The majority of participants (97%) reported being worried some (18%) or a lot (79%) about having enough food and most (87%) reported being worried some (24%) or a lot (63%) about income loss. Only worry about family or friends getting COVID-19 was significantly correlated with rurality. ($x^2(2) = 7.687, p = 0.021$) Among rural participants, 80% reported being worried some (52%) or a lot (28%) about family and friends getting COVID-19, while 67% of non-rural participants worried some (50%) or a lot (17%) about family and friends getting COVID-19.

*3.3. Perceptions on the Effectiveness of Individual Behaviors for Staying Safe from COVID-19*

We found significant correlations between rurality and perceptions of effectiveness for the behaviors of wearing a face mask ($x^2(2) = 9.997, p = 0.007$), limiting time spent indoors in public spaces ($x^2(2) = 13.903, p = 0.001$), avoiding large gatherings ($x^2(2) = 10.006, p = 0.007$), and limiting the frequency of necessary errands ($x^2(2) = 9.015, p = 0.011$). When asked whether wearing a facemask was "effective for keeping you safe from COVID-19", 82% of rural participants reported wearing a facemask was moderately (39%) or highly (43%) effective for protecting against COVID-19, while 75% of non-rural participants reported a facemask was moderately (50%) or highly (25%) effective. When asked about limiting time spent indoors in public spaces, 69% of rural participants perceived this behavior as moderately (42%) or highly (27%) effective for keeping them safe from COVID-19. Among non-rural participants, 55% perceived this behavior as moderately (45%) or highly (10%) effective. In regards to avoiding large gatherings, 68% of rural participants perceived this behavior as moderately (40%) or highly (28%) effective, while 56% of non-rural participants perceived this behavior as moderately (43%) or highly (13%) effective. Among rural participants, 77% reported "limiting frequency of necessary errands requiring public places (e.g., grocery shopping)" was moderately (50%) or highly (27%) effective at keeping them safe from COVID-19, while 65% of non-rural participants reported this behavior as moderately (51%) or highly (14%) effective. We did not find significant associations between rurality and perceptions on the effectiveness of consulting a health care provider, avoiding outdoor public spaces, and avoiding contact with at-risk populations.

*3.4. Perception on the Effectiveness of Public Health Measures for Preventing COVID-19*

When assessing participant perceptions for the effectiveness of public health measures to mitigate COVID-19 transmission, we found significant correlations between rurality and public health measures for guidelines recommending the wearing of facemasks ($x^2(2) = 16.486, p < 0.001$), closing non-essential businesses ($x^2(2) = 14.324, p = 0.001$), recommending people aged 70 and over or with a medical condition stay at home except for essential needs ($x^2(2) = 9.344, p = 0.009$), and for non-essential workers to stay at home except to do basic shopping or because urgent medical care is required ($x^2(2) = 13.116, p = 0.001$). For guidelines recommending the wearing of face masks, 78% of rural participants perceived this public health measure as moderately (33%) or highly effective (45%), while 62% of non-rural participants viewed this public health measure as moderately (39%) or highly (23%) effective. When asked about the closure of non-essential businesses, 91% of rural participants viewed this measure as moderately (29%) or highly (62%) effective, while 88% of non-rural participants reported this public health measure was moderately (49%) or highly (39%) effective. Among rural participants, 73% felt recommendations for those aged 70 and older or with a medical condition to stay home were moderately (48%) or highly (25%) effective. Among non-rural participants, 63% reported this was a moderately (52%) or highly (11%) effective public health measure. Seventy-nine percent of rural participants perceived public health measures recommending non-essential workers stay at home as moderately (38%) or highly (48%) effective. Among non-rural participants, 77% felt this was a moderately (50%) or highly (27%) effective public health measure for mitigating the spread of COVID-19. We did not find significant correlations between rurality and perceptions on the effectiveness of the public health measures of closing schools.

## 4. Discussion

Rurality was significantly associated with perceptions of the effectiveness of public health mitigation strategies including the wear of facemasks, limiting time indoors, avoiding large gatherings, closing non-essential businesses, and elderly and non-essential workers staying home unless required to go out. Further, rural areas demonstrated more concern for the wellbeing of family and friends compared to more urban areas. There appears to be a paradox whereby our findings suggest rural people think mitigations are effective; however, they may not actually partake in the same mitigations they deem effective. Prior research has found rural communities may not adhere to mitigations at the same rate as their urban counterparts [24,33–35]. There may be a disconnect between rural residents' perceptions and risk. Perhaps they deem the risk low since rural areas are dispersed, or perhaps it is related to social media misinformation [36]. Whatever the case may be, public health nurses may be the answer [37].

The higher the percentage of people reporting COVID-19 negatively impacting their work, financial security, mental health, physical health, and having enough food, the higher their perceived impact (severity) of the disease. In this instance, it may not be the severity of the disease process itself, but rather the implications surrounding being ill with the disease (i.e., not being able to work or loss of job). Those participants with higher percentages of worry related to contracting and transmitting COVID-19 correlated with an increased perception of susceptibility to the disease. In other words, they perceived themselves to be susceptible to contracting or transmitting the disease to others. The assessment finding related to the participants' perceptions of the effectiveness of individual behaviors for staying safe from COVID-19 parallels the HBMs construct of perceived benefits to the mitigation strategies. Those participants who reported specific mitigation strategies to be effective in curving the spread of the disease were essentially indicating these actions produced benefits in controlling the spread of COVID-19.

Historically, the role of the public health nurse may not have been well understood, until the world was faced with one of the deadliest pandemics in the last 100 years. Public health nurses began doing what they do best by working collaboratively with community partners to educate people on what they can do to control the spread of COVID-19 [38]. Communities learned what they needed to do to protect themselves and others from this disease. Once vaccines became available, public health nurses provided education to community partners in the efficacy of vaccines, proper storage of vaccines, and strategies to track multi-dose vaccine administration. Public health nurses continue to work with communities for vaccine administration and provide ongoing support and education for those still skeptical of the safety of the vaccines. The role of the public health nurse in conjunction with LHDs is to empower people through education. At a time of great uncertainty, one thing is clear—RNs who work within communities have the knowledge and skills to deliver factual and relevant information regarding mitigation strategies [38]. They are the backbone to addressing this nation's need to eradicate COVID-19. LHD nurses could be the link between perceptions of mitigation success and actual behaviors.

Local health departments and public health nurses are often well connected to the available resources in the community and can act as resource hubs for community members. As our study findings suggest, and previous studies have also reported [39,40], many individuals living in rural areas are concerned about not having enough food and income loss throughout the COVID-19 pandemic. Many LHDs maintain current community resource guides including local food pantries, income, utility, transportation, housing assistance programs, and many other social services. Public health nurses and LHDs can leverage their position and connection to these resources to help community members connect to the services they need.

As COVID-19 continues to be a public health crisis in the United States, and with vaccine rates continuing to lag in rural areas and states with large rural populations, findings from this study may provide opportunities to emphasize rural communities' concern for the well-being of others to address vaccine hesitancy. Effective COVID-19 immunization programs are evidence based [27], and previous studies have identified emphasizing the personal risks of failing to get the vaccine and the potential spread to others in the community as effective health communication messaging [41,42]. Further, researchers suggest tailoring messaging to appeal to the opinions and values of a sub-population can increase their effectiveness [43–45]. Therefore, we provide the following recommendations for messaging aimed at rural communities in the United States:

1. Highlight how getting vaccinated and mitigations can help protect your family and friends from becoming sick [46], and a social responsibility to help your community [40].
2. Continue to discuss the importance of wearing a face mask to prevent the spread of COVID-19. Suggest or encourage outdoor gatherings.
3. Messaging that is from the local community, about the local community (e.g., public health nurses) [47]. Emphasize public health nurses and local health departments as valuable resources in the community, both for answering questions about COVID-19 and for their connections to community resources (food pantries/banks, utility assistance programs, SNAP, WIC, etc.).

*Limitations*

One limitation of the study was the cross-sectional nature in which data were collected; therefore, the results are correlational and causation cannot be determined. A second limitation was the relatively small sample size. A third limitation was that the sample was relatively small and a majority of white females who have reported higher threat perceptions of COVID-19 [46,48]. Although perceived barriers to COVID-19 transmission mitigation strategies were not assessed, future studies should be explored using this construct to gain a greater understanding to address these barriers for greater adherence to disease prevention. Using a qualitative approach to understanding the barriers could be beneficial in understanding specific communities' unique situations to reduce or eliminate recognized barriers. Another limitation to the current study was the fact that rural communities here had abnormally high income—likely due to the recruitment methodology (i.e., online). Lastly, we did not survey people about their actual behavior, only their perceptions of the effectiveness of mitigation strategies.

## 5. Conclusions

For decades, public health professionals have relied on and continue to use the HBM to understand peoples' health behaviors. Whether it is receiving the COVID-19 vaccine and booster or wearing a mask in public places, understanding the public's view in their susceptibility of contracting the disease, the severity the disease will have on their personal lives, and the value placed on mitigation strategies, greatly assists public health nurses and health departments. They are able to align their educational and resource outreach programs to those who may have low perceptions of the severity COVID-19 can have on their lives, their low perceptions of the susceptibility they may have in contracting or spreading the disease, and most importantly, those who may not perceive the mitigation strategies to be beneficial to themselves and those in their family or community. In this study, we found that rural people consider mitigations strategies more effective as compared to their urban/suburban counterparts. While other studies have found rural areas tend to partake in mitigation strategies at a lower clip, we posit those same rural areas might still believe in the efficacy of the strategies. One under-resourced yet passionate messenger to close the gap between mitigation perceptions and partaking in the mitigation strategy is the local public health nurse. Public health nurses have a plethora of information as well as the passion to serve their communities. Understanding their community's perceptions of COVID-19 is the first step in addressing the ongoing need for further education and disease prevention strategies. Finally, after years of divestment, it is recommended to bolster funding to rural LHD's in order to hire more RN's. LHD RN's in rural areas are the lifeblood and key to success in navigating the pandemic now and in the future.

**Author Contributions:** Conceptualization, A.M.B., A.G., E.M.W. and A.J.P.; methodology, A.M.B. and A.G.; formal analysis, A.G. and A.M.B.; investigation, A.M.B., A.J.P., A.G. and E.M.W.; writing—original draft preparation, A.M.B.; writing—review and editing, A.M.B., A.J.P., A.G. and E.M.W.; project administration, A.M.B.; funding acquisition, A.M.B. All authors have read and agreed to the published version of the manuscript.

**Funding:** The National Cancer Institute of the National Institutes of Health funded this research, grant number R01CA211323. The National Cancer Institute of the National Institutes of Health funded the APC. Dr. Wiedenman is supported by a training grant from the National Cancer Institute of the National Institutes of Health under award number T32CA190194. Amanda Gilbert is supported by a training grant of the National Heart, Lung, and Blood institute grant number T32HL130357.

**Institutional Review Board Statement:** The Institutional Review Board at Washington University in St. Louis approved the study with an exempt status (IRB#202008147). The study was conducted according to the guidelines of the Declaration of Helsinki, and approved by the Institutional Review Board (or Ethics Committee) of Washington University in St. Louis (protocol code 202008147 and date of approval 25 August 2020).

**Informed Consent Statement:** Informed consent was obtained from all subjects involved in the study.

**Data Availability Statement:** The data are not publicly available due to privacy concerns.

**Acknowledgments:** The authors would like to thank Ross C. Brownson and the faculty and staff at the CDC funded Prevention Research Center at Washington University in St. Louis (U48DP006395) for their support. The authors would also like to thank Mary Adams and Linda Dix for their administrative support.

**Conflicts of Interest:** The authors declare no conflict of interest. The funders had no role in the design of the study; in the collection, analyses, or interpretation of data; in the writing of the manuscript, or in the decision to publish the results.

# References

1. Duca, L.M.; Coyle, J.; McCabe, C.; McLean, C. COVID-19 Stats. *Morb. Mortal. Wkly. Rep.* **2020**, *69*, 1753.
2. Leatherby, L. The Worst Virus Outbreaks in the US Are Now in Rural Areas. *New York Times*, 22 October 2020.
3. U.S. Department of Agriculture, Economic Research Service. Rural Death Rates from COVID-19 Surpassed Urban Death Rates in Early September 2020. 2021. Available online: https://www.ers.usda.gov/data-products/chart-gallery/gallery/chart-detail/?chartId=100740 (accessed on 24 August 2021).
4. Ullrich, F.; Mueller, K. The Rural Policy Research Institute, Rural Data Brief, December 2021: Confirmed COVID-19 Cases, Metropolitan and Nonmetropolitan Counties. 2021. Available online: https://rupri.public-health.uiowa.edu/publications/policybriefs/2020/COVID%20Data%20Brief.pdf (accessed on 25 August 2021).
5. Beatty, K.; Erwin, P.C.; Brownson, R.C.; Meit, M.; Fey, J. Public Health Agency Accreditation among Rural Local Health Departments: Influencers and Barriers. *J. Public Health Manag. Pract.* **2018**, *24*, 49–56. [CrossRef] [PubMed]
6. Harris, J.K.; Beatty, K.; Leider, J.; Knudson, A.; Anderson, B.L.; Meit, M. The Double Disparity Facing Rural Local Health Departments. *Annu. Rev. Public Heal.* **2016**, *37*, 167–184. [CrossRef]
7. Meit, M.; Knudson, A.; Gilbert, T. *The 2014 Update of the Rural-Urban Chartbook*; The Rural Health Reform Policy Research Center: Chicago, IL, USA, 2014; pp. 1–153.
8. O'Campo, P.; Burke, J.G.; Culhane, J.; Elo, I.T.; Eyster, J.; Holzman, C.; Messer, L.C.; Kaufman, J.S.; Laraia, B.A. Neighborhood Deprivation and Preterm Birth among Non-Hispanic Black and White Women in Eight Geographic Areas in the United States. *Am. J. Epidemiol.* **2007**, *167*, 155–163. [CrossRef]
9. Merchant, J.A.; Stromquist, A.M.; Kelly, K.M.; Zwerling, C.; Reynolds, S.J.; Burmeister, L.E. Chronic Disease and Injury in an Agricultural County: The Keokuk County Rural Health Cohort Study. *J. Rural Health* **2002**, *18*, 521–535. [CrossRef]
10. Doescher, M.P.; Jackson, J.E.; Jerant, A.; Hart, L.G. Prevalence and Trends in Smoking: A National Rural Study. *J. Rural Health* **2006**, *22*, 112–118. [CrossRef] [PubMed]
11. E Cronk, C.; Sarvela, P.D. Alcohol, tobacco, and other drug use among rural/small town and urban youth: A secondary analysis of the monitoring the future data set. *Am. J. Public Health* **1997**, *87*, 760–764. [CrossRef]
12. Bekemeier, B.; Jones, M. Relationships Between Local Public Health Agency Functions and Agency Leadership and Staffing. *J. Public Health Manag. Pract.* **2010**, *16*, e8–e16. [CrossRef]
13. Bhandari, M.W.; Scutchfield, F.D.; Charnigo, R.; Riddell, M.C.; Mays, G.P. New Data, Same Story? Revisiting Studies on the Relationship of Local Public Health Systems Characteristics to Public Health Performance. *J. Public Health Manag. Pract.* **2010**, *16*, 110–117. [CrossRef]
14. Brownson, R.C.; Reis, R.; Allen, P.; Duggan, K.; Fields, R.; Stamatakis, K.A.; Erwin, P.C. Understanding Administrative Evidence-Based Practices. *Am. J. Prev. Med.* **2014**, *46*, 49–57. [CrossRef]

15. Hale, N.L.; Smith, M.; Hardin, J.; Brock-Martin, A. Rural Populations and Early Periodic Screening, Diagnosis, and Treatment Services: Challenges and Opportunities for Local Public Health Departments. *Am. J. Public Health* **2015**, *105*, S330–S336. [CrossRef]
16. Beatty, K.E.; Hale, N.; Meit, M.; Masters, P.; Khoury, A. Local health department clinical service delivery along the urban/rural continuum. *Front. Public Health Serv. Syst. Res.* **2016**, *5*, 21–27.
17. National Association of County and City Health Officials. 2019 National Profile of Local Health Departments. 2019. Available online: https://www.naccho.org/uploads/downloadable-resources/Programs/Public-Health-Infrastructure/NACCHO_2019_Profile_final.pdf (accessed on 25 August 2021).
18. Centers for Disease Control and Prevention. How to Protect Yourself & Others. 2021. Available online: https://www.cdc.gov/coronavirus/2019-ncov/prevent-getting-sick/prevention.html (accessed on 23 August 2021).
19. Centers for Disease Control and Prevention. Quarantine and Isolation. 2021. Available online: https://www.cdc.gov/coronavirus/2019-ncov/if-you-are-sick/quarantine.html (accessed on 23 August 2021).
20. Centers for Disease Control and Prevention. Science Brief: Community Use of Cloth Masks to Control the Spread of SARS-CoV-2. 2021. Available online: https://www.cdc.gov/coronavirus/2019-ncov/science/science-briefs/masking-science-sars-cov2.html (accessed on 23 August 2021).
21. Stutt, R.O.; Retkute, R.; Bradley, M.; Gilligan, C.A.; Colvin, J. A modelling framework to assess the likely effectiveness of facemasks in combination with 'lock-down' in managing the COVID-19 pandemic. *Proc. R. Soc. A Math. Phys. Eng. Sci.* **2020**, *476*, 20200376. [CrossRef] [PubMed]
22. Leung, N.H.; Chu, D.K.; Shiu, E.Y.; Chan, K.H.; McDevitt, J.J.; Hau, B.J.; Yen, H.L.; Li, Y.; Ip, D.K.; Peiris, J.S.; et al. Respiratory virus shedding in exhaled breath and efficacy of face masks. *Nat. Med.* **2020**, *26*, 676–680. [CrossRef] [PubMed]
23. Czeisler, M.; Tynan, M.A.; Howard, M.E.; Honeycutt, S.; Fulmer, E.B.; Kidder, D.P.; Robbins, R.; Barger, L.K.; Facer-Childs, E.R.; Baldwin, G.; et al. Public Attitudes, Behaviors, and Beliefs Related to COVID-19, Stay-at-Home Orders, Nonessential Business Closures, and Public Health Guidance—United States, New York City, and Los Angeles, 5–12 May 2020. *MMWR Morb. Mortal. Wkly. Rep.* **2020**, *69*, 751–758. [CrossRef] [PubMed]
24. Haischer, M.H.; Beilfuss, R.; Hart, M.R.; Opielinski, L.; Wrucke, D.; Zirgaitis, G.; Uhrich, T.D.; Hunter, S.K. Who is wearing a mask? Gender-, age-, and location-related differences during the COVID-19 pandemic. *PLoS ONE* **2020**, *15*, e0240785. [CrossRef]
25. Qeadan, F.; Mensah, N.A.; Tingey, B.; Bern, R.; Rees, T.; Talboys, S.; Singh, T.P.; Lacey, S.; Shoaf, K. What Protective Health Measures Are Americans Taking in Response to COVID-19? Results from the COVID Impact Survey. *Int. J. Environ. Res. Public Health* **2020**, *17*, 6295. [CrossRef]
26. Mayo Clinic. U.S. COVID-19 Vaccine Tracker: See Your State's Progress. 2021. Available online: https://www.mayoclinic.org/coronavirus-covid-19/vaccine-tracker (accessed on 25 August 2021).
27. Khubchandani, J.; Sharma, S.; Price, J.H.; Wiblishauser, M.J.; Sharma, M.; Webb, F.J. COVID-19 Vaccination Hesitancy in the United States: A Rapid National Assessment. *J. Community Health* **2021**, *46*, 270–277. [CrossRef]
28. Qualtrics. *Qualtrics: Survey Research Suite*; Qualtrics: Chicago, IL, USA, 2014. Available online: https://www.qualtrics.com/education/student-and-faculty-research/ (accessed on 25 August 2021).
29. Skinner, C.S.; Tiro, J.; Champion, V.L. The Health Belief Model. In *Health Behavior and Health Education: Theory, Research, and Practice*, 5th ed.; Glanz, K., Rimer, B.K., Viswanath, K., Eds.; Jossey-Bass: San Francisco, CA, USA, 2015; pp. 75–94.
30. Parker, T. *Rural-Urban Continuum Codes*; United States Department of Agriculture Economic Research Service: Washington, DC, USA, 2013.
31. University of Montana, Research & Training Center on Disability in Rural Communities—Defining Rural. Available online: https://www.umt.edu/rural-institute/rtc/focus-areas/research-methods/defining-rural.php (accessed on 25 January 2022).
32. Beck, A.; Gilbert, A.; Duncan, D.; Wiedenman, E. A Cross-Sectional Comparison of Physical Activity during COVID-19 in a Sample of Rural and Non-Rural Participants in the US. *Int. J. Environ. Res. Public Health* **2021**, *18*, 4991. [CrossRef]
33. Callaghan, T.; Lueck, J.A.; Trujillo, K.L.; Ferdinand, A.O. Rural and Urban Differences in COVID-19 Prevention Behaviors. *J. Rural Health* **2021**, *37*, 287–295. [CrossRef]
34. Hutchins, H.J.; Wolff, B.; Leeb, R.; Ko, J.Y.; Odom, E.; Willey, J.; Friedman, A.; Bitsko, R.H. COVID-19 Mitigation Behaviors by Age Group—United States, April–June 2020. *MMWR. Morb. Mortal. Wkly. Rep.* **2020**, *69*, 1584–1590. [CrossRef] [PubMed]
35. Probst, J.C.; Crouch, E.L.; Eberth, J.M. COVID-19 risk mitigation behaviors among rural and urban community-dwelling older adults in summer, 2020. *J. Rural Health* **2021**, *37*, 473–478. [CrossRef] [PubMed]
36. Cuello-Garcia, C.; Pérez-Gaxiola, G.; van Amelsvoort, L. Social media can have an impact on how we manage and investigate the COVID-19 pandemic. *J. Clin. Epidemiol.* **2020**, *127*, 198–201. [CrossRef] [PubMed]
37. Edmonds, J.K.; Kneipp, S.M.; Campbell, L. A call to action for public health nurses during the COVID-19 pandemic. *Public Health Nurs.* **2020**, *37*, 323–324. [CrossRef] [PubMed]
38. National Academies of Science, Engineering and Medicine. *The Future of Nursing 2020–2030: Charting a Path to Achieve Health Equity*; Flaubert, J.L., Le Menestrel, L., Williams, D.R., Eds.; National Academies Press: Washington, DC, USA, 2021.
39. Hertz-Palmor, N.; Moore, T.M.; Gothelf, D.; DiDomenico, G.E.; Dekel, I.; Greenberg, D.M.; Brown, L.A.; Matalon, N.; Visoki, E.; White, L.K.; et al. Association among income loss, financial strain and depressive symptoms during COVID-19: Evidence from two longitudinal studies. *J. Affect. Disord.* **2021**, *291*, 1–8. [CrossRef]
40. Fitzpatrick, K.M.; Harris, C.; Drawve, G.; Willis, D.E. Assessing Food Insecurity among US Adults during the COVID-19 Pandemic. *J. Hunger Environ. Nutr.* **2021**, *16*, 1–18. [CrossRef]

41. Motta, M.; Sylvester, S.; Callaghan, T.; Lunz-Trujillo, K. Encouraging COVID-19 Vaccine Uptake Through Effective Health Communication. *Front. Political Sci.* **2021**, *3*, 1. [CrossRef]
42. Barello, S.; Palamenghi, L.; Graffigna, G. Looking inside the 'black box' of vaccine hesitancy: Unlocking the effect of psychological attitudes and beliefs on COVID-19 vaccine acceptance and implications for public health communication. *Psychol. Med.* **2021**, *2021*, 1–2. [CrossRef]
43. Jamieson, K.H. Messages, Micro-targeting, and New Media Technologies. *Forum* **2013**, *11*, 429–435. [CrossRef]
44. Trujillo, K.L.; Motta, M.; Callaghan, T.; Sylvester, S. Correcting Misperceptions about the MMR Vaccine: Using Psychological Risk Factors to Inform Targeted Communication Strategies. *Political Res. Q.* **2021**, *74*, 464–478. [CrossRef]
45. Callaghan, T.; Moghtaderi, A.; Lueck, J.A.; Hotez, P.J.; Strych, U.; Dor, A.; Franklin Fowler, E.; Motta, M. Correlates and Disparities of COVID-19 Vaccine Hesitancy. *SSRN Electron. J.* **2020**. [CrossRef]
46. Perrotta, D.; Grow, A.; Rampazzo, F.; Cimentada, J.; Del Fava, E.; Gil-Clavel, S.; Zagheni, E. Behaviours and attitudes in response to the COVID-19 pandemic: Insights from a cross-national Facebook survey. *EPJ Data Sci.* **2021**, *10*, 17. [CrossRef] [PubMed]
47. Lennon, R.P.; Small, M.L.; Smith, R.A.; Van Scoy, L.J.; Myrick, J.G.; Martin, M.A. Data4 Action Research Group Unique Predictors of Intended Uptake of a COVID-19 Vaccine in Adults Living in a Rural College Town in the United States. *Am. J. Heal. Promot.* **2021**, *36*, 180–184. [CrossRef] [PubMed]
48. Galasso, V.; Pons, V.; Profeta, P.; Becher, M.; Brouard, S.; Foucault, M. Gender differences in COVID-19 attitudes and behavior: Panel evidence from eight countries. *Proc. Natl. Acad. Sci. USA* **2020**, *117*, 27285–27291. [CrossRef] [PubMed]

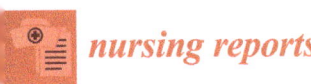 

*Article*

# Stress and Coping Strategies among Nursing Students in Clinical Practice during COVID-19

Hanadi Y Hamadi [1,*], Nazik M. A. Zakari [2], Ebtesam Jibreel [2,*], Faisal N. AL Nami [2], Jamel A. S. Smida [2] and Hedi H. Ben Haddad [3]

1. Brooks College of Health, University of North Florida, Jacksonville, FL 32224, USA
2. College of Applied Sciences, Al Maarefa University, Riyadh 11597, Saudi Arabia; nzakari@mcst.edu.sa (N.M.A.Z.); fnalnami@kfmc.med.sa (F.N.A.N.); jsmida@mcst.edu.sa (J.A.S.S.)
3. Department of Finance and Investment, College of Economics and Administrative Sciences, Imam Mohammad Ibn Saud Islamic University, Riyadh 13318, Saudi Arabia; hhalhaddad@imamu.edu.sa
* Correspondence: h.hamadi@unf.edu (H.Y.H.); ijibreel@mcst.edu.sa (E.J.)

**Citation:** Hamadi, H.Y.; Zakari, N.M.A.; Jibreel, E.; AL Nami, F.N.; Smida, J.A.S.; Ben Haddad, H.H. Stress and Coping Strategies among Nursing Students in Clinical Practice during COVID-19. *Nurs. Rep.* **2021**, *11*, 629–639. https://doi.org/10.3390/nursrep11030060

Academic Editors: Richard Gray and Sonia Udod

Received: 23 July 2021
Accepted: 7 August 2021
Published: 11 August 2021

**Publisher's Note:** MDPI stays neutral with regard to jurisdictional claims in published maps and institutional affiliations.

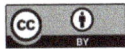

**Copyright:** © 2021 by the authors. Licensee MDPI, Basel, Switzerland. This article is an open access article distributed under the terms and conditions of the Creative Commons Attribution (CC BY) license (https://creativecommons.org/licenses/by/4.0/).

**Abstract:** Stress is common among nursing students and it has been exacerbated during the COVID-19 pandemic. This study examined nursing students' stress levels and their coping strategies in clinical practice before and during the COVID-19 pandemic. A repeated-measures study design was used to examine the relationship between nursing students' stress levels and coping strategies before and during the pandemic. Confirmatory factor analyses were conducted to validate the survey and a student T-test was used to compare the level of stress and coping strategies among 131 nursing students. The STROBE checklist was used. During COVID-19, there was a reliable and accurate relationship between stress and coping strategies. Furthermore, both stress and coping strategy scores were lower before COVID-19 and higher during COVID-19. Nursing students are struggling to achieve a healthy stress-coping strategy during the pandemic. There is a need for the introduction of stress management programs to help foster healthy coping skills. Students are important resources for our health system and society and will continue to be vital long term. It is now up to both nursing educators and health administrators to identify and implement the needed improvements in training and safety measures because they are essential for the health of the patient as well as future pandemics.

**Keywords:** COVID-19; nursing; students; clinical practice; stress; coping skills

## 1. Introduction

Nursing is a practice-based profession, in the sense that the performance of nursing students depends largely on their clinical practicum; therefore, the quality of clinical training practice is crucial to the nursing education and profession. Furthermore, nursing students' opinions regarding the quality of clinical training practices need to be strongly taken into consideration because of the demanding nature of the occupation. Nursing students are exposed to many sources of stress during clinical training and must handle stressful situations accordingly. Stressful situations can vary, including working with and handling breakout infections, where students assume an integral role in infection control measures and come into direct contact with infectious microorganisms. Becoming aware of and understanding students' clinical practice stressors and coping strategies during clinical training in different situations provides educators with valuable information to maximize their students' learning opportunities [1].

During a(n) pandemic/endemic, nursing students find themselves under additional stress factors such as the fear of being infected and infecting their close family members [2]. Two studies during the SARS (2003) and MERS outbreaks (2016) found that nursing students perceived themselves to be at a higher risk of infection and were reluctant to work in healthcare facilities due to inadequate safety and disease control measures [3,4].

Increased stress levels during the 2003 MERS outbreak in South Korea were negatively linked with nursing students' intention to provide care to patients during future emerging infectious diseases [5].

Nursing students and staff are situated on the frontlines to combat infectious diseases and provide care and support to patients. They play a crucial role in providing effective infection control measures and ensuring the de-escalation of the spread of infectious microorganisms. Therefore, along with other medical staff and healthcare workers, nursing students and staff rushed to aid patients suffering from the most recent, fast-emerging, and rapidly spreading virus COVID-19 [6].

The COVID-19 pandemic spread to hospitals and nurses, putting them under enormous pressure in terms of workload and healthcare duties [7]. As a result, the lives and health of nurses and nursing students on the frontline, who are actively fighting the virus and are under great risk of contracting the disease, face dangerous repercussions [8]. COVID-19 studies and findings provide further evidence in regard to the anxiety experienced by nursing students and their response to treating this global pandemic [9].

Due to its extremely infectious and hazardous features, and the drastic lack of medication and treatment for the virus, COVID-19 has resulted in increased stress levels for nursing students and staff, which has consequently affected their coping strategies [8]. Therefore, understanding the relationship between stress levels and coping strategies of nursing students is critical. In non-pandemic times, the findings in Khater, Akhu-Zaheya [10], and Hamaideh [11] suggested that the most common coping behavior utilized by nursing students was problem-solving, followed by staying optimistic and transference.

It is essential to evaluate the quality of the clinical practices and identify stressors that arise from different clinical settings according to nursing students' perspectives. Therefore, this study aimed to examine nursing students' stress levels and their coping strategies in clinical practice before and during the COVID-19 pandemic.

*Theoretical Framework*

Stress has different definitions related to formulated theoretical models. It can be defined either as a stimulus, a response, or a combination of the two [12,13]. The definition of stress as a response was discovered by Selye (1976), who defines stress as the non-specific response of the body to any kind of demand [14,15]. On the other hand, Holmes and Rahes define stress as a stimulus without consideration to any response [16], stating that stress is: "an independent variable stimulus or load produced in an organism, creating discomfort, in such a way that whether tolerance limits are surpassed, stress becomes insufferable, appearing then psychological and physical problems".

The definition that is most relevant to and can be appropriately adopted in this study to explain the reality of nursing student's stress during clinical practice is Lazarus and Folkman's theoretical framework. Based on Lazarus' theory regarding the difficulty in differentiating between response and stimulus as the definition of stress, he conceptualizes an apparent stress definition that can reconcile differences between the separate theories of stress as a response or stress as a stimulus. He defines stress as "A particular relationship between the person and the environment that is appraised by the person as taxing and/or exceeding his or her resources and endangering his or her well-being" [17]. This is because it describes stress as a transactional relationship between the person and their surrounding environment [17]. Stress is not a singular facet, but rather arises due to influencing factors that affect the individual and, in turn, impact their response in such situations. For example, one of these stressful situations can occur during students' clinical practice once the students face a new environment and establish new relationships with staff nurses, patients, and an instructor and/or supervisor [18]. A study found that the most stressful clinical settings identified by the study were the intensive care unit followed by the emergency room, then the surgical units, while the area that was considered the least stressful was the medical units [19]. Therefore, this study uses this working definition of stress to examine nursing students' stress levels and their coping strategies in clinical practice before and during the COVID-19 pandemic.

## 2. Materials and Methods

### 2.1. Setting

The study was conducted in the nursing department at a private University to evaluate and compare the students' perspectives of clinical practice stressors and the coping strategies used to respond to these stressors before the COVID-19 pandemic and during the first wave of the COVID-19 pandemic. The findings from this study will be utilized to improve the learning and the educational process in their current situation, reflecting on the level of the students who will graduate from nursing school in the future.

### 2.2. Design and Sample

A repeated-measures study design was used. The sample nursing students were all undergraduate academic nursing students studying at a private University who are participating in clinical training. Students not in clinical training were excluded from the study.

### 2.3. Data Collection Tool

This survey was developed using two previously validated surveys, the Perceived Stress Scale (PSS) and the Coping Behavior Inventory (CBI) survey. The PSS was developed by Sheu and Lin [20] and measures both the types of stressful events and the degree of stressors within clinical practices. This survey also included three demographic questions: The gender of the participant, their clinical training area, and their academic year of study. The PSS consists of 29 items (See Table 1) on a 5-point Likert scale (from 0 to 4) that are grouped into 6 stress/stressor categories. Those groups are stress from taking care of patients; teachers, and nursing personnel; assignments and workload; peers and daily life; the clinical environment; and lack of professional knowledge and skills.

**Table 1.** The Perceived Stress Scale (PSS) and Coping Behavior Inventory (CBI) questions.

| Subscales | Subscale Questions |
|---|---|
| Stress | |
| Stress from taking care of patients | 1. Lack of experience and ability in providing nursing care and in making judgments<br>2. Do not know how to help patients with physio-psycho-social problems<br>3. Unable to reach one's expectations<br>4. Unable to provide responses to doctors', teachers', and patients' questions<br>5. Worry about not being trusted or accepted by patients or patients' family<br>6. Unable to provide patients with good nursing care<br>7. Do not know how to communicate with patients<br>8. Experience difficulties in changing from the role of student to that of a nurse |
| Stress from teachers and nursing staff | 1. Experience discrepancy between theory and practice<br>2. Do not know how to discuss patients' illnesses with teachers, and medical and nursing personnel<br>3. Feel stressed that teacher's instruction is different from one's expectations<br>4. Medical personnel lack empathy and are not willing to help<br>5. Feel that teachers do not give a fair evaluation on students<br>6. Lack of care and guidance from teachers |

Table 1. Cont.

| Subscales | Subscale Questions |
|---|---|
| Stress from assignments and workload | 1. Worry about bad grades<br>2. Experience pressure from the nature and quality of clinical practice<br>3. Feel that one's performance does not meet teachers' expectations<br>4. Feel that the requirements of clinical practice exceed one's physical and emotional endurance<br>5. Feel that dull and inflexible clinical practice affects one's family and social life |
| Stress from peers and daily life | 1. Experience competition from peers in school and clinical practice<br>2. Feel pressure from teachers who evaluate students' performance by comparison<br>3. Feel that clinical practice affects one's involvement in extracurricular activities<br>4. Cannot get along with other peers in the group |
| Stress from lack of professional knowledge and skills | 1. Unfamiliar with medical history and terms<br>2. Unfamiliar with professional nursing skills<br>3. Unfamiliar with patients' diagnoses and treatments |
| Stress from the environment | 1. Feel stressed in the hospital environment where clinical practice takes place<br>2. Unfamiliar with the ward facilities<br>3. Feel stressed from the rapid change in patient's condition |
| Coping Strategy | |
| Avoidance | 1. To avoid difficulties during clinical practice<br>2. To avoid teachers<br>3. To quarrel with others and lose temper<br>4. To expect miracles so one does not have to face difficulties<br>5. To expect others to solve the problem<br>6. To attribute to fate |
| Problem-solving | 1. To adopt different strategies to solve problems<br>2. To set up objectives to solve problems<br>3. To make plans, list priorities, and solve stressful events<br>4. To find the meaning of stressful incidents<br>5. To employ past experience to solve problems<br>6. To have confidence in performing as well as senior schoolmates |
| Stay optimistic | 1. To keep an optimistic and positive attitude in dealing with everything in life<br>2. To see things objectively<br>3. To have confidence in overcoming difficulties<br>4. To cry, to feel moody, sad, and helpless |
| Transference | 1. To feast and take a long sleep<br>2. To save time for sleep and maintain good health to face stress<br>3. To relax via TV, movies, a shower, or physical exercise (playing, jogging) |

A score of 2.67 and higher was indicative of a high level of stress, a score between 1.34 and 2.66 was indicative of a moderate level of stress, and a score of less than 1.34 indicated a low level of stress [21]. The instrument's reliability showed Cronbach's alpha values of 0.86 and 0.89 [20,22] and a content validity index of 0.94 [22].

The CBI survey was first developed by Sheu and Lin [20] and measures the coping methods nursing students are more likely to utilize and their perceived effectiveness. The CBI survey consists of 19 items (See Table 1) all on a 5-point Likert Scale (from 0 to 4) that are grouped into 4 categories: Avoidance, Transference, Problem-solving, and Stay optimistic. A score of 2.67 and higher was indicative of a high level of coping strategies, a score between 1.34 and 2.66 was indicative of a moderate level of coping strategies, and a score of less than 1.34 indicated a low level of coping strategies. The instrument's reliability showed a Cronbach's alpha coefficient ranging from 0.76 to 0.80 [20,22].

*2.4. Data Collection Procedure*

Prior to data collection, the study protocol was approved by the Institutional Review Board (IRB) of the university. A researcher approached all eligible nursing students at the end of in-person lectures and explained to them the purpose of the study. They were informed that participation in this study is voluntary, and they could withdraw from it at any time. A refusal to participate would not affect their learning process and academic results. Students who were interested in the study were asked to sign a paper or digital consent form, fill in the questionnaire, and immediately return it to the researcher. Other eligible students who did not have in-person lectures were sent the survey via a Google Form to invite them to participate and complete the survey. The survey was sent out to a total of 180 students. Nursing students completed the survey on paper and online between 1 January 2019, and 2 February 2019, for the period before COVID-19 and 30 September 2020, and 30 October 2020, for the period during COVID-19.

*2.5. Participants*

Overall, 75 students were enrolled in clinical practice before and during COVID-19. One hundred and thirty-one nursing student responses were provided, resulting in about an 82% response rate before and during COVID-19. Out of the responses, 99 (75.6%) identified as female and 32 (24.4%) identified as male (See Table 2). The majority (60.3%) of the nursing students were in the Medical-Surgical clinical training area. In addition, 36 (27.5%) nursing students were in Level 5 (first year of clinical practice) of their academic year, and 32 (24.4%) were in Level 10 (last year of clinical practice also known as internship year) of their academic year. Nursing students in Level 5 participate in up to 2 clinical practice courses while Level 9 and 10 nursing students are in full clinical practice internships. The higher the level, the higher the clinical practice competency needed and the higher the necessary complexity. Only surveys that were fully completed were calculated in our response rate, therefore we had no missing data within the response for our analysis.

*2.6. Ethical Considerations*

Before using the PSS and CBI tools, the researcher obtained permission from the original authors. The data collection tool contained a cover page that explained the aim of the study. All principles of ethics were adhered during the study. Therefore, anonymity and confidentiality of each individual's data were also assured during the data collection stage. Participation in the survey was entirely optional and was at the discretion of each receiving the survey.

*2.7. Statistical Analysis*

The nursing student sample in this study was used to test the reliability and validity of the combined survey using confirmatory factor analysis. To analyze the results of the survey, means and standard deviations were utilized to examine the level of stress and coping strategies subscales and total scores. The Student T-test was used to compare the subscales and mean scores for the level of stress and coping strategies before and during the COVID-19 pandemic. We also used the Kolmogorov–Smirnov test to check the cumulative distributions of our two samples. All analyses were conducted in Stata 16, and significance was determined at $p < 0.05$.

**Table 2.** Nursing student demographic characteristics, $n = 131$.

| Variable | Total | | Before COVID-19 ($n = 61$) | | During COVID-19 ($n = 70$) | |
|---|---|---|---|---|---|---|
| | Frequency | Percent | Frequency | Percent | Frequency | Percent |
| **Gender** | | | | | | |
| Male | 32 | 24.4 | 8 | 13% | 24 | 34% |
| Female | 99 | 75.6 | 53 | 87% | 46 | 66% |
| **Clinical Training Area** | | | | | | |
| Medical-surgical | 79 | 60.3 | 36 | 59% | 43 | 61% |
| Critical care | 16 | 12.2 | 7 | 11.5% | 9 | 13% |
| Psychiatric | 6 | 4.6 | 6 | 10% | 0 | 0% |
| Maternity | 12 | 9.2 | 7 | 11.5% | 5 | 7% |
| all areas | 18 | 13.7 | 5 | 8% | 13 | 19% |
| **Academic Year of Study** | | | | | | |
| Level 4 | 13 | 9.9 | 9 | 15% | 4 | 6% |
| Level 5 | 36 | 27.5 | 12 | 20% | 24 | 34% |
| Level 6 | 7 | 5.3 | 2 | 2% | 5 | 7% |
| Level 7 | 10 | 7.6 | 7 | 11% | 3 | 4% |
| Level 8 | 15 | 11.5 | 9 | 15% | 6 | 9% |
| Level 9 | 18 | 13.7 | 6 | 10% | 12 | 17% |
| Level 10 | 32 | 24.4 | 16 | 26% | 16 | 23% |

## 3. Results

The results from the comprehensive confirmatory factor analysis based on the varimax rotation factors of the entire sample results, the sample results before COVID-19, and the sample results after COVID-19 can be viewed in Table 2. Although not shown, the covariance between stress and coping strategies was positive and significant for all the sample (covariance = 0.4; $p < 0.001$), both the sample results before (covariance = 0.28; $p < 0.001$) and after (covariance = 0.58; $p < 0.001$) COVID-19. When examining the entire sample responses factor loading show in Table 3, all factor loadings were above 0.40 [23].

**Table 3.** Unstandardized estimated for all-sample, before and after COVID-19.

| Measurement | All ($n = 131$) | | Before COVID-19 ($n = 61$) | | During COVID-19 ($n = 70$) | |
|---|---|---|---|---|---|---|
| | Standardized Factor Loading | $mc^2$ | Standardized Factor Loading | $mc^2$ | Standardized Factor Loading | $mc^2$ |
| **Stress** | | | | | | |
| Stress from taking care of patients | 0.79 | 0.62 | 0.83 | 0.68 | 0.69 | 0.47 |
| Stress from teachers and nursing staff | 0.86 | 0.74 | 0.84 | 0.71 | 0.84 | 0.70 |
| Stress from assignments and workload | 0.88 | 0.77 | 0.87 | 0.75 | 0.87 | 0.76 |
| Stress from peers and daily life | 0.87 | 0.77 | 0.83 | 0.79 | 0.89 | 0.79 |
| Stress from lack of professional knowledge and skills | 0.78 | 0.61 | 0.74 | 0.54 | 0.75 | 0.56 |
| Stress from the environment | 0.82 | 0.67 | 0.76 | 0.59 | 0.83 | 0.7 |
| **Coping Strategy** | | | | | | |
| Avoidance | 0.59 | 0.35 | 0.62 | 0.38 | 0.53 | 0.28 |
| Problem Solving | 0.87 | 0.76 | 0.86 | 0.74 | 0.88 | 0.77 |
| Stay optimistic | 0.91 | 0.83 | 0.97 | 0.95 | 0.86 | 0.75 |
| Transference | 0.73 | 0.53 | 0.76 | 0.58 | 0.71 | 0.51 |
| LR test | chi2(34)/df = 3.94 | | chi2(34)/df = 2.08 | | chi2(34)/df = 3.88 | |

Notes: LR test is the Wheaton et al. (1977) relative/normed chi-square ($\chi^2$/df), mc is the correlation between the dependent variable and its prediction, and $mc^2 = mc^2$ is the Bentler-Raykov squared multiple correlation coefficient.

The overall average score of stress before COVID-19 was 1.32 (low stress) and 1.95 (moderate stress) during COVID-19 (See Table 4). Across all six stress categories, the average stress score was lower before COVID-19 than during COVID-19. The largest change was found in the stress category "lack of professional knowledge and skills" where the average stress score before COVID-19 was 0.95 (low stress) and 1.78 (moderate stress) during COVID-19 with a 0.83 change. The smallest change was found in the stress category "the environment" from an average stress level of 1.16 (low stress) before COVID-19 and 1.70 (moderate stress) during COVID-19. The overall average score of coping strategies before COVID-19 was 1.84 (moderate coping) and 2.17 (moderate coping) during COVID-19. Across all four coping strategies categories, the average coping strategies score is lower before COVID-19 than during COVID-19. The largest change was found in the coping strategy category "Transference" where the average coping strategy score before COVID-19 was 1.87 (moderate) and 12.41 (moderate) during COVID-19 with a 0.54 change. The smallest change was found in the coping strategy category "stay optimistic" from an average coping strategy level of 2.06 (low) before COVID-19 and 2.15 (moderate) during COVID-19.

**Table 4.** Means and std. deviation and T-test for subscales items of stress experienced by nursing students and coping strategies in their clinical practice before and during the COVID-19 pandemic.

| Item | Before COVID-19 ($n$ = 61) | | | During COVID-19 ($n$ = 70) | | | Sig. |
| --- | --- | --- | --- | --- | --- | --- | --- |
| | Mean | Std. Deviation | Levels | Mean | Std. Deviation | Levels | |
| Mean score of stress | 1.32 | 0.80 | low | 1.95 | 0.76 | moderate | 0.000 * |
| Stress from taking care of patients | 1.30 | 0.91 | low | 1.95 | 0.80 | moderate | 0.001 * |
| Stress from teachers and nursing staff | 1.36 | 0.95 | moderate | 1.93 | 0.88 | moderate | 0.000 * |
| Stress from assignments and workload | 1.59 | 0.94 | moderate | 2.21 | 0.85 | moderate | 0.000 * |
| Stress from peers and daily life | 1.33 | 0.87 | low | 1.93 | 0.92 | moderate | 0.000 * |
| Stress from lack of professional knowledge and skills | 0.95 | 0.94 | low | 1.78 | 1.03 | moderate | 0.004 * |
| Stress from the environment | 1.16 | 1.01 | low | 1.70 | 1.09 | Moderate | 0.000 * |
| Mean score of coping strategies | 1.84 | 0.85 | moderate | 2.17 | 0.75 | moderate | 0.019 * |
| Avoidance | 1.47 | 0.89 | moderate | 1.90 | 0.91 | moderate | 0.007 * |
| Problem-solving | 2.09 | 1.09 | moderate | 2.32 | 0.93 | moderate | 00.20 |
| Stay optimistic | 2.06 | 0.99 | moderate | 2.15 | 0.87 | moderate | 00.55 |
| Transference | 1.87 | 0.95 | moderate | 2.41 | 1.04 | moderate | 0.02 * |

\* $p$-value for Chi-squared test < 0.05.

The results from the T-tests (See Table 4) show that there are statistically significant differences in both average stress scores and average coping strategies before and during COVID-19 across the majority of the categories. This statistical difference shows that both stress and coping strategy scores were lower before COVID-19 and higher during COVID-19. However, there was no statistically significant difference in the coping strategy category "Problem-solving" and "Stay optimistic" with a before-COVID-19 average coping strategy score of 2.09 and 2.06, and during scores of 2.32 and 2.15, respectively.

## 4. Discussion

Through the development of this survey, we have built upon previous research indicating the importance of understanding nursing students' well-being through examining their stress levels and coping strategies. We have developed and tested a measurement scale that is reliable and accurately measures all identified in the Perceived Stress Scale (PSS) and the Coping Behavior Inventory (CBI) survey individually. However, our findings show that when the study is conducted on nurses in Saudi Arabia, there is not a strong reliable relationship between perceived stress and coping strategies (loading factor 0.4 and less) for the entire sample and the before COVID-19 sample. However, interestingly during COVID-19, there was a reliable and accurate relationship between stress and the use of coping strategies. A recent 2020 article regarding students' coping strategies during the COVID-19 pandemic found that approximately 35% of students experienced some level of anxiety and used four types of coping strategies: Seeking social support, avoidance/acceptance, mental disengagement, and humanitarian [24].

The current study aimed to analyze the impact of the COVID-19 pandemic on nursing students' stress levels and coping strategies. Through the combination of these two surveys, were have built upon previous research indicating the importance of stress and coping strategies among nursing students during unprecedented times. We have utilized a measurement scale that reliably and accurately measures stress and coping strategies before and during the COVID-19 pandemic. These findings can help inform nursing curricula developers on how to incorporate the needed skills and resources to prepare nurses for future infectious outbreaks. This is important as the Saudi Vision 2030 framework, released in 2017, has set a path to increase nurse graduates over the next 10 years and enhance the health delivery system to be community-focused. To meet this goal, Saudi Arabia has committed to increasing the nursing workforce by graduating and hiring 10,000 new nurses annually [25].

While multiple studies have reported on the psychological well-being of healthcare workers during COVID-19 [26–34], our study is one of the first to examine the influence of the pandemic by controlling for before the pandemic in nursing students in Saudi Arabia. Data collection occurred during the first wave of the pandemic in the country. The results of this study reflect an increased level of stress and coping strategies among nursing students during the continuing COVID-19 pandemic than before the pandemic. We found that, overall, across all subscales of stress there was a significant increase in stress relating to taking care of patients, teachers and nursing staff, assignments and workload, peers and daily life, lack of professional knowledge and skills, and the environment. These stressors can be attributed to multiple factors such as the unpreparedness to care for COVID-19 patients, increases in safety protocols in the clinical setting and decreases in safety personal protective equipment, relying heavily on simulation for training, and added assignments in an online learning environment to keep up with skill development. The stressful learning environment hinders student success. The completion of clinical practice and a precursor to licensure adds even more added pressure on students to complete an excessive workload to meet the non-direct care hours required [34].

According to previous research, even in normal circumstances, nursing students experience stress and must utilize several coping strategies to reduce both stress and anxiety. A study conducted in Bahrain found that almost all nursing students experience moderate to severe levels of stress while in their clinical practice [35]. Furthermore, another study found that over 99% of nursing students reported the level of perceived stress moderate or high. Several studies have revealed that the cause of clinical stress can be attributed to fear and uncertainty of unknown events, fear of medical errors, working with unfamiliar equipment, and gaps between theory and practice [36]. The additional increase in the level of stress among nursing students due to COVID-19 can have both internal and external consequences [37]. It can cause students to perform poorly and may lead to a withdraw from the program as self-doubt sets in, changes in mental and physical health, and can eventually affect the quality of care provided to patients. Several studies have shown that due to the demand and utilization of personal protective equipment across the globe, many direct care workers such as nurses and nursing students lacked the proper protective equipment, which increased their vulnerability to contracting COVID-19 [38,39]. As a result, many nurses have lost their lives to COVID-19, while others continue to fight against the deadly virus. Consequently, nurses perceive an increased risk of catching COVID-19 [40], which has increased turnover intentions [41]. However, a study conducted in China during the COVID-19 pandemic found that only 3% of their sample believed clinical nursing work to be "too dangerous to engage in" and have an increased intention of leaving the nursing profession [42].

The COVID-19 pandemic is currently the biggest threat to the lives and health of nurses and nursing students and has been shown to impact their emotional response and coping strategies. Our study shows that nursing students' use of Avoidance and Transference as coping strategies and overall coping strategies increased during the COVID-19 pandemic in comparison to before the pandemic. However, our study did not identify a statistical difference between nursing students' use of problem-solving or staying optimistic as coping strategies. This is in contradiction to a recent study that found that nursing students were more willing to use coping strategies that focused on problem-solving [8]. Our study findings can be explained by examining Gan and Liu's [43] study, which found that undergraduate students who regarded stressful events as controllable were more likely to apply problem-focused coping strategies; however, since COVID-related events were uncontrollable during the study period, students might have relied on emotion-focused coping strategies such as Avoidance and Transference, which contradict some priory studies [44,45]. A study conducted before the pandemic found that the most common coping behavior used by nursing students was transference, followed by staying optimistic and problem-solving, while the least used was Avoidance [46]. These findings are important for both nursing schools and hospitals, where they must focus on providing psychological support to nurses as well as training them in all available coping strategies to improve their ability to manage their emotions and effective coping tools to improve the lives of the nursing student, their families, and ultimately their patients.

*Limitations*

The study focused on nursing students in Saudi Arabia from a single private university. Due to the correlational nature of our study, no causal conclusions can be made; however, our findings may lead to a greater understanding of stress and coping strategies of nursing students involved in the COVID-19 pandemic. Hence, the findings should not be generalized to the overall student population.

## 5. Conclusions

The psychological impact of the pandemic on nursing students should not be ignored. The well-being of these students is affected by high levels of stress and emotional-based coping strategies. To alleviate the degree of impact, guidelines and strategies should be adopted into current nursing curricula even before the student is in clinical practice. Prioritizing research and policy effort on mental health, stress, and coping strategies of students needs to occur to equip future nursing students with the tools needed to be successful in the field of nursing. However, future research needs to replicate this study on a greater scale across multiple universities across multiple countries. Moreover, using in-depth data collection strategies, such as qualitative interviews or focus groups, in future research would significantly help explain the rationales behind why students adopted one coping strategies over another.

*Relevance to Clinical Practice*

Our study highlights that there was a strong, reliable, and accurate relationship between stress and the use of coping strategies during the COVID-19 pandemic compared to before. We anticipate that this relationship will only continue. Students are important resources for our health system and society and will continue to be vital long term. It is now up to both nursing educators and health administrators to identify and implement the needed improvements in training and safety measures because they are essential for the health of the patient, but also future pandemics.

**Author Contributions:** Study design: H.Y.H., E.J., N.M.A.Z., and J.A.S.S.; data collection and analysis: F.N.A.N. and H.H.B.H.; manuscript writing: H.Y.H., E.J., N.M.A.Z., F.N.A.N., H.H.B.H., and J.A.S.S.; agrees to be accountable for all aspects of work: H.Y.H., E.J., N.M.A.Z., F.N.A.N., H.H.B.H., and J.A.S.S. All authors have read and agreed to the published version of the manuscript.

**Funding:** This research received no external funding.

**Institutional Review Board Statement:** The study was conducted according to the guidelines of the Declaration of Helsinki and approved by the Institutional Review Board (or Ethics Committee) of AlMaarefa University (protocol code 07-20062021 and 21 June 2019).

**Informed Consent Statement:** Informed consent was obtained from all subjects involved in the study.

**Data Availability Statement:** The data that support the findings of this study are available on request from the corresponding author. The data are not publicly available due to privacy or ethical restrictions.

**Acknowledgments:** The authors would like to thank Almaarefa University for its financial support of this research. The authors would also like to thank the University of North Florida, and all the participants in who took part of the study.

**Conflicts of Interest:** The authors declare no conflict of interest.

# References

1. Chapman, R.; Orb, A. Coping strategies in clinical practice: The nursing students' lived experience. *Contemp. Nurse* **2001**, *11*, 95–102. [CrossRef] [PubMed]
2. Masha'al, D.; Rababa, M.; Shahrour, G. Distance Learning–Related Stress among Undergraduate Nursing Students during the COVID-19 Pandemic. *J. Nurs. Educ.* **2020**, *59*, 666–674. [CrossRef]
3. Wong, J.G.; Cheung, E.P.; Cheung, V.; Cheung, C.; Chan, M.T.; Chua, S.E.; McAlonan, G.M.; Tsang, K.W.; Ip, M.S. Psychological responses to the SARS outbreak in healthcare students in Hong Kong. *Med. Teach.* **2004**, *26*, 657–659. [CrossRef]
4. Elrggal, M.E.; Karami, N.A.; Rafea, B.; Alahmadi, L.; Al Shehri, A.; Alamoudi, R.; Koshak, H.; Alkahtani, S.; Cheema, E. Evaluation of preparedness of healthcare student volunteers against Middle East respiratory syndrome coronavirus (MERS-CoV) in Makkah, Saudi Arabia: A cross-sectional study. *Z. Gesundh. Wiss.* **2018**, *26*, 607–612. [CrossRef] [PubMed]
5. Oh, N.; Hong, N.; Ryu, D.H.; Bae, S.G.; Kam, S.; Kim, K.Y. Exploring Nursing Intention, Stress, and Professionalism in Response to Infectious Disease Emergencies: The Experience of Local Public Hospital Nurses during the 2015 MERS Outbreak in South Korea. *Asian Nurs. Res. Korean Soc. Nurs. Sci.* **2017**, *11*, 230–236. [CrossRef]
6. Shaheen, S.R.; Moussa, A.A.; Khamis, E.A.R. Knowledge and Attitude of Undergraduate Nursing Students toward COVID 19 and their Correlation with Stress and Hope Level. *Assiut Sci. Nurs. J.* **2021**, *9*, 73–83.
7. Fernandez, R.; Lord, H.; Halcomb, E.; Moxham, L.; Middleton, R.; Alananzeh, I.; Ellwood, L. Implications for COVID-19: A systematic review of nurses' experiences of working in acute care hospital settings during a respiratory pandemic. *Int. J. Nurs. Stud.* **2020**, *111*, 103637. [CrossRef]
8. Huang, L.; Lei, W.; Xu, F.; Liu, H.; Yu, L. Emotional responses and coping strategies in nurses and nursing students during Covid-19 outbreak: A comparative study. *PLoS ONE* **2020**, *15*, e0237303.
9. Bauchner, H.; Fontanarosa, P.B.; Livingston, E.H. Conserving Supply of Personal Protective Equipment—A Call for Ideas. *JAMA* **2020**, *323*, 1911. [CrossRef]
10. Khater, W.; Akhu-Zaheya, L.; Shaban, I. Sources of stress and coping behaviours in clinical practice among baccalaureate nursing students. *Int. J. Humanit. Soc. Sci.* **2014**, *4*, 194–202.
11. Hamaideh, S.H. Sources of Knowledge and Barriers of Implementing Evidence-Based Practice among Mental Health Nurses in Saudi Arabia. *Perspect. Psychiatr. Care* **2016**, *53*, 190–198. [CrossRef]
12. Charlton, B.G. Stress. *J. Med. Ethics* **1992**, *18*, 156–159. [CrossRef]
13. Papathanasiou, I.V.; Tsaras, K.; Neroliatsiou, A.; Roupa, A. Stress: Concepts, theoretical models and nursing interventions. *Am. J. Nurs. Sci.* **2015**, *4*, 45–50. [CrossRef]
14. Selye, H. *The Stress of Life, Rev. ed.*; McGraw-Hill: New York, NY, USA, 1976; p. xxvii. 515p.
15. Fitzgerald, A.; Konrad, S. Transition in learning during COVID-19: Student nurse anxiety, stress, and resource support. *Nurs. Forum* **2021**, *56*, 298–304. [CrossRef] [PubMed]
16. López Rodríguez, I.; Morales Ruiz, L.; Simón Gómez, Á. Stress perception in nursing students facing their clinical practices. *Enferm. Glob.* **2013**, *31*, 244.
17. Lazarus, R.S.; Folkman, S. *Stress, Appraisal, and Coping*; Springer Publishing Company: Berlin/Heidelberg, Germany, 1984.
18. Madian, A.E.; Abdelaziz, M.; Ahmed, H. Level of stress and coping strategies among nursing students at Damanhour University, Egypt. *Am. J. Nurs. Res.* **2019**, *7*, 684–696. [CrossRef]
19. Aedh, A.I.; Elfaki, N.K.; Mohamed, I.A. Factors associated with stress among nursing students (Najran University-Saudi Arabia). *IOSR J. Nurs. Health Sci. IOSR-JNHS* **2015**, *4*, 33–38.
20. Sheu, S.; Lin, H.-S.; Hwang, S.-L. Perceived stress and physio-psycho-social status of nursing students during their initial period of clinical practice: The effect of coping behaviors. *Int. J. Nurs. Stud.* **2002**, *39*, 165–175. [CrossRef]
21. Labrague, L.J. Stress, Stressors, and stress Responses of Student Nurses in a Government Nursing School. *Health Sci. J.* **2014**, *7*, 424–435.
22. Chan, C.K.; So, W.K.; Fong, D.Y. Hong Kong baccalaureate nursing students' stress and their coping strategies in clinical practice. *J. Prof. Nurs.* **2009**, *25*, 307–313. [CrossRef]

23. Perry, J.L.; Nicholls, A.R.; Clough, P.J.; Crust, L. Assessing model fit: Caveats and recommendations for confirmatory factor analysis and exploratory structural equation modeling. *Meas. Phys. Educ. Exerc. Sci.* **2015**, *19*, 12–21. [CrossRef]
24. Khoshaim, H.B.; Al-Sukayt, A.; Chinna, K.; Nurunnabi, M.; Sundarasen, S.; Kamaludin, K.; Baloch, G.M.; Hossain, S.F.A. How students in the Kingdom of Saudi Arabia are coping with COVID-19 pandemic. *J. Public Health Res.* **2020**, *9*, 1898. [CrossRef] [PubMed]
25. Alsufyani, A.M.; Alforihidi, M.A.; Almalki, K.E.; Aljuaid, S.M.; Alamri, A.A.; Alghamdi, M.S. Linking the Saudi Arabian 2030 vision with nursing transformation in Saudi Arabia: Roadmap for nursing policies and strategies. *Int. J. Afr. Nurs. Sci.* **2020**, *13*, 100256. [CrossRef] [PubMed]
26. Du, J.; Dong, L.; Wang, T.; Yuan, C.; Fu, R.; Zhang, L.; Liu, B.; Zhang, M.; Yin, Y.; Qin, J. Psychological symptoms among frontline healthcare workers during COVID-19 outbreak in Wuhan. *Gen. Hosp. Psychiatry* **2020**, *67*, 144. [CrossRef]
27. Hu, D.; Kong, Y.; Li, W.; Han, Q.; Zhang, X.; Zhu, L.X.; Wan, S.W.; Liu, Z.; Shen, Q.; Yang, J. Frontline nurses' burnout, anxiety, depression, and fear statuses and their associated factors during the COVID-19 outbreak in Wuhan, China: A large-scale cross-sectional study. *EClinicalMedicine* **2020**, *24*, 100424. [CrossRef]
28. Lai, J.; Ma, S.; Wang, Y.; Cai, Z.; Hu, J.; Wei, N.; Wu, J.; Du, H.; Chen, T.; Li, R. Factors associated with mental health outcomes among health care workers exposed to coronavirus disease 2019. *JAMA Netw. Open* **2020**, *3*, e203976. [CrossRef]
29. Pearman, A.; Hughes, M.L.; Smith, E.L.; Neupert, S.D. Mental health challenges of United States healthcare professionals during COVID-19. *Front. Psychol.* **2020**, *11*, 2065. [CrossRef] [PubMed]
30. Canestrari, C.; Bongelli, R.; Fermani, A.; Riccioni, I.; Bertolazzi, A.; Muzi, M.; Burro, R. Coronavirus disease stress among Italian healthcare workers: The role of coping humor. *Front. Psychol.* **2021**, *11*, 3962. [CrossRef]
31. McFadden, P.; Ross, J.; Moriarty, J.; Mallett, J.; Schroder, H.; Ravalier, J.; Manthorpe, J.; Currie, D.; Harron, J.; Gillen, P. The role of coping in the wellbeing and work-related quality of life of UK health and social care workers during COVID-19. *Int. J. Environ. Res. Public Health* **2021**, *18*, 815. [CrossRef]
32. Hicks-Roof, K.K.; Xu, J.; Zeglin, R.J.; Bailey, C.E.; Hamadi, H.Y.; Osborne, R. Covid-19 Impacts on Florida's Healthcare Professionals. *Hosp. Top.* **2021**, 1–12. [CrossRef] [PubMed]
33. Engelbrecht, M.C.; Heunis, J.C.; Kigozi, N.G. Post-Traumatic Stress and Coping Strategies of South African Nurses during the Second Wave of the COVID-19 Pandemic. *Int. J. Environ. Res. Public Health* **2021**, *18*, 7919. [CrossRef] [PubMed]
34. Majrashi, A.; Khalil, A.; Nagshabandi, E.A.; Majrashi, A. Stressors and Coping Strategies among Nursing Students during the COVID-19 Pandemic: Scoping Review. *Nurs. Rep.* **2021**, *11*, 444–459. [CrossRef]
35. John, B.; Al-Sawad, M. Perceived stress in clinical areas and emotional intelligence among baccalaureate nursing students. *J. Indian Acad. Appl. Psychol.* **2015**, *41*, 75–84.
36. Pourafzal, F.; Seyedfatemi, N.; Inanloo, M.; Haghani, H. Relationship between Perceived Stress with Resilience among Undergraduate Nursing Students. *Hayat* **2013**, *19*, 1–12.
37. Wyatt, T.; Baich, V.A.; Buoni, C.A.; Watson, A.E.; Yurisic, V.E. Clinical Reasoning: Adapting Teaching Methods During the COVID-19 Pandemic to Meet Student Learning Outcomes. *J. Nurs. Educ.* **2021**, *60*, 48–51. [CrossRef]
38. Liu, M.; Cheng, S.-Z.; Xu, K.-W.; Yang, Y.; Zhu, Q.-T.; Zhang, H.; Yang, D.-Y.; Cheng, S.-Y.; Xiao, H.; Wang, J.-W. Use of personal protective equipment against coronavirus disease 2019 by healthcare professionals in Wuhan, China: Cross sectional study. *BMJ* **2020**, *369*, m2195. [CrossRef]
39. Wang, J.; Zhou, M.; Liu, F. Reasons for healthcare workers becoming infected with novel coronavirus disease 2019 (COVID-19) in China. *J. Hosp. Infect.* **2020**, *105*, 100–101. [CrossRef]
40. Ng, K.; Poon, B.H.; Kiat Puar, T.H.; Shan Quah, J.L.; Loh, W.J.; Wong, Y.J.; Tan, T.Y.; Raghuram, J. COVID-19 and the risk to health care workers: A case report. *Ann. Intern. Med.* **2020**, *172*, 766–767. [CrossRef] [PubMed]
41. Irshad, M.; Khattak, S.A.; Hassan, M.M.; Majeed, M.; Bashir, S. How perceived threat of Covid-19 causes turnover intention among Pakistani nurses: A moderation and mediation analysis. *Int. J. Ment. Health Nurs.* **2020**. [CrossRef]
42. Shengxiao, N.; Chao, S.; Lei, W.; Xia, W. The Professional Identity of Nursing Students and Their Intention to Leave the Nursing Profession During the Coronavirus Disease (COVID-19) Pandemic. *J. Nurs. Res.* **2021**, *29*, e139.
43. Gan, Y.; Liu, Y.; Zhang, Y. Flexible coping responses to severe acute respiratory syndrome-related and daily life stressful events. *Asian J. Soc. Psychol.* **2004**, *7*, 55–66. [CrossRef]
44. Labrague, L.J.; McEnroe-Petitte, D.M.; Gloe, D.; Thomas, L.; Papathanasiou, I.V.; Tsaras, K. A literature review on stress and coping strategies in nursing students. *J. Ment. Health* **2017**, *26*, 471–480. [CrossRef] [PubMed]
45. Savitsky, B.; Findling, Y.; Ereli, A.; Hendel, T. Anxiety and coping strategies among nursing students during the covid-19 pandemic. *Nurse Educ. Pract.* **2020**, *46*, 102809. [CrossRef] [PubMed]
46. Zhao, F.F.; Lei, X.L.; He, W.; Gu, Y.H.; Li, D.W. The study of perceived stress, coping strategy and self-efficacy of Chinese undergraduate nursing students in clinical practice. *Int. J. Nurs. Pract.* **2015**, *21*, 401–409. [CrossRef] [PubMed]

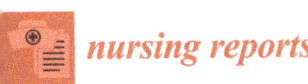 

*Article*

# Healthcare Management and Quality during the First COVID-19 Wave in a Sample of Spanish Healthcare Professionals

Patricia Torrent-Ramos [1,2], Víctor M. González-Chordá [2,*], Desirée Mena-Tudela [2], Laura Andreu Pejó [2], Celia Roig-Marti [3], María Jesús Valero-Chillerón [2] and Águeda Cervera-Gasch [2]

1. Preventive Medicine Service, Hospital General de Castellón, 12071 Castellón, Spain; ptorrent@uji.es
2. Nursing Department, Universitat Jaume I, 12071 Castellón, Spain; dmena@uji.es (D.M.-T.); pejo@uji.es (L.A.P.); chillero@uji.es (M.J.V.-C.); cerveraa@uji.es (Á.C.-G.)
3. Internal Medicine Service, Hospital General de Castellón, 12071 Castellón, Spain; celia.roig.marti@gmail.com
* Correspondence: vchorda@uji.es

**Abstract:** The aim of this study was to assess how the healthcare professionals in the Castellón Province (Spain) perceive healthcare quality and management during the first COVID-19 wave. A cross-sectional study was carried out. An online survey on healthcare quality and management during the first COVID-19 wave was sent to healthcare professionals. Almost half of the sample believed that healthcare quality worsened during the first COVID-19 wave (45.3%; $n = 173$). Heavier workload (m = $4.08 \pm 1.011$) and patients' complexity (m = $3.77 \pm 1.086$) were the factors that most negatively impacted healthcare quality. Health department 3, primary care center, and other doctors assessed human and material resources management as significantly worse ($p < 0.05$). Human and material resources management and the healthcare organization negatively affected healthcare quality during the first COVID-19 wave. Significant differences were observed according to departments, services, and professionals.

**Keywords:** COVID-19 pandemic; coronavirus; nursing; medical staff; healthcare quality; human resources; primary care; hospitals; nursing home

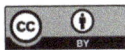

## 1. Introduction

Spain has one of the best health systems in the world [1] and occupies position 15 in the Global Health Security Index ranking [2]. Nevertheless, data indicate Spain as one of the countries to be most affected by the COVID-19 pandemic, and some experts stress the need to individually evaluate how Spain has responded to this pandemic [3]. While waiting for this evaluation to be made, healthcare professionals lived the consequences of the taken measures first-hand and have witnessed the possible impact on healthcare quality.

COVID-19 is an infectious disease caused by a new kind of coronavirus known as SARS-CoV-2 [4]. This virus is transmitted via direct contact or when an infected person releases droplet while talking, coughing or sneezing [5], and possibly via aerosols [6]. Although some cases are asymptomatic, the virus is initially manifested by mild respiratory symptoms after 4–8 incubation days, and can become clinically serious with pneumonia, multisystem failure, and even death, which occur mainly in people with previous diseases [7].

The first cases of COVID-19 disease were detected in the Hubei Province (China) at the end of 2019. The new coronavirus rapidly spread to other Asian countries and had reached Europe by the end of January 2020. The World Health Organization (WHO) declared a pandemic by SARS-CoV-2 on 11 March 2020, with 118,000 cases in 114 countries [8]. There were more than 152 million infected people and almost 3 million worldwide on 1 May 2021 [9].

SARS-CoV-2 has a limited capacity to produce serious disease and its mortality is estimated at 4.8% (95% CI: 1.00–11.4) [7]. However, its marked capacity to transmit this virus and the rapid growing number of cases in a short time led to an unforeseeable increase in the demand and requirement of infrastructures, as well as human and material resources. This meant that healthcare systems all over the world came to a standstill, which compromised healthcare quality [10].

In Spain, the first imported COVID-19 case was notified on 30 January 2020. The increasing number of COVID-19 cases led the Spanish Government to declare a state of alarm that lasted 3 months and 7 days, from 14 March to 21 June [11]. The state of alarm is a legislative instrument contemplated by the Spanish Constitution, which temporarily concentrates power in governments and allows them to make unilateral decisions. This measure can be taken in exceptional situations, such as natural catastrophes or healthcare crises [12].

The intention of this state of alarm was to stop the virus from spreading and to flatten the curve of contagions [13]. To do so, and according to how the curve of contagions progressed, different physic-social distancing measures were taken while the state of alarm lasted, such as restricting the population's movements to shop and purchase medicines, closing public spaces, wearing masks, confining the population, and not performing any non-essential occupational activity during a 15-day period.

Apart from taking these measures to prevent the virus from spreading, other measures were taken to avoid blocking health services, and to ensure that infrastructures and human and material resources were available [14]. Another approved measure was for public health services to manage private health services. The Spanish Government also centralized purchases of the material resources and personal protective equipment (PPE) needed to prevent professionals from catching the virus while attending COVID-19 patients. Retired healthcare professionals were also authorized to return to work, and final-year nursing and medicine students were contracted to work [15].

All these measures have implied relevant changes in the organization of health services and, specifically, in nursing services. Despite the limited literature available so far on how nursing managers and registered nurses are dealing with the organization of health services to cope with the pandemic, recent studies in Spain show the magnitude of decisions and the speed with which they are being taken. This is due to the overwhelming need to increase the nursing workforce, reorganize the organizational model of care, and ensure the availability of material resources [16,17].

Despite all these measures, accumulated cases went from 4231 to 246,835 in 3 months [18], which pushed the operational capacity of Spanish health services to the limit. Recent studies informed how inpatient units were transformed into intensive care units [19] or how healthcare professionals caught the virus because they had no PPE [20]. Hence, the objective of this study was to assess how healthcare professionals from the Castellón Province (Spain) perceive healthcare quality and management during the first COVID-19 wave.

## 2. Materials and Methods

### 2.1. Design and Setting

A cross-sectional study with an online survey was conducted in the Castellón Province (E Spain), where the health system is organized into three health departments, each with a reference hospital and different primary care centers that each cover populations between 200,000 and 250,000 inhabitants. One of the health departments has two other hospitals: one specializes in oncology and mental health, while the other is used for chronic patients and rehabilitation. This province has 40 nursing homes for the elderly and disabled. Of these, 60% ($n = 24$) are private homes and the rest are public. Private healthcare is limited to one hospital, with rooms for medical specialists and hemodialysis clinics.

## 2.2. Participants and Sample

Our study population included the healthcare professionals who worked in the various services offered in the Castellón Province in both private and public healthcare. According to the most recently available data, in 2019 there were 2959 registered nurses and 2667 medical practitioners (doctors). No data are available about other groups, such as nursing assistants, and data do not differ between public and private systems or between the different types of center and service [21]

## 2.3. Variables

An online survey devised with Google Docs was forwarded. It included 28 questions arranged into different blocks. The first block of seven questions asked the professionals if they thought that healthcare quality had worsened, remained the same, or had improved during the state of alarm. They were also asked to assess the impact of different factors on healthcare quality (workload, human resources, material resources, teamwork, patients' clinical complexity, and healthcare organization). These questions were answered on a 5-point Likert-type scale (1: Strong negative impact; 5: Strong positive impact).

The second block contained 11 questions about managing human and material resources. The professionals were asked to assess on an ascending 5-point Likert-type scale (1: Not at all appropriate; 5: Most appropriate) the staff reinforcement contracts signed and contract duration. They were also asked to assess on an ascending 5-point Likert-type scale the availability of different material resources (surgical gloves, protective face shields, impermeable gowns, cleaning and disinfecting products, and other material resources). Two questions were included about the training received in handling PPE and cleaning/disinfecting products.

The third block comprised 10 questions about how health care was organized during the state of alarm. They were asked to specifically assess on an ascending 5-point Likert-type scale (1: Not very appropriate; 5: Most appropriate) how centers' management responded, supervisors' direct concern about work teams' well-being, how work was organized, the clarity of protocols, and the suitability of the circuits set up to attend to COVID-19 patients. Two questions were also included about the training received in the new organization of both work and teamwork. The professionals were also requested to assess if their occupational rights and conditions were respected during the state of alarm. Finally, they were asked to assess if the health system was ready to face a new outbreak.

We collected socio-demographic variables: age, gender, and family responsibilities (children, elderly people, dependent people), as well as perceived health status (very good, good, normal, bad). Occupational variables were also included, such as type of center (public; private), the health department they belonged to (HD1; HD2; HD3), healthcare service (primary care center; hospital; nursing home; others (healthcare transport or private offices, among others)), their professional category (doctor; nurse; nursing assistant; others (hospital porter or technicians, among other)), their contract type (temporary; permanent; contracted specially for the pandemic; substitution; resident in training; other), years of experience (less than 5; between 5 and 10; between 10 and 15; more than 15), and other variable related to COVID-19 exposure (positive case, diagnosis technique, isolation).

## 2.4. Data Collection

Data collection took place between 1 and 15 July 2020. The online survey was diffused on social networks like Facebook, Twitter, Instagram, or WhatsApp as they are the most widely used in Spain. The recommendations by Pedersen and Kurz [22] about using social networks for data collection were followed.

## 2.5. Data Analysis

A descriptive analysis was carried out of the variables included in this study in line with their nature. The comparison of the results according to health service, health department, and professional category was made using the Kruskal–Wallis H test after confirming that groups did not follow normal distribution. The categories nursing homes and other services were grouped for poor representativeness. A chi-squared test (X2) was used with the qualitative variables. It was not necessary to address missing data. The statistical analysis was done by the SPSS V21 software (IBM, New York, EEUU). The level of significance was set at $p < 0.05$.

### 2.6. Ethical Considerations

This study was designed in accordance with Spanish Organic Law 03/2018 on Personal Data Protection and Guaranteeing Digital Rights. Additional provision 17 on processing of health data, paragraph 2g, specifies that studies with pseudomized or anonymized data must be submitted for evaluation by an ethics and research committee. This study did not experiment with human beings and the participants answered voluntarily and anonymously and no personal data that could identify each participant, email, or IP address were collected to guarantee confidentiality, so it did not need approval by an ethics and research committee. The first page of the survey included information on the study objective and methodology, along with a box with which the participants gave their informed consent, confirming that their participation was voluntary and anonymous. Moreover, Declaration of Helsinki Principles were respected (charity, non-maleficence, autonomy, justice).

## 3. Results

### 3.1. Sample Characteristics

We collected 382 surveys. The participants' mean age was 42.97 (95% CI: 41.94–44.00) years; 82.2% ($n = 314$) were female and 53.7% ($n = 205$) considered that their health status was good; 63.4% ($n = 242$) had children, and 21.7% ($n = 83$) looked after elderly people. Most of the participants in our sample were registered nurses (56.8%; $n = 217$); 54.7% ($n = 209$) of the sample had more than 15 years of experience and 52.4% ($n = 209$) had temporary contracts. Most of the participants belonged to the public health system (96.9%; $n = 370$), specifically from HD2 (74.6%; $n = 285$), they worked in a hospital (74.6%; $n = 285$), and 84.8% ($n = 324$) had been in contact with COVID-19 patients. Only 15.7% ($n = 60$) stated that they had had a diagnosis test and 18.3% ($n = 70$) had been isolated. The prevalence of COVID-19 cases in the study sample was 7.6% ($n = 29$). Table 1 shows the analysis of the socio-demographic, occupational, and COVID-19 exposure-related variables.

### 3.2. Healthcare Quality

Healthcare quality was perceived by 45.3% ($n = 173$) of our sample as becoming worse during the first COVID-19 wave, while the other respondents stated that the same conditions remained (43.7%; $n = 167$) or improved (11%; $n = 42$). No significant differences were found for health department (H = 4.007; $p = 0.405$) or service type (H = 7.355; $p = 0.499$). Nevertheless, significant differences appeared according to professional category because doctors (60.9%; $n = 42$) and registered nurses (44.7%; $n = 97$) were the professional groups that mainly thought that healthcare quality worsened during the state of alarm (H = 14.36; $p = 0.026$).

Workload was assessed as the factor with the most negative impact on healthcare quality (m = 1.92 ± 1.011) (H = 4.189; $p = 0.123$), followed by patients' clinical complexity (m = 2.23 ± 1.086) (H = 0.02; $p = 0.99$), but no significant differences were found according to healthcare service. Another factor with a negative impact on healthcare quality was material resources management (m = 2.35 ± 1.228), mostly in primary care centers (m = 1.88 ± 1.045) as opposed to nursing homes and other services (m = 2.29 ± 1.243) and hospitals (m = 2.46 ± 1.243), with significant differences (H = 12.616; $p = 0.002$).

Table 1. Socio-demographic, occupational, and COVID-19 exposure-related variables.

| Title 1 | Title 2 | %(n) |
|---|---|---|
| Gender | Man | 17.3 (68) |
| | Woman | 82.2 (314) |
| Have children | Yes | 63.4 (242) |
| | No | 36.6 (140) |
| Look after elderly people | Yes | 21.7 (83) |
| | No | 78.3 (299) |
| Look after dependent people | Yes | 11.5 (44) |
| | No | 88.5 (338) |
| Health status | Very good | 34.8 (133) |
| | Good | 53.7 (205) |
| | Normal | 11 (42) |
| | Bad | 0.5 (2) |
| Health department | HD1 | 5.2 (20) |
| | HD2 | 74.6 (285) |
| | HD3 | 20.2 (77) |
| Type of center | Public | 96.9 (370) |
| | Private | 2.9 (11) |
| Professional category | Doctors | 18.1 (69) |
| | Registered nurses | 56.8 (217) |
| | Nursing assistants | 18.1 (69) |
| | Others (hospital porters, technicians) | 7.1 (27) |
| Years of experience | <5 | 12.6 (48) |
| | 5–10 | 13.6 (52) |
| | 10–15 | 19.1 (73) |
| | >15 | 54.7 (209) |
| Type of contract | Temporary | 52.4 (200) |
| | Permanent | 27.2 (104) |
| | Reinforcement for pandemic | 8.4 (32) |
| | Substitution | 6.0 (23) |
| | Resident in training | 4.5 (4.5) |
| | Other | 1.6 (6) |
| Service | Health center | 17.3 (66) |
| | Hospital | 74.6 (285) |
| | Nursing home and others | 8.1 (31) |
| Contact with COVID-19 patients | Yes | 84.8 (324) |
| | No | 15.2 (58) |
| Positive COVID-19 | Yes | 7.6 (29) |
| | No | 89.5 (342) |
| | I'd rather not answer | 2.9 (11) |
| Isolation | Yes | 18.3 (70) |
| | No | 80.9 (309) |

Human resources management was assessed at 2.38 (±1.180) points. The professionals who worked in primary care centers (m = 2.11 ± 1.069), as well as nursing homes and other services (m = 2.1 ± 1.012), indicated that this factor had the stronger negative impact versus those professionals who worked in hospitals (m = 2.48 ± 1.209), with significant differences (H = 6.655; $p$ = 0.036). Health service organizations obtained a score of 2.77 (±1.278) points, and no significant differences were found according to health service (H = 0.65; $p$ = 0.723).

Finally, teamwork was considered to be the only factor with a positive impact on healthcare quality (m = 3.60 ± 1.255), mainly in hospitals (m = 3.70 ± 1.255) vs. primary care centers (m = 3.26 ± 1.281) and nursing homes and other services (m = 3.35 ± 1.05), with significant differences (H = 0.65; $p$ = 0.011). Table 2 offers these results for health department and professional category.

**Table 2.** Factors that negatively affected healthcare quality according to health department and professional category.

| Factors | Health Department (m; sd) | | | | Professional Category (m; sd) | | | | |
|---|---|---|---|---|---|---|---|---|---|
| | HD1 | HD2 | HD3 | $p$ | Nurses | Doctors | Assistants | Others | $p$ [1] |
| Workload | 2.25 (1.209) | 1.97 (1.026) | 1.64 (0.842) | 0.017 | 1.98 (1.056) | 1.67 (0.918) | 1.90 (0.91) | 2.11 (1.05) | 0.078 |
| Human resources | 2.75 (1.517) | 2.40 (1.181) | 2.25 (1.066) | 0.383 | 2.60 (1.229) | 1.84 (1.038) | 2.23 (1.002) | 2.44 (1.086) | <0.001 |
| Material resources | 2.65 (1.387) | 2.39 (1.242) | 2.10 (1.107) | 0.135 | 2.53 (1.277) | 1.91 (1.011) | 2.26 (1.221) | 2.22 (1.086) | 0.005 |
| Teamwork | 3.70 (1.174) | 3.53 (1.263) | 3.83 (1.229) | 0.134 | 3.73 (1.21) | 3.48 (1.313) | 3.43 (1.377) | 3.22 (1.013) | 0.065 |
| Clinical complexity | 2.55 (1.05) | 2.23 (1.082) | 2.14 (1.109) | 0.261 | 2.22 (1.051) | 2.26 (1.066) | 2.22 (1.223) | 2.30 (1.103) | 0.950 |
| Healthcare organization | 3.00 (1.622) | 2.75 (1.224) | 2.77 (1.385) | 0.828 | 2.69 (1.266) | 2.97 (1.35) | 2.83 (1.224) | 2.70 (1.325) | 0.468 |

[1] Level of significance was set at $p < 0.05$.

*3.3. Managing Human and Material Resources*

In general terms, human resources management during the state of alarm obtained 3.07 (±1.210) points and no significant differences appeared for health services (H = 3.053; $p$ = 0.217). The number of staff reinforcement contracts obtained 3.16 (±1.343) points, with a worse score for primary care centers (m = 2.42 ± 1.29) and nursing homes and other services (m = 2.97 ± 1.449) than for hospitals (m = 3.35 ± 1.285), with significant differences (H = 25.231; $p$ < 0.001). The time that reinforcement staff contracts lasted (2.95 ± 1.379) was scored worse in primary care centers (m = 2.36 ± 1.211) and nursing homes and other services (m = 2.45 ± 1.457) than in hospitals (m = 3.14 ± 1.359), with significant differences (H = 21.422; $p$ < 0.001).

Availability of protective face shields scored 2.88 (±1.446) points, and the score given by the professionals for working in hospitals was statistically higher (m = 3.06 ± 1.438) than in primary care centers (m = 2.36 ± 1.32) and nursing homes and other services (m = 2.42 ± 1.455) (H = 15.956; $p$ < 0.001). The availability of impermeable gowns (m = 2.91 ± 1.358) and masks (m = 2.94 ± 1.336) obtained a significantly higher score in hospitals (gowns m = 3.12 ± 1.332; masks m = 3.11 ± 1.31) than in primary care centers (gowns m = 2.24 ± 1.151; masks m = 2.41 ± 1.24) and in nursing homes and other services (gowns m = 2.45 ± 1.457; masks m = 2.48 ± 1.411) (gowns H = 26.277, $p$ < 0.001; masks H = 18.209, $p$ < 0.001). Similar results were found for the availability of cleaning and disinfecting materials (m = 3.65 ± 1.234), which were significantly better assessed in hospitals (m = 3.76 ± 1.211) (H = 9.899; $p$ = 0.007).

Finally, no significant differences were observed for healthcare professionals' assessments according to the health service about the availability of other material resources required to attend to patients (m = 3.26 ± 1.148) (H = 2.801; $p$ = 0.247) and the availability of surgical gloves (m = 3.6 ± 1.276) (H = 0.38; $p$ = 0.827). Nor were significant differences observed for training in handling PPE (m = 2.80 ± 1.294) (H = 1.747; $p$ = 0.418) and training in the use of cleaning and disinfecting products (m = 2.84 ± 1.282) (H = 2.972; $p$ = 0.226). Table 3 shows the results of human/material resources management according to health department and professional category.

**Table 3.** Results of human/material resources management according to health department and professional category.

| Questions | Health Department (m; sd) | | | | Professional Category (m; sd) | | | | |
|---|---|---|---|---|---|---|---|---|---|
| | HD1 | HD2 | HD3 | p | Nurses | Doctors | Assistants | Others | p [1] |
| Human resources management | 3.65 (1.268) | 3.04 (1.204) | 3 (1.192) | 0.102 | 3.2 (1.172) | 2.68 (1.169) | 2.99 (1.3) | 3.19 (1.21) | 0.023 |
| Reinforcement contracts | 3.7 (1.525) | 3.13 (1.319) | 3.13 (1.370) | 0.143 | 3.44 (1.228) | 2.04 (1.130) | 3.46 (1.313) | 2.96 (1.344) | <0.001 |
| Contract duration | 3.65 (1.755) | 2.94 (1.339) | 1.79 (1.380) | 0.51 | 3.17 (1.389) | 2.07 (1.048) | 3.2 (1.279) | 2.78 (1.423) | <0.001 |
| Availability of masks | 3.20 (1.399) | 3.02 (1.317) | 2.55 (1.333) | 0.015 | 3.16 (1.306) | 2.68 (1.312) | 2.48 (1.335) | 3 (1.301) | 0.001 |
| Availability of surgical gloves | 3.9 (1.294) | 3.58 (1.263) | 3.57 (1.322) | 0.468 | 3.84 (1.177) | 3.32 (1.388) | 3.12 (1.334) | 3.59 (1.152) | <0.001 |
| Availability of gowns | 3.1 (1.334) | 3.06 (1.318) | 2.34 (1.373) | 0.001 | 3.12 (1.329) | 2.49 (1.324) | 2.70 (1.354) | 2.85 (1.406) | 0.003 |
| Availability of face shields | 3.6 (1.603) | 2.88 (1.428) | 2.70 (1.433) | 0.053 | 3.16 (1.465) | 2.38 (1.373) | 2.57 (1.323) | 2.78 (1.311) | <0.001 |
| Availability of other material resources | 3.5 (1.235) | 3.28 (1.138) | 3.13 (1.162) | 0.317 | 3.44 (1.104) | 2.83 (1.2) | 3.19 (1.154) | 3.19 (1.075) | 0.001 |
| Availability of cleaning products | 4.05 (1.317) | 3.69 (1.191) | 3.42 (1.341) | 0.034 | 3.85 (1.161) | 3.2 (1.208) | 3.64 (1.317) | 3.26 (1.318) | 0.004 |
| Training in PPE | 3.4 (1.667) | 2.83 (1.284) | 2.53 (1.165) | 0.063 | 2.93 (1.345) | 2.51 (1.066) | 2.94 (1.282) | 2.15 (1.167) | <0.001 |
| Training in cleaning/disinfecting products | 3.15 (1.663) | 2.93 (1.213) | 2.39 (1.339) | 0.002 | 2.86 (1.030) | 2.58 (1.218) | 3.1 (1.274) | 2.63 (1.214) | 0.091 |

[1] Level of significance was set at $p < 0.05$.

### 3.4. Healthcare Organisation

The whole sample gave 3.36 (±1.147) points for the response of healthcare centers' management to the COVID-19 pandemic. The professionals who worked in primary care gave a significantly better score (m = 3.61 ± 1.456) than those who worked in hospitals (m = 3.21 ± 1.169) and in nursing homes and other services (m = 2.97 ± 1.169) (H = 10.552; $p$ = 0.005). Supervisors' concern for work teams' well-being was scored 3.74 (±1.316) points, and there were no significant differences for health services (H = 2.862; $p$ = 0.239).

How work was organized obtained a mean score of 3.57 (±1.175) points and was significantly better assessed in primary care centers (m = 3.89 ± 1.125) than in hospitals (m = 3.53 ± 1.179) and nursing homes and other services (m = 3.26 ± 1.125) (H = 8.747; $p$ = 0.013). No significant differences appeared in the assessments of either the healthcare protocols set up (m = 2.70 ± 1.281) (H = 1.853; $p$ = 0.396) or the suitability of the circuits set up to attend to COVID-19 patients (m = 3.20 ± 1.091; $p$ = 0.65).

No significant differences were found in the assessments of either training received (m = 2.71 ± 1.203) (H = 1.824; $p$ = 0.402) or teamwork (m = 4.13 ± 1.115) (H = 3.418; $p$ = 0.402) according to healthcare service. However, primary care professionals (m = 2.59 ± 1.425) assessed respect for their occupational rights as being significantly worse than those professionals from hospitals (m = 3.06 ± 1.336) and nursing homes and other services (m = 2.74 ± 1.483) (H = 6.661; $p$ = 0.36); primary care professionals (m = 2.61 ± 1.402) assessed their working conditions as being significantly worse than those from nursing homes and other services (m = 2.9 ± 1.446) and hospitals (m = 3.04 ± 1.365) (H = 3.04 ± 1.365).

Finally, preparing health services to face a new COVID-19 outbreak obtained a score of 2.99 (±1.234) points, and significant differences were found depending on the service that the professionals worked for (H = 6.262; $p$ = 0.027). Primary care professionals gave a lower score (m = 2.68 ± 1.23), followed by the professionals from hospitals (m = 3.02 ± 1.217), and finally nursing homes and other services (m = 3.32 ± 1.301). Table 4 shows the analysis done of these matters according to health department and professional category.

Table 4. Healthcare organization according to health department and professional category.

| Questions | Health Department (m; sd) | | | | Professional Category (m; sd) | | | | |
|---|---|---|---|---|---|---|---|---|---|
| | HD1 | HD2 | HD3 | p | Nurses | Doctors | Assistants | Others | p [1] |
| Management's response | 3.8 (1.152) | 3.19 (1.121) | 3.38 (1.023) | 0.034 | 3.19 (1.297) | 3.61 (1.297) | 3.07 (1.048) | 3.37 (1.275) | 0.006 |
| Concern about work teams | 4.45 (1.05) | 3.68 (1.308) | 3.75 (1.368) | 0.02 | 3.79 (1.035) | 3.84 (1.302) | 3.61 (1.297) | 3.33 (1.468) | 0.267 |
| How work was organized | 3.95 (1.146) | 3.49 (1.174) | 3.78 (1.154) | 0.036 | 3.59 (1.132) | 3.87 (1.123) | 3.33 (1.291) | 3.3 (1.203) | 0.025 |
| Clarity of protocols | 3.35 (1.348) | 2.68 (1.213) | 2.62 (1.170) | 0.071 | 2.7 (1.258) | 2.74 (1.159) | 2.65 (1.161) | 2.81 (1.241) | 0.928 |
| COVID-19 circuits | 3.60 (1.046) | 3.15 (1.098) | 3.29 (1.062) | 0.087 | 3.24 (1.092) | 3.22 (0.998) | 3.10 (1.113) | 3.11 (1.281) | 0.837 |
| Training | 3.35 (1.599) | 2.67 (1.185) | 2.68 (1.117) | 0.019 | 2.66 (1.249) | 2.86 (1.102) | 2.72 (1.123) | 2.67 (1.301) | 0.585 |
| Teamwork | 4.35 (1.268) | 4.06 (1.124) | 4.32 (1.019) | 0.046 | 4.23 (1.042) | 4.12 (1.182) | 4.01 (1.266) | 3.67 (1) | 0.027 |
| Occupational rights | 3.45 (1.504) | 3.03 (1.350) | 2.53 (1.334) | 0.005 | 3.09 (1.322) | 2.33 (1.268) | 2.88 (1.44) | 3.59 (1.338) | <0.001 |
| Working conditions | 3.20 (1.576) | 3.02 (1.378) | 2.66 (1.334) | 0.1 | 3.13 (1.344) | 2.10 (1.214) | 3.14 (1.320) | 3.26 (1.059) | <0.001 |
| Ready for a new outbreak | 2.95 (1.538) | 2.98 (1.163) | 3.04 (1.409) | 0.886 | 3.02 (1.215) | 2.64 (1.2) | 3.09 (1.280) | 3.37 (1.214) | 0.039 |

[1] Level of significance was set at $p < 0.05$.

## 4. Discussion

A well-organized and prepared health system should have the capacity to maintain reasonable access to high-quality health services during a healthcare emergency. This capacity depends on a coordinated response from health authorities, having contingency plans that allow for health services to be organized, clear protocols to attend to patients, and suitable human and material resources management [23]. Today the COVID-19 pandemic challenges the operation and sustainability of health systems worldwide, with differences among countries as far as measures taken and the obtained results [24]. Initially in Spain, a virus containment model was adopted and the national government centralized decision-making [13]. However, subsequent decisions seem to have been taken from a perspective of living with the virus and decision-making returned to the regional governments. It is convenient to remember that Spain is a decentralized country where health competences, among others, are transferred to regional governments. The measures adopted by the central government have an impact at the regional level and this can be observed in the interregional differences in the evolution of the pandemic [25], although the magnitude of this impact must be confirmed in future studies.

Nearly 50% of the healthcare professionals who participated in this study believed that healthcare quality worsened during the first COVID-19 wave. Doctors and registered nurses were the groups that assessed healthcare quality as worse during this period, probably because they were the professionals who worked in the first healthcare line of attention, and who endured a very heavy physical, psychological, and social load [26]. Indeed, more than 80% stated having been in contact with COVID-19 patients, although only 15.7% of the surveyed professionals had diagnostic tests. The prevalence of the healthcare professionals with COVID-19 in Spain was 20% but was 7.6% in this study. Nonetheless, the quantity of infected professionals varied from one region of Spain to another, and official data for provinces are not available to compare these results [27].

Workload was assessed as the factor that most impacted healthcare quality. In fact, a recent study indicates how the nursing workload was heavier when working with COVID-19 patients than with non-COVID-19 patients in an intensive care unit [28]. Nevertheless, it is striking that registered nurses were not the professional group that assessed human resources management, hiring staff, or respecting occupational rights as worse, according to the large body of evidence for occupational precariousness and shortage of registered nurses in Spain, with a nurse-patients ratio below the mean reported by the OECD [29]. Despite the current situation of the nursing workforce in Spain, which has been tremendously complicated by the pandemic, it is very possible that the humanistic values of the profession, its willingness to serve people who need it, and its capacity of resilience can explain these results, coinciding with other studies [20,30].

The differences encountered in health departments on the impact that workload had on healthcare quality, as well as other aspects on human and material resources management and organizing health care, can be explained by high healthcare pressure due to COVID-19 cases on HD2 and HD3 compared to HD1 [31]. Nevertheless, benchmarking techniques will help to detect the possible differences in the strategies adopted in the three health departments [32].

Moreover, those professionals who worked in primary care, nursing homes, and other services assessed human and material resources management worse. Spain's initial response came late and primary care strategies were not developed to contain SARS-CoV-2 from spreading, which coincided with the seasonal flu epidemic [33]. Moreover, the pandemic evidenced the precarious situation of nursing homes in Spain [34]. Therefore, all efforts had to center on supplying hospitals in order to attend to the increasing general number of cases and serious cases.

The healthcare organization assessment can be considered appropriate. Nonetheless, the primary care professionals better assessed their organization than that in hospitals, nursing homes, and other services. As previously mentioned, hospitals received most of the patients with this new disease caused by the virus that had recently appeared. Modes of viral transmission, its risk factors, clinical evolution, symptoms, or treatments for this disease are being investigated as the pandemic advances. These factors could have had an influence when setting up suitable circuits and clear protocols to attend to these patients, which could have made healthcare organization difficult. Another point to stress is the poor assessment that the professionals made of previous training in using PPE, disinfection, cleaning, and the new work organization. The WHO considers that training and supporting professionals are fundamental in this healthcare emergency [24].

The results of this work must be taken cautiously. On the one hand, this study was conducted only about the healthcare professionals working in one province in Spain and the impact of the first COVID-19 wave was variable. Professionals from other Spanish regions may have different views about healthcare management and quality. Even the opinion and perception of the same group of professionals may vary depending on their field of work. For example, there could be differences between the perception of registered nurses who work in hospitals, health centers, or nursing homes. However, our sample was limited and not randomized, which prevents some variables from being compared, e.g., if services were public or private. These types of analyses should be addressed in future studies, with representative and larger samples. In addition, there are not enough data available to determine the representativeness of the sample on the population studied according to the type of health system, department, center, or service. Another important aspect is related to the data collection instrument, since a survey was used instead of a validated questionnaire. This can affect the reliability of the results.

Other studies carried out in Spain, with online surveys and similar limitations, focused on studying the quality of life of healthcare professionals during the first COVID-19 wave [35] or the factors related to SARS-CoV-2 infection in healthcare professionals [36]. However, despite these limitations, our results are interesting because no previous studies about how Spanish healthcare professionals assess healthcare management and quality during an epidemic outbreak were found, possibly because Spain has not recently been affected by serious epidemic outbreaks. Knowing how healthcare professionals assess healthcare quality and management during the first COVID-19 wave is important. The outcomes of this study can help to detect aspects that can improve when preparing the health system for a new wave of COVID-19 or other infectious diseases. Specifically, it was observed how the emergency situation caused by the COVID-19 pandemic increased the needs of the workforce and material resources, in addition to requiring a new organization of patient care. Decision makers and managers of health services should seriously consider these factors when preparing contingency plans.

## 5. Conclusions

Overall, 45% of the healthcare professionals from the Castellón Province (Spain) consider that healthcare quality worsened during the first COVID-19 wave. The factors that negatively impacted healthcare quality were heavier workload and patients' complexity, both of which are related to human/material resources management and healthcare organization. Significant differences were observed according to health department, type of health service, and type of professional, and studies with bigger samples should deal with these variables in the future.

**Author Contributions:** Conceptualization, V.M.G.-C. and P.T.-R.; methodology, V.M.G.-C., D.M.-T., Á.C.-G. and L.A.P.; formal analysis, D.M.-T. and V.M.G.-C.; data curation, P.T.-R. and C.R.-M.; writing—original draft preparation, V.M.G.-C. and M.J.V.-C.; writing—review and editing, D.M.-T., L.A.P., Á.C.-G., P.T.-R. and C.R.-M. All authors have read and agreed to the published version of the manuscript.

**Funding:** This research received no external funding.

**Institutional Review Board Statement:** Not applicable.

**Informed Consent Statement:** The first page of the survey included information on the study objective and methodology, along with a box with which the participants gave their informed consent, confirming that their participation was voluntary and anonymous.

**Data Availability Statement:** Data are available upon request to the authors.

**Conflicts of Interest:** The authors declare no conflict of interest.

## References

1. GBD 2016 Healthcare Access and Quality Collaborators. Measuring performance on the Healthcare Access and Quality Index for 195 countries and territories and selected subnational locations: A systematic analysis from the Global Burden of Disease Study 2016. *Lancet* **2018**, *391*, 2236–2271. [CrossRef]
2. GHS Index Country Profile for Spain. Available online: https://www.ghsindex.org/country/spain/ (accessed on 11 May 2021).
3. García-Basteiro, A.; Alvarez-Dardet, C.; Arenas, A.; Bengoa, R.; Borrell, C.; Del Val, M.; Franco, M.; Gea-Sánchez, M.; Otero, J.; Valcárcel, B.; et al. The need for an independent evaluation of the COVID-19 response in Spain. *Lancet* **2020**, *396*, 529–530. [CrossRef]
4. International Committee on Taxonomy of Viruses. Naming the 2019 Coronavirus. Available online: https://talk.ictvonline.org/ (accessed on 11 May 2021).
5. Rothan, H.A.; Byrareddy, S.N. The epidemiology and pathogenesis of coronavirus disease (COVID-19) outbreak. *J. Autoimmun.* **2020**, *109*, 102433. [CrossRef]
6. Wax, R.S.; Christian, M.D. Practical recommendations for critical care and anaesthesiology teams caring for novel coronavirus (2019-nCoV) patients. *Can. J. Anaesth.* **2020**, *67*, 568–576. [CrossRef]
7. Park, M.; Cook, A.R.; Lim, J.T.; Sun, Y.; Dickens, B.L. A systematic review of COVID-19 epidemiology based on current evidence. *J. Clin. Med.* **2020**, *9*, 967. [CrossRef]
8. World Health Organization. Coronavirus Disease (COVID-19) Outbreak. Available online: https://www.who.int/emergencies/diseases/novel-coronavirus-2019 (accessed on 11 May 2021).
9. Johns Hopkins. Coronavirus Resource Center. 2020. Available online: https://coronavirus.jhu.edu/map.html (accessed on 11 May 2021).
10. Leite, H.; Lindsay, C.; Kumar, M. COVID-19 outbreak: Implications on healthcare operations. *TQM J.* **2020**, *33*, 247–256. [CrossRef]
11. Spanish Government. Real Decreto 463/2020, de 14 de Marzo, por el que se Declara el Estado de Alarma Para la Gestión de la Situación de Crisis Sanitaria Ocasionada por el COVID-19. 2020. Available online: https://boe.es/boe/dias/2020/03/11/pdfs/BOE-A-2020-3434.pdf#BOEn (accessed on 11 May 2021).
12. Catoira, A.A. El estado de alarma en España. *Teor. Y Real. Const.* **2011**, *28*, 313–341. [CrossRef]
13. Thunström, L.; Newbold, S.C.; Finnoff, D.; Ashworth, M.; Shogren, J.F. The Benefits and Costs of Using Social Distancing to Flatten the Curve for COVID-19. *J. Benefit-Cost Anal.* **2020**, 1–17. [CrossRef]
14. Legido-Quigley, H.; Mateos-García, J.T.; Campos, V.R.; Gea-Sánchez, M.; Muntaner, C.; McKee, M. The resilience of the Spanish health system against the COVID-19 pandemic. *Lancet Public Health* **2020**, *5*, e251–e252. [CrossRef]
15. Cervera-Gasch, Á.; González-Chordá, V.M.; Mena-Tudela, D. COVID-19: Are Spanish medicine and nursing students prepared? *Nurse Educ. Today* **2020**, *92*, 104473. [CrossRef] [PubMed]

16. Martinez Estalella, G.; Zabalegui, A.; Sevilla Guerra, S.; en nombre del Comité Técnico de la Dirección Enfermera (CTDE). Gestión y liderazgo de los servicios de Enfermería en el plan de emergencia de la pandemia COVID-19: La experiencia del Hospital Clínic de Barcelona [Management and leadership of nursing services in the emergency plan for the pandemic COVID-19: The experience of the Clinic Hospital of Barcelona]. *Enferm. Clin. (Engl. Ed.)* **2021**, *31*, S12–S17. [CrossRef] [PubMed]
17. Fernández Sánchez, S.P.; Rodríguez Muñoz, F.; Laiz, A.; Castellví, I.; Magallares, B.; Corominas, H. Impact of the COVID-19 Pandemic on Rheumatology Nursing Consultation. Impacto de la COVID-19 en la consulta de enfermería reumatológica. *Reumatol. Clin. (Engl. Ed.)* **2021**. published online ahead of print. [CrossRef]
18. World Health Organization. WHO Coronavirus Disease (COVID-19) Dashboard. Available online: https://covid19.who.int/ (accessed on 11 May 2021).
19. Rosello Sancho, J.; Gámez García, S.; Roel Fernández, A.; Martínez-Estalella, G. Transformar una planta de hospitalización en una unidad de críticos para la pandemia de COVID-19 [Transform a conventional ward into a critical care unit for the COVID-19 pandemic]. *Tesela* **2020**, *27*, e12926.
20. Santana López, B.N.; Santana-Padilla, Y.G.; González-Martín, J.M.; Santana-Cabrera, L. Attitudes and beliefs of Spanish healthcare professionals during the COVID-19 pandemic. *Sci. Prog.* **2021**, *104*, 368504211003775. [CrossRef]
21. Instituto Nacional de Estadística. Home. Available online: https://www.ine.es/index.htm (accessed on 11 May 2021).
22. Pedersen, E.R.; Kurz, J. Using Facebook for health-related research study recruitment and program delivery. *Curr. Opin. Psychol.* **2016**, *9*, 38–43. [CrossRef]
23. World Health Organization. COVID-19: Operational Guidance for Maintaining Essential Health Services during an Outbreak Interim Guidance. 25 March 2020. Available online: https://apps.who.int/iris/handle/10665/331561 (accessed on 11 May 2021).
24. Greer, S.L.; King, E.J.; Da Fonseca, E.M.; Peralta-Santos, A. The comparative politics of COVID-19: The need to understand government responses. *Global Public Health* **2020**, *15*, 1413–1416. [CrossRef]
25. Pérez-Arnal, R.; Conesa, D.; Alvarez-Napagao, S.; Suzumura, T.; Català, M.; Alvarez-Lacalle, E.; Garcia-Gasulla, D. Comparative Analysis of Geolocation Information through Mobile-Devices under Different COVID-19 Mobility Restriction Patterns in Spain. *ISPRS Int. J. Geo-Inf.* **2021**, *10*, 73. [CrossRef]
26. Shaukat, N.; Ali, D.M.; Razzak, J. Physical and mental health impacts ofCOVID-19 on healthcare workers: A scoping review. *Int. J. Emerg. Med.* **2020**, *13*, 40. [CrossRef]
27. Centro Nacional de Epidemiología. Informes Sobre la Situación de COVID-19. Available online: https://www.isciii.es/QueHacemos/Servicios/VigilanciaSaludPublicaRENAVE/EnfermedadesTransmisibles/Paginas/InformesCOVID-19.aspx (accessed on 11 May 2021).
28. Lucchini, A.; Giani, M.; Elli, S.; Villa, S.; Rona, R.; Foti, G. Nursing Activities Score is increased in COVID-19 patients. *Intensive Crit. Care Nurs.* **2020**, *59*, 102876. [CrossRef]
29. Esteban-Sepúlveda, S.; Moreno-Casbas, M.T.; Fuentelsaz-Gallego, C.; Ruzafa-Martinez, M. The nurse work environment in Spanish nurses following an economic recession: From 2009 to 2014. *J. Nurs. Manag.* **2019**, *27*, 1294–1303. [CrossRef]
30. Luceño-Moreno, L.; Talavera-Velasco, B.; García-Albuerne, Y.; Martín-García, J. Symptoms of Posttraumatic Stress, Anxiety, Depression, Levels of Resilience and Burnout in Spanish Health Personnel during the COVID-19 Pandemic. *Int. J. Environ. Res. Public Health* **2020**, *17*, 5514. [CrossRef]
31. Generalitat Valenciana. COVID-19 C. *Valenciana: Monitoratge de la situación.* Available online: http://coronavirus.san.gva.es/es/estadisticas (accessed on 11 May 2021).
32. George, B.; Verschuere, B.; Wayenberg, E.; Zaki, B.L. A Guide to Benchmarking COVID-19 Performance Data. *Public Adm. Rev.* **2020**, *80*, 696–700. [CrossRef]
33. Coma, E.; Mora, N.; Prats-Uribe, A.; Fina, F.; Prieto-Alhambra, D.; Medina, M. Excess cases of influenza and the coronavirus epidemic in Catalonia: A time-series analysis of primary-care electronic medical records covering over 6 million people. *BMJ Open* **2020**, *10*, e039369. [CrossRef]
34. Rada, A.G. COVID-19: The precarious position of Spain's nursing homes. *BMJ* **2020**, *369*, m1554. [CrossRef]
35. Ruiz-Fernández, M.D.; Ramos-Pichardo, J.D.; Ibáñez-Masero, O.; Cabrera-Troya, J.; Carmona-Rega, M.I.; Ortega-Galán, Á.M. Compassion fatigue, burnout, compassion satisfaction and perceived stress in healthcare professionals during the COVID-19 health crisis in Spain. *J. Clin. Nurs.* **2020**, *21*, 4321–4330. [CrossRef]
36. Moreno-Casbas, M.T. Factors related to SARS-CoV-2 infection in healthcare professionals in Spain. The SANICOVI project. *Enferm. Clin.* **2020**, *30*, 360–370. [CrossRef]

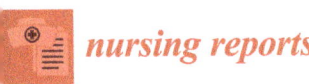 

*Review*

# Stressors and Coping Strategies among Nursing Students during the COVID-19 Pandemic: Scoping Review

Aisha Majrashi [1,*], Asmaa Khalil [2,3], Elham Al Nagshabandi [2] and Abdulrahman Majrashi [4]

1. Medical-Surgical Nursing Department, King Abdulaziz University, Jeddah 21589, Saudi Arabia
2. Faculty of Nursing, King Abdulaziz University, Jeddah 21589, Saudi Arabia; akhleel@kau.edu.sa (A.K.); elham@kau.edu.sa (E.A.N.)
3. Faculty of Nursing, Ain Shams University, Cairo 11566, Egypt
4. Critical Care Medicine, Queen Mary University of London, London E14NS, UK; emsabood@gmail.com
* Correspondence: AHASSANMAJRASHI@stu.kau.edu.sa

**Abstract:** COVID-19 has impacted every aspect of life around the world. Nursing education has moved classes online. Undoubtedly, the period has been stressful for nursing students. The scoping review aimed to explore the relevant evidence related to stressors and coping strategies among nursing students during the COVID-19 pandemic. The scoping review methodology was used to map the relevant evidence and synthesize the findings by framing the research question using PICOT, determining the keywords, eligibility criteria, searching the CINAHL, MEDLINE, and PubMed databases for the relevant studies. The review further involved study selection based on the PRISMA flow diagram, charting the data, collecting, and summarizing the findings. The critical analysis of findings from the 13 journal articles showed that the COVID-19 period has been stressful for nursing students with classes moving online. The nursing students feared the COVID-19 virus along with experiencing anxiety and stressful situations due to distance learning, clinical training, assignments, and educational workloads. Nursing students applied coping strategies of seeking information and consultation, staying optimistic, and transference. The pandemic affected the psychological health of learners as they adjusted to the new learning structure. Future studies should deliberate on mental issues and solutions facing nursing students during the COVID-19 pandemic.

**Keywords:** coping strategies; COVID-19 pandemic; nursing students; stressors

**Citation:** Majrashi, A.; Khalil, A.; Nagshabandi, E.A.; Majrashi, A. Stressors and Coping Strategies among Nursing Students during the COVID-19 Pandemic: Scoping Review. *Nurs. Rep.* **2021**, *11*, 444–459. https://doi.org/10.3390/nursrep11020042

Academic Editors: Richard Gray and Sonia Udod

Received: 16 April 2021
Accepted: 27 May 2021
Published: 3 June 2021

**Publisher's Note:** MDPI stays neutral with regard to jurisdictional claims in published maps and institutional affiliations.

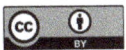

**Copyright:** © 2021 by the authors. Licensee MDPI, Basel, Switzerland. This article is an open access article distributed under the terms and conditions of the Creative Commons Attribution (CC BY) license (https://creativecommons.org/licenses/by/4.0/).

## 1. Introduction

The coronavirus disease 2019 (COVID-19) pandemic is the latest global health disaster of the century with high morbidity and mortality rates. In December 2019, a new infectious respiratory disease appeared in Wuhan, China. The World Health Organization (WHO) named the disease "COVID-19" after confirming its pandemic level potential. According to WHO, on 18 April 2020, the current outbreak of COVID-19 had affected over 2,164,111 people, and more than 146,198 deaths had been confirmed in more than 200 countries worldwide [1]. COVID-19 is one of the fastest spreading viral infections, which WHO declared a pandemic after affirming the high infectious levels. The disease spread from person to person through infected air droplets released through coughing or sneezing. Additionally, people spread the virus through physical contact, such as greetings or touching infected surfaces. Countries have sought vaccines and treatment protocols for COVID-19 vaccines and treatments amidst the implementation of various containment measures worldwide to combat the disease. Such containment measures have included the closure of public places, schools, universities, imposing curfews, and other physical distancing measures, such as the cancelation of large events [2].

The COVID-19 pandemic has forced political leaders and universities to take drastic measures to safeguard citizens' and students' lives. As many universities have suspended classroom teaching and switched to online teaching, the lives of students have changed completely and students have become prone to developing stressors, such as fear about physical health, family, and a loss of control related to the change in the educational environment [3].

Stress refers to a "situation in which internal demands, external demands, or both, are appraised as taxing or exceeding the adaptive or coping resources of an individual or group" [4]. Nursing students can suffer from a high level of stress during their education program. Specifically, there are two significant sources of stress among nursing students, academic and clinical stressors. The stressors related to academia include heavy assignments, examinations, and workloads. Other sources of stress related to the clinical area for nursing students include a lack of professional nursing skills and unfamiliarity with patients' diagnoses, medical history, or treatment [4].

The specific stressors related to the impact of COVID-19 among nursing students are stress from COVID-19 infection and a lack of preventive measures in clinical training [1]. This period has been undoubtedly stressful for learners; with classes moving online, nursing students face difficulties, such as being unable to concentrate and having difficulties participating, writing assignments, taking exams, and meeting the deadlines of academic assignments [5].

Coping strategies are stabilizing methods for helping individuals maintain psychological adaption during stressful events [6]. Coping strategies are classified as problem-based or emotion-based coping. The problem-solving approach is the most common coping strategy employed by nursing students to adjust to stressors, while an avoidance approach is the coping behavior least used by nursing students [4]. Nursing students use strong resilience, as one of the coping strategies during COVID-19 has been strong resilience. The learners have used humor, which studies associate with lower to moderate anxiety levels. Additionally, other coping strategies, such as mental disengagement, have led to high levels of anxiety [7]. This study sought to unearth the specific stressors and coping strategies employed by nursing students in universities during the COVID-19 pandemic.

*Aim of the Study*

This scoping review aimed to explore the relevant evidence related to stressors and coping strategies among nursing students during the COVID-19 pandemic.

## 2. Materials and Methods

A scoping review methodology was used to map the relevant evidence and synthesize the findings. The 6 steps of scoping review by Pérez et al. [8] guided the study. The steps involved the identification of the research question, determining the keywords, inclusion and exclusion criteria, searching the databases for the relevant studies, the study selection, charting the data, collecting, and summarizing the findings.

*2.1. Research Question Formulation Using PICOT*

The PICOT framework was used to develop and frame the research question "What are the stressors and coping strategies during the COVID-19 pandemic among nursing students?" The PICOT Framework in Table 1 generated the keywords used to undertake the research process in the selected electronic databases.

**Table 1.** PICOT framework.

| PICOT | Content | Question |
|---|---|---|
| P | Nursing students | What are the stressors and coping strategies during the COVID-19 pandemic among nursing students? |
| I | Not applicable | |
| C | Not applicable | |
| O | Stressors and coping strategies | |
| T | During the COVID-19 pandemic | |

### 2.2. Key Words

A combination of the following terms was used to search the databases, using Boolean operators ("and", "or"): "Nursing students", "COVID-19", "coronavirus", "stressors", "coping strategies", "pandemic", and "outbreak".

### 2.3. Inclusion Criteria

The inclusion criteria for the searched articles were full-text articles in the English language from 2010 to 2020. The review further included studies that addressed stressors and coping strategies among students in line with the research question. Studies with quantitative methods were included in the review. Peer-reviewed and scholarly articles published within 5 years between 2016 and 2021 were included in the study.

### 2.4. Exclusion Criteria

The exclusion criteria for the articles included letters, reports, conference abstracts, dissertations, book chapters, and unpublished manuscripts.

### 2.5. Search Strategies

Various electronic databases, including CINAHL, MEDLINE, and PubMed, were searched using the pre-determined keywords to find the relevant articles that explore stressors and coping strategies among nursing students during the COVID-19 pandemic. After searching in the 3 databases, 15 articles were found in CINAHL, 20 articles in MEDLINE, and 24 articles in PubMed. Other databases utilized in this process generated 24 studies. Out of the 24 articles, 13 were from Google Scholar, 6 from JSTOR, 3 from ERIC, and 2 from Gale. In addition, Google Scholar was also used to locate open access articles. The keywords used in the search process include "Nursing students", "COVID-19", "stressors", "coping strategies", and "pandemic and outbreak". The Boolean operators "AND" and "OR" were used to combine the keywords to create a focused search in each database.

### 2.6. Study Selection Process

The search strategy on the electronic database generated many articles. Inclusion and exclusion criteria were developed to guide the study selection and screening process. The inclusion criteria comprised articles that were full-text articles published in the English language from 2010 to 2020. The articles used quantitative research designs and journals that addressed the stressors as well as coping strategies during the COVID-19 pandemic among the nursing students. The exclusion criteria featured articles in the form of letters, reports, conference abstracts, dissertations, and unpublished manuscripts. The selection excluded articles that failed to address the concept of stressors and coping mechanisms among nursing students during the COVID-19 pandemic. Journals that lacked quantitative research designs, or were published in other languages besides English before 2010, were excluded in the final count.

The PRISMA flow diagram guided the process of retrieval and the screening of studies (see Figure 1) after the most relevant articles were identified through the search process. In the article retrieval and screening process, a total of 83 studies were initially retrieved. Out of these articles, the screening process commenced, and 58 articles were removed due to duplication. The remaining 25 studies were subjected to the full-text examination to check their objective and relevance to the research question and a further 11 were excluded, and 1 article was removed.

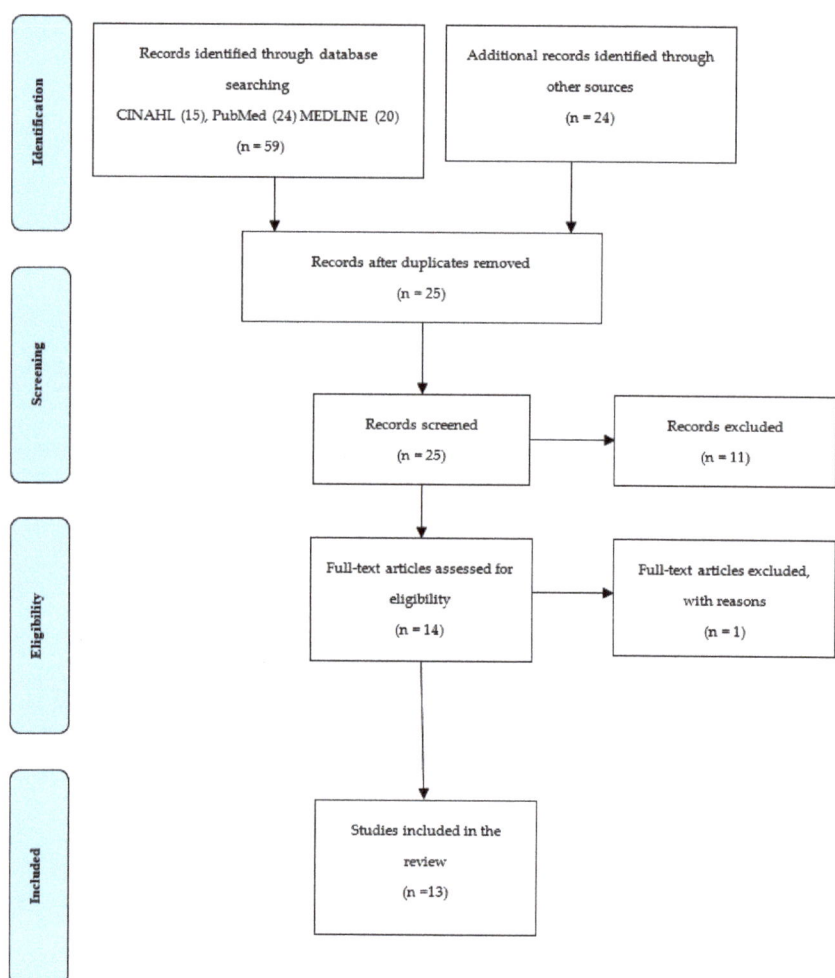

**Figure 1.** PRISMA flow diagram.

*2.7. Quality Assessment*

The 13 studies that meet the eligibility criteria of the scoping review were assessed using separately using Hawker's Quality assessment tool. The quality assessment tool evaluates the abstract, title, introduction, aims, methods, data, sampling procedure, data analysis, ethics and bias, as well as findings and results [9]. The assessment further focuses on the transferability, different implications, and usefulness of each study using a 36-points scale where each point received a maximum of 4 points ranging from 1 to 4 to signify poor and good quality respectively. The overall quality grades we used the following definitions were good (4), fair (3), poor (2), and very poor (1). Table 2 shows the quality appraisal for the studies in this review.

Table 2. Quality-approved total score allocation. Maximum score = 36.

| Author (s) | 1 Abstract/Title | 2 Introduction/Aims | 3 Method/Data | 4 Sampling | 5 Data Analysis | 6 Ethics/Bias | 7 Results | 8 Transferability | 9 Implications | Total |
|---|---|---|---|---|---|---|---|---|---|---|
| Deo et al. (2020) [10] | 4 | 3 | 3 | 4 | 4 | 3 | 4 | 3 | 2 | 30 |
| Begam and Devie (2020) [11] | 4 | 3 | 3 | 1 | 3 | 3 | 3 | 3 | 1 | 24 |
| Masha'al et al. (2020) [12] | 4 | 3 | 4 | 4 | 4 | 3 | 4 | 3 | 3 | 32 |
| Fitzgerald and Konrad (2021) [5] | 4 | 3 | 4 | 4 | 4 | 4 | 4 | 4 | 4 | 35 |
| Hussien et al. (2020) [13] | 4 | 4 | 4 | 4 | 4 | 4 | 4 | 3 | 4 | 35 |
| Begum (2020) [14] | 4 | 2 | 2 | 1 | 2 | 4 | 4 | 3 | 1 | 23 |
| Savitsky et al. (2020) [7] | 3 | 3 | 4 | 4 | 4 | 3 | 4 | 3 | 2 | 30 |
| Zeynep (2020) [15] | 4 | 3 | 4 | 4 | 4 | 3 | 4 | 3 | 1 | 30 |
| Lovrić et al. (2020) [16] | 4 | 3 | 4 | 4 | 4 | 3 | 3 | 3 | 4 | 32 |
| Gallego-Gomez et al. (2020) [17] | 3 | 3 | 4 | 4 | 4 | 3 | 4 | 2 | 1 | 28 |
| Subedi et al. (2020) [18] | 4 | 3 | 4 | 4 | 4 | 3 | 3 | 2 | 2 | 29 |
| Aslan and Pekince (2020) [19] | 3 | 2 | 4 | 3 | 4 | 4 | 4 | 3 | 4 | 31 |
| Kochuvilayil et al. (2020) [20] | 4 | 3 | 4 | 4 | 4 | 4 | 3 | 3 | 3 | 32 |

## 2.8. Charting of the Data

This phase comprised the extraction of the appropriate data from the selected literature to compile important insights to answer the research question, as recommended [21,22]. The extraction of the appropriate data assisted in identifying the relevant variables for answering the primary review question. According to [8], the data extraction process reduces bias and improves the overall reliability and validity of the review. The recorded information comprised the characteristics of the study, such as the authors, the sample size and setting, the country of study, the study design, the measurement tools, and the quality assessment. A thematic framework guided the presentation of the narrative accounts of the 13 studies, which then initiated the collection, summaries, and descriptions of the main findings (see Table 3).

Table 3. Characteristics of the reviewed studies.

| Author (s) | Sample Size and Setting | Country of Study | Study Design | Measurement Tool | Main Findings |
|---|---|---|---|---|---|
| Deo et al. (2020) [10] | 148 nursing students at Nobel college | Nepal | Cross-sectional, survey-based study | A digitalized structured questionnaire contained a total of 45 questions to assess sociodemographic characteristics, associative factors, DASS (Depression, anxiety, stress scale) and ISI (Insomnia Index Scale). | The study found out that the COVID-19 pandemic presents significant effects on nursing students in Nepal. Some of the COVID-19-related stressors among this population include the fear of delayed graduation. |
| Begam and Devi e (2020) [11] | 244 nursing students in an online mode in three schools of nursing, Assam | India | Cross-sectional study | Google Form that contained Tool I for collecting sociodemographic data and Tool II for the Perceived Stress Scale (10) by Cohen Sheldon with 5-Point Likert Scale | The study found out that they had experienced moderate levels of stress due to COVID-19. |
| Masha'al et al. (2020) [12] | 335 nursing students in an online platform through Jordan universities | Jordan | Mixed methods | Online survey in Google Forms that contained the students' sociodemographic characteristics and the Higher Education Stress Inventory | According to this study, COVID-19 presents particularly stressful experiences for nursing students doing distance learning. |
| Fitzgerald and Konrad (2021) [5] | 50 nursing students participating in a web-based platform | USA | Descriptive study | Web-based survey developed through Qualtrics Software to develop a checklist based on a 10-item anxiety Symptoms Checklist | The study sought to unearth the stress and anxiety experienced by nursing students during COVID-19, nursing students feeling anxious and overwhelmed from handling the academic workload and stress from a lack of PPE in the workplace. |
| Hussien et al. (2020) [13] | 284 nursing students at the Faculty of Nursing, Zagazig University, Egypt, Faculty of Applied Medical Science, Taibah University, and Al-Ghad International Colleges, KSA | Saudi Arabia and Egypt | Descriptive cross-sectional design | Questionnaire with a sociodemographic datasheet, the Emotional Intelligence Scale, and the Intolerance of Uncertainty Scale | Hussien et al. (2020) study found out that emotional intelligence is an important coping strategy for nursing students in these two countries during the COVID-19 pandemic. Comparing the two sets of students, Saudi nursing students demonstrated higher levels of emotional intelligence than their Egyptian counterparts. |

Table 3. Cont.

| Author(s) | Sample Size and Setting | Country of Study | Study Design | Measurement Tool | Main Findings |
|---|---|---|---|---|---|
| Begum (2020) [14] | 124 nursing students participating in online research during lockdown | Saudi Arabia | Quantitative cross-sectional study | Adapted questionnaire from a Chinese study that detailed demographic variables of age and gender, and 15 knowledge-based, 10 attitude-based, and 5 practice-based questions | According to this study, Saudi nursing students have a satisfactory level of knowledge about COVID-19. In addition, these students also possessed a positive attitude towards the pandemic and the possibility of overcoming it. |
| Savitsky et al. (2020) [7] | 244 nursing students at a nursing department during a national lockdown | Israel | Cross-sectional study | Generalized Anxiety Disorder 7-Item Scale that outlined a cut-off point of 10 for moderate anxiety and of 15 for severe anxiety levels | The study found that the most common coping mechanisms among nursing students during the pandemic were resilience, seeking information, mental disengagement, humor, and the use of spiritual support. |
| Zeynep (2020) [15] | 316 nursing students at a university in the Eastern Black Sea region, Turkey | Turkey | Cross-sectional study | Personal information form Generalized Anxiety Disorder-7 Scale Stress Coping Strategies Scale | The COVID-19 pandemic has affected the overall performance of nursing students. Nevertheless, the study found that the participants were demonstrating moderate levels of anxiety. |
| Lovrić et al. (2020) [16] | 33 nursing students at the Faculty of Dental Medicine and Health, Osijek | Croatia | Qualitative study | Online form with two major questions | All students were aware and concerned about the issues of misinformation on social media and the risky behavior of the population. Additionally, most of them were worried about getting infected and were concerned about their families' well-beings. Therefore, they constantly applied protective measures. Moreover, the students understood their responsibility to the community and the importance and risks of the nursing profession. They also described negative experiences with public transportation and residing in the student dorm. |
| Gallego-Gomez et al. (2020) [17] | 142 students at the Faculty of Nursing of the Catholic University of Murcia (UCAM) located in Murcia, Spain | Spain | Observational | Student Stress Inventory–Stress Manifestations (SSI-SM) questionnaire with 19 items in a 5-point Likert-type score | The nursing students experienced an increase in stress levels during the lockdown. They also experienced family and financial problems during this period. Their main coping strategy was engaging in physical exercise. |

**Table 3.** *Cont.*

| Author (s) | Sample Size and Setting | Country of Study | Study Design | Measurement Tool | Main Findings |
|---|---|---|---|---|---|
| Subedi et al. (2020) [18] | 1116 nursing students at different nursing colleges in Nepal | Nepal | Descriptive cross-sectional online survey | Self-administered questionnaire in an online survey | Close to half of the teachers (42.3%) indicated that they witnessed disturbances to their online classes due to electricity issues. Moreover, 48.1% of them stated that they had challenges with internet access. Over half of the students polled (63.2%) stated that their online learning was affected by electricity and 63.6% had internet problems; only 64.4% of the students had internet access for their online classes. |
| Aslan and Pekince (2020) [19] | 662 nursing students at Inonu, Kilis, and Bingol Universities | Turkey | Cross-sectional design | Information form and perceived stress scale | Stress was prevalent among many nursing students during the COVID-19 pandemic. Nursing students between the ages of 18 and 20 years and female students reported higher levels of stress. The study also found out that the most important stressors among these students included watching the news, worrying about the risk of infection, and the imposed curfew. |
| Kochuvilayil et al. (2020) [20] | 99 Australian and 113 Indian nursing students at NSW and Kerala | Australia and India | Cross-sectional study a comparative study | Online survey prepared through Survey Monkey | Student nurses inevitably experience heightened anxiety. |

## 3. Results

### 3.1. Results of the Search

This section outlines the evidence gathered from the selected literature for the review. It highlights the characteristics of the review study, the key results, and themes arising from the thirteen journal articles.

### 3.2. Characteristics of the Reviewed Studies

All the studies met the inclusion criteria and were published between 2010 and 2021. The review of the studies revealed the deployment of three key research designs of cross-sectional studies [7,10,11,13–15,18–20], mixed-methods [12] observational prospective studies [17], descriptive designs [5], and qualitative designs [16]. The sample comprised nursing exclusively, which fostered the generalizability to other nursing studies. Furthermore, the reviewed findings were from different geographical locations, including developing and advanced healthcare systems. The countries included Australia, India, Turkey, Egypt, Saudi Arabia, Spain, the United States, Israel, Croatia, and Jordan. Table 2 outlines the measurements and sample sizes gathered in each study.

### 3.3. Main Findings

Thirteen articles were selected and subjected to thematic analysis, showing different themes. The discussion used seven themes based on the information retrieved from them. Those seven themes fall into the broad categories of stressors and coping strategies. The first four themes are related to the nursing students' stressors, while the last three are related to the coping strategies employed by those students.

#### 3.3.1. Theme 1: Nursing Students' Stressors

Nine articles were concerned with studies on COVID-19-related stressors, from which four subthemes emerged. The first subtheme is "stress from distance learning", in which issues such as remote learning's psychological impacts are covered. The second subtheme is "stress from assignments and workload". The third subtheme is "stress from clinical training". The fourth subtheme is "fear of infection", and it covers issues such as feeling isolated and worrying about getting infected.

Stress from Distance Learning

Eight articles provided a link between the COVID-19 pandemic and nursing students' stress, with a focus on various stressors, including distance learning. During the COVID-19 pandemic, distance learning is a significant source of stress for nursing students. A cross-sectional study was conducted in 13 different nursing colleges in Nepal on 1116 participants [18]. The study aimed to assess the impact of E-learning during the COVID-19 pandemic among nursing students. The study found that many students suffered from the disruption of online classes related to the technological issues that occurred since higher learning institutions had moved to online classes. More than 63.2% of nursing students suffered from electricity problems, while 63.6% of nursing students suffered from internet problems, and only 64.4% of nursing students had internet access in the home for their online classes. Another cross-sectional study by [7] in Israel on 244 nursing students at Ashkelon Academic College assessed the levels of anxiety and coping strategies among nursing students during the COVID-19 pandemic. The study discovered that nursing students suffered significantly high levels of anxiety due to challenges presented by distance learning.

A qualitative study by [16] on 33 nursing students in Croatia explored how nursing students perceived the COVID-19 pandemic and their studying experience during the period. Distance learning presented many challenges to nursing students, including difficulties concentrating, as opposed to what they would do in a typical lecture room or face-to-face environment. The study also noted that nursing students found it difficult to remember and develop the motivation to undertake distance learning.

An observational and prospective study by [17] was on 142 nursing students in their second year in Murcia, Spain. The study's purpose was to assess the levels of stress among nursing students before and during the COVID-19 lockdown and its influence on taking online exams. The study established that levels of stress significantly increased among nursing students after lockdown. In addition, the study noted that the students who failed the online exam had higher levels of stress compared to those who passed.

The perceived stress levels and poor concentration emerged in another cross-sectional study by [19]. The study on 662 nursing students in Turkey evaluated nursing students' views on the COVID-19 pandemic and their perceived stress levels. The study proved that the nursing students suffered from moderate stress levels, but they had higher levels of stress than students assessed in the previous year. Nursing students expressed concerns about their clinical practice and inadequate clinical skills related to the interruption of education and moving to online learning during the pandemic.

Another cross-sectional descriptive study by [10] recruited 184 nursing students from universities in Nepal. The study assessed the factors associated with perceived stress, anxiety, and insomnia during the COVID-19 pandemic among nursing students. The study showed that 29.9% of the nursing students were afraid of delayed graduation, 36.4% suffered from costly mobile data and the necessity of spent money on mobile charging devices for their online classes, 17.4% had difficulties attending online access, 29.3% had difficulties concentrating, and 15.2% they were afraid of failure because they were unable to understand the online classes. The findings were confirmed in another study by [11], where they undertook a cross-sectional descriptive study on 244 nursing students in India. The authors assessed the perceived stress among nursing students during the COVID-19 lockdown. The study established that nursing students had moderate levels of stress related to a lack of resources and distance learning challenges.

Moreover, in a mixed-methods study by [12] that was conducted in Jordan on 335 nursing students, they analyzed the stress levels and sources of stressors related to distance learning and experienced by nursing students during the COVID-19 pandemic. It became evident that overall stress levels were higher among nursing students with low family income; 84.2% of the participants had a financial burden from paying for internet services. Furthermore, the Jordanian study found that distance learning has presented many stressors to nursing students, including difficulties concentrating because of distracting environments and no private areas for studying, limited resources, unorganized workloads, and a lack of strategies for standardized distance learning.

Stress from Assignments and Workload

Three articles reported that during the COVID-19 pandemic, assignments and workloads were a vital stress source for nursing students. One of these was the study conducted by [10], which reported that the global pandemic has affected university students in many ways. For nursing students working in a hospital, 44.4% suffered from long hours of duty, and 16.7% experienced increased workloads related to increased numbers of patients infected with the COVID-19 virus. Correspondingly, a study conducted by [7] reported that, in relation to the increase in the number of cases of the COVID-19 virus, there was a need to hire nursing students due to labor shortages in hospitals and in the community during the pandemic. Approximately 69% of the nursing students employed by hospitals had increased levels of anxiety. According to a descriptive study by [5], conducted in the United States among nursing students, learners showed difficulties in handling assignments, too. The study found that of the 84% of nursing students feeling anxious and overwhelmed, 62% had difficulty handling the academic workload, while 20% of nursing students had stress and difficulty writing assignments.

Stress from Clinical Training

Moreover, four articles found that stress from clinical training is one of the stressors that affected nursing students from around the world during the COVID-19 pandemic. In the first article by [7], which was conducted in Israel at Ashkelon Academic College, 50% of participants reported that they suffered from a lack of personal protective equipment (PPE) at the workplace. According to the study among nursing students, a lack of PPE was associated with higher anxiety scores in comparison with those students who did not suffer from a lack of PPE at the workplace.

Another study by [19] found that the main stressors for student nurses during this pandemic include adhering to COVID-19 precautions due to lack of adequate preparation. The third study was conducted in Nepal by [10]. According to the cross-sectional study, the pandemic presented more stressors to nursing students who were working in the hospital and worried about the necessity of adhering to COVID-19 precautions. In agreement, the pandemic caused anxiety and stress, according to another study by [5]. The authors conducted the study in the United States among 50 nursing students to explore anxiety and stress experienced by nursing students and identify sources of support during the transition to online learning. The study points out, anxiety and stress were evident due to a lack of PPE among nursing students who work in the hospital during the pandemic.

Stress from COVID-19 Infection

Four articles reported on the issue of stress from COVID-19 infection. The first study by [7], which was conducted in Israel on 244 nursing students, found that a high level of anxiety was related to a fear of getting infected by the COVID-19 virus; the anxiety score was 13.7 out of 14 according to generalized anxiety disorder 7- item scale. The second study by [16] in Croatia on 33 nursing students pointed out that 19 of the students felt stress and fear about the elderly members of their families getting infected by COVID-19. At the same time, 15 of them worried about getting infected by COVID-19 in the clinical setting.

The third study by [19] was also conducted in Turkey on 662 nursing students. A total of 68% of them worried about being infected by the COVID-19 virus, and 78.9% of the students apply adequate precautions against infection to protect themselves, 97% wash their hands frequently, 82.3% wear a mask, and 92.9% maintain a social distance. The fourth study by [10] involved 184 nursing students from universities in Nepal. The study reported that 21% of the students worried about their families being infected by the COVID-19 virus, while 8.2% worried about themselves being infected by the virus. Additionally, the studies established the coping mechanisms of the nursing students during the pandemic.

3.3.2. Theme 2: Coping Strategies

Six articles identified various coping mechanisms used by nursing students. The three most prominent subthemes are addressed in the following section. The first subtheme is seeking information and consultations. In addition, developing a positive attitude has emerged as one of the most used coping strategies by nursing students. The second subtheme is staying optimistic, whereby the nursing students showed tendencies of having generalized positive expectations for the outcome. The third subtheme is getting transference by employing efforts to transfer one's attention from stressful situations. Examples of transferring attention included eating well, exercising, and getting enough sleep. The topic assesses how distancing from the challenges associated with the virus, such as anger and frustration, has helped or can help nursing students in universities worldwide to mitigate the negative impacts of COVID-19 on their social life and enhance their academic experience.

Seeking Information and Consultation

Seeking information and consultation is a possible coping strategy for nursing students during the COVID-19 pandemic. The cross-sectional study conducted by [7] on 244 nursing students discovered that COVID-19 increased concerns among many nursing students, not just about this disease but also about the disruption of their daily routines, financial challenges, spending much time away from their friends and family, and the new paradigm of moving academics online with remote learning. The study further noted that maintaining a positive attitude in seeking information and consultation was a positive coping strategy associated with better mental outcomes among nursing students.

Staying Optimistic

The importance of staying optimistic was evident in another study in Saudi Arabia. Another author [14] conducted a cross-sectional study on 124 participants in Saudi Arabia to find 79% of nursing students in the country understood that by staying optimistic, they had a viable strategy for coping with COVID-19-related stressors, such as fear of getting infected and the deaths of patients as a result of this disease. Therefore, optimism has emerged as a positive coping strategy that urged nursing students to stabilize and gain psychological adaptation during this period.

Transference

Four articles emphasized the importance of transference as a coping strategy for COVID-19 by nursing students. Another author [17] conducted a study in Spain and noted the effect of the COVID-19 pandemic on nursing students' challenging daily lifestyles. The pandemic created fear, anxiety, and stress among Spanish nursing students. Consequently, transference, such as doing regular exercise and talking with other people, positively reduced stress among nursing students. Authors [13] agreed with [17] on transference behaviors among nursing students after a descriptive cross-sectional study conducted in Egypt and Saudi Arabia. The authors noted that getting social support from peers was one of the most effective coping strategies for nursing students during the COVID-19 pandemic.

The third study was a cross-sectional study by [15], conducted on 316 nursing students in Turkey to evaluate anxiety levels and coping strategies during the pandemic. According to the authors, nursing students suffered from moderate anxiety levels as a result of COVID-19. The study further found out that 48.1% of the students used the eating coping method, and 77.8% spend time on the internet; this indicates ineffective coping strategies, which are associated with stressful events during the pandemic.

The fourth article by [20] underlined the importance of transference after conducting another study in Australia and India. The comparative study assessed anxiety levels and coping strategies among nursing students. The cross-sectional study indicated that these student nurses inevitably experience heightened anxiety. Therefore, one of the coping strategies applied by Indian nursing students to reduce stress levels is exercise and talking to other people.

## 4. Discussion

The scoping review explored the relevant evidence on the stressors and coping strategies of nursing students during the COVID-19 pandemic. The review relied on evidence from 13 studies. The inclusion of the 13 studies and subsequent critical comparison of the evidence revealed compelling stressors of the nursing students and the various mechanisms for coping with the disruption of the pandemic on the learning process.

The nursing students cited distance learning as a source of stress. The new technological-based option of delivering nursing education brings technical issues, internet problems, and poor management of online classes. Challenges arise for the nursing students because they prefer conventional learning as opposed to the online distance learning options [23]. Distance learning might not enhance more student-centered learning, monitoring, and teaching assessments than the conventional classroom does during a lockdown.

Assignments and workload emerged as compelling stressors for the nursing students as COVID-19 created a newly structured learning process. The online learning environment compels educators to provide assignments to keep up with skill development as they do in the normal classroom setting. The stressful learning circumstances may not translate into quality skills, as the students require real-life demonstrations or simulations [24]. The completion of the pre-licensure nursing students becomes difficult because they rely on the excessive workload to meet the non-direct care hours as well as optimizing virtual clinical experience with their supervisors.

The review further revealed that clinical training has created anxiety and stress among nursing students during the pandemic. The pre-licensure students are among healthcare workers without access to PPE at times, so they face the risk of contracting the virus. According to [24], the students might lack proper preparation through mentorship or preceptorship to handle the challenging active care environment with positivity rates of COVID-19 increasing every day. The fears, anxiety, and stress arise from the virus as well as students' inability to reach a proper learning trajectory [25]. The nursing students lack proper familiarity with self-efficacy, communication, and resilience-oriented mechanisms.

The stress of clinical training underscores the impact of the COVID-19 infections without proper clinical skills, treatment mechanisms, and overall response repertoire. The review emphasized the effort of social distancing, wearing masks, and washing hands besides taking other necessary precautions against the virus. The students face micro-aggressions and a limited chance of making choices for the safety of their physical as well as psychological health as they do in the active care setting or virtual learning environment [26]. The universities or nursing colleges contribute to the challenge by allowing nursing students to enter high-risk health environments without the proper skills.

The stress and anxiety from the learning or high-risk environments have necessitated the adoption of coping mechanisms by the nursing students. The review ascertains the wide-ranging use of information and consultations to develop the right attitude during the COVID-19 pandemic. The information is critical in overcoming confinements, eliminating uncertainties, and teaching new methodologies for overcoming COVID-19 mental health challenges among learners [27]. The information and consultation of supervisors in schools or high-risk environments should eliminate uncertainty about COVID-19 as well as the completion of a nursing curriculum in readiness for registration.

Optimism emerges as the critical coping tool for nursing students hoping to complete their courses through virtual learning. The review affirms the method as a psychological adaptation to the new learning structure created by the pandemic. Optimism underlines the hopes for better eventualities for the learning environment as the nursing transitions to the professional nursing practice [28]. The findings ascertain continued efforts by nursing students to adopt behaviors that promote their well-being while hoping for a restoration of the normal learning approach.

Transference is another effective coping mechanism for nursing students who have hopeful prospects about the trajectory of their nursing education. The nursing students deal with the virtual learning environment, clinical training in a high-risk environment, and workloads with exercises or socialization. Social support is critical due to the overall life interruptions and hopeful prospects of completing nursing programs despite the COVID-19 pandemic [29]. The newly structured learning environment provides nursing students with challenging choices and has immense implications for the nursing practice.

Nursing education should adopt other impactful and interactive methods, such as video-simulated options. The nursing students could reduce fears and anxiety or stress by working with interactive modalities more than working on theoretical tasks without the capacity to enhance their practical nursing skills. On the other hand, continuous counseling and social support are essential in the communities, as universities and colleges seek better engagement for the pre-licensure nursing students. The strategies will complement the coping mechanisms of transference, seeking information or consultation, and optimism because nursing students anticipate a smooth transition to the practice during the COVID-19 pandemic.

However, the scoping review had several limitations. The review pointed towards available studies in stressors and coping mechanisms of nursing students during COVID-19 that opposite the research that allows searching of new findings. The method further lacked the articulation of the risk of bias that reduced the reliability of the outcomes. The results are based on the relatively novel COVID-19 topic, which continues to evolve over time, and thus, the overall reliability remains contentious.

COVID-19 painted a grim picture of the world's lack of preparedness for a pandemic such as this. In this review about stressors and coping strategies, it was discovered that nursing students suffered from stressors during this pandemic in their academic journeys. There are various stressors that nursing students face, including stress from distance learning, stress from assignments and workloads, stress from clinical training, and stress from COVID-19 infection. In response to these stressors, nursing students have developed coping strategies that were employed to adjust to these COVID-19-related stressors, such as seeking information and consultation, staying optimistic, and transference.

## 5. Recommendation

The review contends that using different mechanisms improves the quality of nursing education delivered to the nursing students during the pandemic. The coping mechanisms discussed in the study imply the importance of creating a structured learning environment to enhance the outcomes of the nursing students while minimizing their susceptibility to anxiety and stress. Further studies will suffice to deliberate on mental issues and solutions facing nursing students during the COVID-19 pandemic.

**Author Contributions:** Conceptualization A.M. (Aisha Majrashi), A.K., E.A.N. and A.M. (Abdulrahman Majrashi); methodology, A.M. (Aisha Majrashi), A.K., E.A.N. and A.M. (Abdulrahman Majrashi); software A.M. (Aisha Majrashi), A.K., E.A.N. and A.M. (Abdulrahman Majrashi); validation, A.M. (Aisha Majrashi), A.K., E.A.N. and A.M. (Abdulrahman Majrashi); formal analysis, A.M. (Aisha Majrashi), A.K., E.A.N. and A.M. (Abdulrahman Majrashi); investigation, A.M. (Aisha Majrashi), A.K., E.A.N. and A.M. (Abdulrahman Majrashi); resources, A.M. (Aisha Majrashi), A.K., E.A.N. and A.M. (Abdulrahman Majrashi); data curation, A.M. (Aisha Majrashi), A.K., E.A.N. and A.M. (Abdulrahman Majrashi); writing—original draft preparation, A.M. (Aisha Majrashi), A.K., E.A.N. and A.M. (Abdulrahman Majrashi); writing—review and editing, A.M. (Aisha Majrashi), A.K., E.A.N. and A.M. (Abdulrahman Majrashi); supervision, A.K., E.A.N.; All authors have read and agreed to the published version of the manuscript.

**Funding:** This research received no external funding.

**Institutional Review Board Statement:** The study was conducted according to the guidelines of the Declaration of Helsinki, and approved by the Chair of Nursing Research Ethical Committee of King Abdulaziz University (protocol code Ref No 1M. 21 and approval on 20/9/2020).

**Informed Consent Statement:** Not applicable.

**Data Availability Statement:** No new data were created or analyzed in this study. Data sharing is not applicable to this article.

**Acknowledgments:** We recognize the additional administrative and technical support offered by the school for editing the manuscript for further review.

**Conflicts of Interest:** The authors declare no conflict of interest.

## References

1. Cooke, J.E.; Eirich, R.; Racine, N.; Madigan, S. Prevalence of posttraumatic and general psychological stress during COVID-19: A rapid review and meta-analysis. *Psychiatry Res.* **2020**, *292*, 113347. [CrossRef] [PubMed]
2. Chakraborty, I.; Maity, P. COVID-19 outbreak: Migration, effects on society, global environment and prevention. *Sci. Total Environ.* **2020**, *728*, 138882. [CrossRef]
3. Elmer, T.; Mepham, K.; Stadtfeld, C. Students under lockdown: Comparisons of students' social networks and mental health before and during the COVID-19 crisis in Switzerland. *PLoS ONE* **2020**, *15*, e0236337. [CrossRef]
4. Labrague, L.J.; McEnroe-Petitte, D.M.; Gloe, D.; Thomas, L.; Papathanasiou, I.V.; Tsaras, K. A literature review on stress and coping strategies in nursing students. *J. Ment. Health* **2017**, *26*, 471–480. [CrossRef] [PubMed]
5. Fitzgerald, A.; Konrad, S. Transition in learning during COVID-19: Student nurse anxiety, stress, and resource support. *Nurs. Forum.* **2021**. [CrossRef]

6. Mariani, R.; Renzi, A.; Di Trani, M.; Trabucchi, G.; Danskin, K.; Tambelli, R. The Impact of Coping Strategies and Perceived Family Support on Depressive and Anxious Symptomatology During the Coronavirus Pandemic (COVID-19) Lockdown. *Front. Psychiatry* **2020**, *11*, 587724. [CrossRef]
7. Savitsky, B.; Findling, Y.; Ereli, A.; Hendel, T. Anxiety and coping strategies among nursing students during the covid-19 pandemic. *Nurse Educ. Pract.* **2020**, *46*, 102809. [CrossRef]
8. Pérez, E.Z.; Canut, M.T.L.; Pegueroles, A.F.; Llobet, M.P.; Arroyo, C.M.; Merino, J.R. Critical thinking in nursing: Scoping review of the literature. *Int. J. Nurs. Pract.* **2014**, *21*, 820–830. [CrossRef]
9. Hawker, S.; Payne, S.; Kerr, C.; Hardey, M.; Powell, J. Appraising the evidence: Reviewing disparate data systematically. *Qual. Health Res.* **2002**, *12*, 1284–1299. [CrossRef]
10. Deo, P.K.; Raut, S.B.J.; Adhikari, B.; Shrestha, J. Factors Associated with Perceived Stress, Anxiety, Depression, Insomnia during COVID-19 Outbreak among Nursing Students. *Int. J. Sci. Res.* **2020**, *9*, 23–29.
11. Begam, B.; Devi, K. A Study to Assess the Perceived Stress among Nursing Students during COVID-19 Lockdown. *Int. J. Sci. Healthc. Res.* **2020**, *5*, 388–393.
12. Masha'al, D.; Rababa, M.; Shahrour, G. Distance Learning-Related Stress Among Undergraduate Nursing Students During the COVID-19 Pandemic. *J. Nurs. Educ.* **2020**, *59*, 666–674. [CrossRef]
13. Hussien, R.M.; Elkayal, M.M.; Shahin, M.A.H. Emotional Intelligence and Uncertainty among Undergraduate Nursing Students during the COVID-19 Pandemic Outbreak: A Comparative Study. *Open Nurs. J.* **2020**, *14*, 220–231. [CrossRef]
14. Begum, D.F. Knowledge, Attitudes, and Practices towards COVID-19 among B.Sc. Nursing Students in Selected Nursing Institution in Saudi Arabia during COVID-19 Outbreak: An Online Survey. *Saudi J. Nurs. Health Care* **2020**, *3*, 194–198. [CrossRef]
15. Zeynep, T. Nursing Students' Anxiety Levels and Coping Strategies during the COVID-19 Pandemic. *Int. Arch. Nurs. Health Care* **2020**, *46*, 102809.
16. Lovrić, R.; Farčić, N.; Mikšić, Š.; Včev, A. Studying During the COVID-19 Pandemic: A Qualitative Inductive Content Analysis of Nursing Students' Perceptions and Experiences. *Educ. Sci.* **2020**, *10*, 188. [CrossRef]
17. Gallego-Gomez, J.I.; Campillo-Cano, M.; Carrion-Martinez, A.; Balanza, S.; Rodriguez-Gonzalez-Moro, M.T.; Simonelli-Munoz, A.J.; Rivera-Caravaca, J.M. The COVID-19 Pandemic and Its Impact on Homebound Nursing Students. *Int. J. Environ. Res. Public Health* **2020**, *17*, 7383. [CrossRef] [PubMed]
18. Subedi, S.; Nayaju, S.; Subedi, S.; Shah, S.K.; Shah, J.M. Impact of E-learning during COVID-19 Pandemic among Nursing Students and Teachers of Nepal. *Int. J. Sci. Healthc. Res.* **2020**, *5*, 68–76.
19. Aslan, H.; Pekince, H. Nursing students' views on the COVID-19 pandemic and their percieved stress levels. *Perspect Psychiatr. Care* **2020**. [CrossRef]
20. Kochuvilayil, T.; Fernandez, R.S.; Moxham, L.J.; Lord, H.; Alomari, A.; Hunt, L.; Middleton, R.; Halcomb, E.J. COVID-19: Knowledge, anxiety, academic concerns and preventative behaviours among Australian and Indian undergraduate nursing students: A cross-sectional study. *J. Clin. Nurs.* **2021**, *30*, 882–891. [CrossRef]
21. Lockwood, C.; Dos Santos, K.B.; Pap, R. Practical Guidance for Knowledge Synthesis: Scoping Review Methods. *Asian Nurs. Res. (Korean Soc. Nurs. Sci.)* **2019**, *13*, 287–294. [CrossRef] [PubMed]
22. Schmidt, B.M.; Colvin, C.J.; Hohlfeld, A.; Leon, N. Defining and conceptualising data harmonisation: A scoping review protocol. *Syst. Rev.* **2018**, *7*, 226. [CrossRef] [PubMed]
23. Bdair, I.A. Nursing students' and faculty members' perspectives about online learning during COVID-19 pandemic: A qualitative study. *Teach. Learn. Nurs.* **2021**, *1*. [CrossRef]
24. Fogg, N.; Wilson, C.; Trinka, M.; Campbell, R.; Thomson, A.; Merritt, L.; Tietze, M.; Prior, M. Transitioning from direct care to virtual clinical experiences during the COVID-19 pandemic. *J. Prof. Nurs.* **2020**, *36*, 685–691. [CrossRef]
25. Ulenaersa, D.; Grosemans, J.; Schrootena, W.; Bergs, J. Clinical placement experience of nursing students during the COVID-19 pandemic: A cross-sectional study. *Nurse Educ. Today* **2020**, *99*, 104746. [CrossRef] [PubMed]
26. Hayter, M.; Jackson, D. Pre-registration undergraduate nurses and the COVID-19 pandemic: Students or workers? *J. Clin. Nurs.* **2020**, *29*, 3115–3116. [CrossRef]
27. Ramos-Morcillo, A.J.; Leal-Costa, C.; Moral-Garcia, J.E.; Ruzafa-Martinez, M. Experiences of Nursing Students during the Abrupt Change from Face-to-Face to e-Learning Education during the First Month of Confinement Due to COVID-19 in Spain. *Int. J. Environ. Res. Public Health* **2020**, *17*, 5519. [CrossRef]
28. Cleofas, J.V. Life Interruptions, Learnings and Hopes among Filipino College Students during COVID-19 Pandemic. *J. Loss Trauma* **2020**, 1–9. [CrossRef]
29. Bahçecioğlu Turan, G.; Köse, S.; Aksoy, M. Analysis of nursing students' obsessive and coping behaviors during the COVID-19 pandemic. *Perspect. Psychiatr. Care* **2021**. [CrossRef]

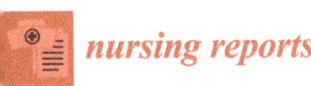 

*Article*

# Novice Nurses' Experiences Caring for Acutely Ill Patients during a Pandemic

Heather Naylor [1,2,*], Cynthia Hadenfeldt [3] and Patricia Timmons [1]

1. College of Nursing, Creighton University, Phoenix, AZ 85012, USA; patriciatimmons@creighton.edu
2. Sinclair School of Nursing, University of Missouri, Columbia, MO 65201, USA
3. College of Nursing, Creighton University, Omaha, NE 68178, USA; cynthiahadenfeldt@creighton.edu
* Correspondence: heathernaylor@creighton.edu

**Abstract:** The Coronavirus pandemic erupted in 2020 and new graduate registered nurses (RNs) found themselves caring for those with devastating illness as they were transitioning into nursing practice. The purpose of this study was to describe the experience of novice nurses working in acute care settings during a pandemic. This qualitative phenomenological study of novice nurses working in facilities providing acute care for COVID-19 patients was conducted in Phoenix, Arizona, USA. Purposive sampling identified 13 participants for interviews. Data were analyzed using thematic analysis. Eight themes emerged: Dealing with death, Which personal protective equipment (PPE) will keep us safe?, Caring for high acuity patients with limited training, Difficulties working short-staffed, Everything is not okay, Support from the healthcare team, Nursing school preparation for a pandemic, I would still choose nursing. Novice nurses felt challenged by the experience and were at times overwhelmed and struggling to cope. Support from peers and coping skills learned during nursing school helped them continue to work during a critical time. Data from this study suggest that some participants may have been experiencing symptoms of anxiety, depression, or post-traumatic stress disorder, and findings provide foundational insights for nursing education and psychological interventions to support the nursing workforce.

**Keywords:** COVID-19; nursing; pandemic; qualitative research; workforce

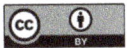

## 1. Introduction

New graduate registered nurses (RNs) face stressful challenges learning their role as novice nurses. New nurses entering into clinical practice can face daunting issues: complex environments with advanced medical technology, high patient-to-nurse ratios requiring high-level skills, the need to advocate for patients and their families while delivering safe, quality care, and extending respect and compassion to individuals and their families. New graduate nurses may struggle with critical thinking skills, patient needs identification, and prioritization of patient care needs [1].

Without appropriate support, many new graduate RNs may experience stress, fatigue, anxiety, and burnout [2–5] and may leave the profession due to difficulty adapting to their role [6]. The stress of role transition accounts for up to 30% attrition of new graduate nurses in their first year [6], and up to 57% in their second year [7].

Undoubtedly, the well-documented stress of role transition is compounded when met with the severe strain of a global pandemic, and as cases of illness rise, the need for a robust workforce becomes paramount. Emerging evidence suggests that nurses have increased risk of stress, depression and burnout during COVID-19, with younger, less experienced female nurses at increased risk for mental health issues [8]. Providing appropriate support and resources during this transition is imperative to the satisfaction and retention of new graduate nurses; however, doing so is highly dependent on understanding the experiences of these key personnel during times of extreme stress. A recent meta-analysis found that a barrier to implementing appropriate interventions is lack of understanding of what staff and organizations need during pandemics to support their mental health [9].

While prior studies document Severe Acute Respiratory Syndrome (SARS) pandemic effects on nursing students [10], and the psychological impact on experienced nurses caring for COVID-19 patients in China [11], the current study captures the experience of novice nurses managing the stress of their professional role transition in a variety of settings during the COVID-19 pandemic which has not been previously reported. Heung and colleagues [10] suggested that working during a pandemic reinforced a strong sense of professional identity for nursing students in Hong Kong, China, during the peak of SARS. The study by Sun and associates [11] found that nurses with a median of 3.5 years of work experience similarly adapted to negative and positive emotions as well as personal growth in response to caring for patients with COVID-19. The purpose of this study was to describe the experience of novice nurses with less than two years experience working in acute care settings during a pandemic.

## 2. Materials and Methods

Phenomenology is a philosophical approach and qualitative research method that can be particularly effective when studying phenomenon where little knowledge has been previously uncovered as in the phenomenon experienced by nurses caring for acutely ill patients during a pandemic. Phenomenology is the study of an individual's lived experiences and helps to develop a better understanding of what the experience means [12,13]. The purpose of the research method is to describe the reality of an experience and the effect that the experience has on the person [12,13]. Phenomenology has a unique approach to data collection in that the researcher is the primary study instrument and the subject's story is the data [12,13]. Data collected through phenomenological methods may be the basis for the development of quantitative measures utilized in future studies. Researchers must bracket their own perceptions and views during data collection and analysis so as not to bias results [12].

### 2.1. COREQ Checklist

Methodological data were presented in this section using the consolidated criteria for reporting qualitative research (COREQ) checklist for qualitative research to ensure explicit and comprehensive reporting. The COREQ checklist is a 32-item checklist for interviews to ensure rigor in reporting in qualitative studies [14].

### 2.2. Participants

Once university institutional review board approval was received, recruitment of novice nurses was conducted in Phoenix, Arizona, a large southwestern city and the fifth-most populous city in the United States. Purposive sampling was employed to recruit novice nurses with invitations via email listserv of one university's accelerated nursing program alumni, and social media posts on a page maintained by those nursing alumni. Participants were invited to respond with their interest via email, call, or text. Participants were recruited to represent a broad sampling of specialties (e.g., medical/surgical intensive care, labor and delivery, inpatient psychiatry). Care was also taken to include participants working in various acute care settings throughout the city with or without direct contact with COVID patients as part of their daily work assignment.

Participants were novice nurses with two years or less experience working full-time in any acute care setting that cared for patients with COVID-19. Six different acute care facilities were represented. Ten nurses worked with COVID patients or patients under investigation (PUIs), and three worked on non-COVID units, with one of these three asked to cross-train to work in a COVID unit. Nurses were graduates of Creighton University College of Nursing's one-year accelerated program who had already completed another Baccalaureate Degree in an unrelated field. Consequently, students were older than traditional nursing students. The program is based in Phoenix, Arizona, and participants graduated with Bachelor of Nursing Science degrees. Specialties represented in the sample included: neurological intensive care unit-turned-COVID unit, emergency, telemetry, medical/surgical, labor and delivery, adolescent psychiatry, neonatal intensive care, trauma step-down, medical oncology, observation, and float pool. The sample included 13 nurses, of which three were male and 10 were female. Two additional participants expressed interest but did not respond to a follow-up inquiry to schedule an interview. All who responded and scheduled were interviewed. The average age of participants was 29 years with a range of 24–41 years. The average time since graduation from nursing school was 13 months, with an average time working of 11 months (range: 6–18 months) (see Table 1).

**Table 1.** Participant Attributes ($n$ = 13).

| Variables | Categories | n | % |
|---|---|---|---|
| Gender | Female | 10 | 76.9 |
|  | Male | 3 | 23.1 |
| Education | Baccalaureate Degree Nursing | 13 | 100 |
|  | Baccalaureate Degree Non-Nursing | 13 | 100 |
| Age | 24–29 | 9 | 69.2 |
|  | >30 | 4 | 30.8 |
| Type of unit | COVID Intensive Care | 3 | 23.1 |
|  | Emergency | 1 | 7.7 |
|  | Medical/Surgical Telemetry | 1 | 7.7 |
|  | Medical Oncology | 1 | 7.7 |
|  | Trauma Step-Down | 1 | 7.7 |
|  | Labor and Delivery | 1 | 7.7 |
|  | Neonatal Intensive Care | 1 | 7.7 |
|  | Adolescent Psychiatry | 1 | 7.7 |
|  | Observation Telemetry | 1 | 7.7 |
|  | Pediatric Float Pool | 1 | 7.7 |
|  | Critical Care Float Pool | 1 | 7.7 |
| Daily exposure to COVID-19 or PUIs | Yes | 10 | 76.9 |
|  | No | 3 | 23.1 |
| Amount of experience as nurse (years) | <1 | 9 | 69.2 |
|  | 1–2 | 4 | 30.8 |
|  | >2 | 0 | 0 |

### 2.3. Interview Procedures

All interviews were conducted by the principal investigator (PI) who is a PhD student at the University of Missouri and an Instructor in the College of Nursing at Creighton University. The PI is also employed as a nurse practitioner on the acute pain service at a large tertiary care facility in Phoenix, AZ. All participants were former students of the PI and one of the co-authors. Though the PI was working at the hospital during the pandemic, she did not provide regular or significant direct patient care to COVID patients. Care was taken to bracket her personal experiences during data collection to minimize bias. The PI shared with participants that she was interested in capturing their unique and important perspective of working during a pandemic as a new nurse with intent to share findings broadly through scholarly presentation and publication because little research exists to describe this experience.

Individual, private interviews were conducted with face-to-face video teleconference technology to allow for appropriate social distancing. Each interview lasted approximately one hour, extending beyond this timeframe at the discretion of the participant. No repeat interviews were conducted. Interviews were recorded via the teleconference technology along with a digital audio voice recorder with participants' permission. A recording feature of the teleconferencing technology was used to capture verbatim dialogue of interviews.

Transcriptions were cross-referenced with the digital recordings for accuracy by the PI. Written field notes were also collected by the PI during the interviews.

A semi-structured interview guide was used to collect demographic information and responses to open-ended questions (see Table 2). Broad questions were asked, such as, "What are your thoughts about working during this pandemic?" and "Has it affected you personally, and if so, how?" Probing follow-up questions were used as appropriate such as, "Tell me more about that." One participant emailed a one-page blog post she authored in advance of her interview that detailed her experience, and offered her permission to include this as an artifact with her interview transcript for analysis. After interviewing 13 participants, no new information emerged, and it was determined that saturation had been reached and data collection was complete. As two methods of recording interviews were used and cross-referenced for accuracy by the PI, transcripts were not returned to participants for correction.

**Table 2.** Semi-Structured Interview Guide.

| Demographic Questions | Open-Ended Questions |
| --- | --- |
| (a) Gender identity?<br>(b) Age?<br>(c) How long have you been out of nursing school?<br>(d) How long have you been working as a nurse?<br>(e) Do you work full-time, part-time, PRN?<br>(f) What type of floor do you work on?<br>(g) Have you used any resilience resources (counseling, mental health webinars, etc.) since the pandemic began?<br>(h) Do you work with COVID-19 patients or PUIs as part of your daily job?<br>(i) Have you been cross-trained or asked to float to COVID units? | (j) What are your thoughts about working during this pandemic? Has is affected you personally? How?<br>(k) What motivates you to work extra shifts offered by your institution during the COVID crisis?<br>(l) What fears do you have about working in a COVID environment?<br>(m) How does your place of employment protect your health?<br>(n) How well do you feel your academic program prepared you to work in this environment? What helped? What more could have been done?<br>(o) What resources would be helpful to you right now?<br>(p) How do you feel about your decision to become a nurse? |

### 2.4. Data Analysis

For the data analysis, a team of three researchers, including the PI, independently examined and coded the 13 de-identified transcripts using Microsoft Word and "track changes" and "comments" features with notes on sidebar. Themes were derived from the data. Transcript data were analyzed using qualitative thematic analysis as described by Castleberry and Nolen [15]. In this approach, data are comprehensively analyzed through a systematic five-step process: compiling, disassembling, reassembling, interpreting, and concluding. Compiling involves transcribing data into a usable form for analysis. Transcription and data organization were completed by the PI, which allowed for an intimate knowledge of transcription data. Disassembling is a process of parsing data and searching for meaningful connections through coding and identification of similarities and differences. This was accomplished through color-coding and highlighting by reviewers. In reassembling, data are analyzed in context with each other, and themes and subthemes begin to emerge. The interpretation phase, which can and should occur throughout the process, involves the discussion of relationships between themes supported by raw data or quotations from transcriptions. Data were analyzed through independent review of transcripts by researchers, then bringing themes to the group for discussion. If a difference in interpretation of the themes arose, the researchers revisited the transcripts and negotiated a common understanding. Concluding is the final phase during which research questions are answered based on the previous data analysis [15]. Member checking was performed by sending the results to the participants, and accuracy of the results was confirmed. Due to the smaller sample size, budget, and time constraints, no qualitative data analysis software was used to manage the data.

## 3. Results

Participants described challenges of dealing with frequency of patient deaths, high-acuity patients, changing personal protective equipment (PPE) requirements, and working short-staffed. They also described positive aspects such as bonding with teammates, satisfaction with their decision to become a nurse, and how nursing school featured in their adaptation to working in a pandemic. Below is a summary of these findings with supporting quotes. All participants were assigned pseudonyms to protect their privacy.

### 3.1. Dealing with Death

Of concern to many participants were the difficulties with increased frequency of experiencing the death of patients despite intense efforts to keep them alive. They felt responsible to be there for their patients during end of life when family were not able to be there. Gabby described, "So most of my patients with COVID die. So if they're in the ICU, they don't leave the ICU alive. So, I think that's a big fear, just knowing I'm the last person to be there with them because most of they don't make it." Participants described being greatly impacted by each passing, but after a while, could not recall each patient in their care who had died. Irena put it this way: "The amount of loss that I've seen since March, at first it was always in front of my mind. I would say, I've lost four patients so far, I've lost six patients so far and now the sad truth is, I can't even keep track anymore."

Emma noted that even her experienced nurse colleagues had never experienced so many deaths, "A lot of the nurses that I worked with have literally never experienced a death, even in five or six years of nursing. Now we're seeing it every shift so it's a big adjustment for us. We're used to having patients have good outcomes." She also noted that the Ethics Committee was needed more frequently to make final, end-of-life decisions for patients. Amy noted the emotional toll of withdrawing care: "When you have to sit there and withdraw care at the bedside, it kind of just takes a little bit of your soul away every time you have to do it."

### 3.2. Which PPE Will Keep Us Safe?

Participants expressed concerns about how to protect themselves in patient rooms, and how the guidelines for personal protective equipment (PPE) changed frequently in the early stages of the pandemic. They sometimes experienced daily changes to PPE protocols. Jane and Hattie shared their perspectives on PPE requirements they described as changing each shift:

Jane noted, "Things were changing every day with their recommendations saying you can wear two masks and then no, it's not a good idea to wear two masks and you can use and reuse these certain types of N95s and things were just changing all the time and it kind of felt like we weren't ever getting the most accurate information which is pretty scary . . . so every shift, things were changing and the protocols were different. So it just kind of felt like chaos."

Hattie said, "I think they're trying their hardest to keep us up to date on the rules, but one day we're wearing safety glasses. The next day, you only wear them if you're in rule-out rooms . . . later everyone would be going to the COVID unit if they're rule-outs and then for a week, rule-outs would come to the floor."

Nurses felt some PPE decisions were made based upon available supplies. Jane said, "It was hard to know if changing PPE requirements were based on new evidence and knowledge or because the hospital has to mitigate low stock of N95s." They worried about personally getting COVID and taking it home to family members. Irena put it this way

"My first reaction I had the first day that I heard that I was going to a COVID unit was sheer fear . . . so much unknown about the virus and how it spreads and how we protect ourselves. They would allow us to go into the patient rooms with just surgical masks on. And we weren't wearing N95s as long as we stood within this box that they had taped off on the floor, because if you were 6 feet away from the patient, they thought you were safe."

*3.3. Caring for High-Acuity Patients with Limited Training*

Participants reported that the medical demands of COVID patients required them to pivot quickly to caring for patients of a much higher acuity. As Emma stated, "the level of acuity of my patients increased exponentially overnight with no training and we just had to go with the flow and figure out how to handle it." Many felt inadequately prepared for this transition, as Irena described, "The reality for us is that we basically had an ICU situation on almost every floor that we were on, so our house supervisor basically said, you're working on an ICU unit without ICU training right now." Nurses mentioned that managing critically ill patients is stressful for new nurses under normal circumstances, but the pandemic compounded the stress. Bill gave an example of caring for a challenging trauma patient with multi-organ system dysfunction who also had COVID, "they're not only a trauma patient but now they've contracted COVID, so where they would otherwise not need aggressive respiratory support, now they're needing respiratory support."

Nurses described an increase in daily code events and uncertainty about code outcomes that added to their stress. Denise noted a particularly difficult two-week time period during the pandemic's peak, "The ER (emergency room) is one of those units where it does happen from time to time . . . I've never had so many codes in one short time frame." Many described uncertainty about whether they would recognize key symptoms that indicate clinical decline. As Irena stated, "It's just always in the back of your mind. Am I doing enough? Did I catch everything? You know, did I miss something . . . I think you're always kind of second-guessing yourself, especially as a new grad because you're still learning what all that stuff sounds like and feels like and presents as." Participants also described uncertainty with the new disease process of COVID itself, and the speed at which symptoms appear and patients deteriorate. As Marie said, "The other thing with COVID is just, it just happens so quickly. These patients are declining so rapidly."

*3.4. Difficulties Working Short-Staffed*

Participants described problems with staffing. Many mentioned staff quit their employment, which participants attributed to fear of working during the pandemic. As Fernando put it,

"You have people that are pregnant, you have people that have small children, you know, everybody has families. Everybody wants to keep safe and so you almost immediately had tons of staffing problems. And you have people calling out because they're scared."

Some of the participants described nurses who quit to take more lucrative travel nursing jobs. Others described colleagues who became burned out and quit. Staffing shortages were not limited to nursing but also patient care technicians and certified nursing assistants, adding to nursing workloads. As Marie noted, "We were kind of forced to take on the role of a tech and a nurse with higher acuity patients. So, I think day in and day out for a few weeks there it was very stressful for those reasons." Because of the shortage, nurse-to-patient ratios increased as did overtime requests. Participants worked extra shifts for a variety of reasons, such as wanting to help the team. Bill described picking up extra hours as, "It's exhausting. But I like what it stands for and being able to help and be there for the rest of my team and the patients." Others worked extra, sometimes excessively, for financial incentives. Emma said, "There used to be all sorts of rules and regulations in place of how many shifts in a row we can work and how many shifts in a pay period you can pick up, but desperate times call for desperate measures, and there were no rules. Some people just did crazy things to make crazy amounts of money."

### 3.5. Everything Is Not Okay

Many individuals described the difficulties in caring for very ill patients, the loss of life, and how it was impacting the nurses' ability to cope. Nurses reported nightmares and difficulties with sleeping, depression, anxiety, and fear as they watched the suffering and took the emotional toll home with them. They expressed that they were not able to get away from COVID. As Emma noted,

> "You leave work and you get in the car and the radio's on and all anybody is talking about is COVID so then you have to turn that off. And then you call somebody to decompress while you're driving home and all they want to talk about is COVID. And then you get home and you turn on the TV and it's COVID."

Participants also worried about their patients long after their shifts ended. Irena admitted, "I'm not doing okay. I'm like, I'm not sleeping. I'm having trouble eating. I'm worrying about my patients all the time. Like I drive home and I am just sobbing like the whole way home. And I just, I don't know what to do." Nurses expressed that the situations they were experiencing are hard to handle emotionally. Layla put it this way: "So I think it is incredibly depressing. Not only from the work aspect, but then trying to go home and pretend everything's fine, it's okay, when it's not." They had difficulty processing the events they had seen and moving on with their lives, and noted that their families were not able to fully understand what they were going through. As Amy described,

> "Being a nurse is hard every day. There are people who die every day and you can't come home and talk to your significant other and spill out all on them, because they didn't sign up for that. That's not fair. And you can't come home and be negative ... and it doesn't feel like they even understand or comprehend or can really be there for you because they don't."

Nurses not working with COVID patients were not immune to the stress as they experienced guilt that their co-workers were overwhelmed and they were not there in the middle of it trying to help them. Karen summed it up: "I almost had some guilt that I know some of my classmates are working on the COVID units and they're just stressed and overwhelmed and I just felt like I needed to be a part of that, too." Irena shared with the authors a blog post that she wrote prior to her interview regarding her experience (see Box 1).

### 3.6. Support from the Health Care Team

Participants talked about the importance of having support from other nurses and health care workers who understood what they were experiencing and the demands of caring for very ill, often terminal, patients. Nurses described strategies that had emerged to provide support such as texting and calling each other throughout the day and after their shift to offer support, establishing a group email to discuss feelings about difficult patient situations, and meeting up for lunch at work. Irena described how the group email strategy helped her cope:

> "On difficult days we would "reply all" to a group email at work and start an open dialogue where there was no judgment ... We would read it and know that we weren't alone in it. Even if it was just a quick email like 'I feel like I'm drowning—I don't even want to go back to work tomorrow it's so bad'. People responded and said 'Hey, I'm working tomorrow, let's meet up for lunch. Let me know when you're taking your break'. Just knowing that you have that kind of support, especially as a new nurse and somebody who's brand new at the hospital ... this kind of helped to bring me into a little circle which felt good to be able to get out feelings and frustrations in a no judgment zone."

Family and friends attempted to be supportive but the nurses did not feel that they understood what the nurse had just experienced. Marie commented, "The support at the hospital has been incredible. The way the team and all the nurses have just really been doing an amazing job of coming together and supporting one another, whether it's going into a room to help with a task or it's some mental support at the end of the day. The last couple months were really tough and I think about how much we all have helped one another."

**Box 1.** Participant Irena's unsolicited blog post received via email in advance of interview.

> 5 August 2020
>
> "Hi,
>
> I thought I would share one of my latest Blog entries with you about my experience with COVID. I share my thoughts and frustrations with a small group of friends and other RNs as I find it helps to be able to have a way to express feelings during this unprecedented time.
>
> Irena (pseudonym)"
>
> "The sweat is running down my back as I blink to try to see through my foggy, streaked face shield. The beeping of the machines just will not relent. My patient is dying, and I know it. I fumble with the phone clipped to my scrubs underneath my paper thin yellow gown, desperate to call for help. I am alone in this isolation room with my patient and COVID 19. The oxygen saturation monitor keeps dropping - 84, 80, 76. I call for help but no one comes right away. Our hospital is bursting at the seams with COVID patients and there is no one to help. After what seems like an eternity, someone enters the room in head to toe protective gear and we start the dance. We begin carefully untangling the lines, tubes, and wires connected to my patient, we need to get him lying on his belly as quickly as we can. The moving is exhausting. My body aches and my patient is in excruciating pain from just turning over because this virus is relentless and unforgiving. I have been doing this for 127 days now. The sweating, the praying, the dancing, and the grieving. My patient is moaning on his belly now, his oxygen is still not improving despite giving him all the oxygen we can. I stroke his arm and tell him to take some deep breaths and that we are going to help him. I know I am lying because I have seen this too many times to count. I make the call to the ICU and when a bed opens up (after someone expires) they will whisk him away to be intubated. I just hope I can keep him alive that long. My other 4 patients are waiting in their own rooms of isolation hell and they are all very sick. They are all on oxygen, COVID positive, struggling to breath, desperate, and all alone. I make the phone call to my patient's family and tell them that their loved one is not improving, and the next step will be intubation. I hear the all too familiar sobbing and begging me to let them speak to the patient, but the patient can't speak through the tight mask blowing life into his lungs.
>
> How did I end up here? A new graduate RN in the middle of a global pandemic. I can only describe it as being on a long, grueling hike up a mountain to finish nursing school and pass the NCLEX exam and when I finally make it to the top, I am thrown off the edge of the cliff. No parachute, no training, no lifeline. Here I am at 41 years old finally working at my dream job of being a Registered Nurse and I am in hell."

### 3.7. Nursing School Preparation for a Pandemic

Each participant expressed both satisfaction and limitations in their nursing education, describing the coursework as sufficient but the application to practice specific to pandemic was missing. Many described feeling unprepared and, at times, powerless as they were required to adhere to standards of care changing rapidly and practices, like reusing PPE and increasing nurse to patient ratios, became commonplace. They recalled learning about pandemics, viruses, and emergency preparedness during their educational program; however, participants were ill equipped to employ related nursing protocols in the context of a large-scale pandemic. This gap was not seen as detrimental to their success because working as a nurse during a pandemic was unknown to all nurses they encountered. Emma describes this imparity:

> "I don't think there's anything that could have fully prepared us for the pandemic. I mean, we learned about pandemics. We learned about viruses, you know, we learned all these things, but I don't think there's anything that can prepare you for just being thrown into it."

Marie praised her program for imparting needed information but was aware of the incongruence between didactic education and bedside practice: "I think the reality of nursing school is that not everything is going to copy over directly onto the job, but I think my, I think our school did a good job of doing their best." Cesar noted his colleagues who were experienced nurses reverted to novice nurses when faced with the uncertain challenges of working during a pandemic. He felt that this was evidence that nursing programs cannot fully prepare you:

> " . . . The veteran nurses on the floor and they're like, yeah, we've kind of seen nothing like this either and they're the people you kind of go to, to ask questions. So, if they didn't know what was going on, and I mean, I don't think there's anything that could have made me more prepared."

Conversely, many believed that aspects of their academic program effectively prepared them to assume the role of the nurse. They noted that clinical experiences were valuable as were post-clinical debriefings, which allowed students to discuss clinical based topics among their peers. Marie believed that hands-on clinical were "the most beneficial" aspect of nursing school, specifically, post-clinical debriefing:

> "I found that to be so helpful, whether it's debriefing regarding a task of medication or whole patient experience that we had to deal with that day . . . just being able to sit down with a group, a smaller group of people and really just talk about things."

Denise echoed this opinion that sharing experiences after a clinical was important: "I would say that definitely helped because even though I didn't have like an experience, it was nice to hear like other people's experience."

Participants described the ability to manage time effectively, employ flexibility, and put into practice new skills was a result of learning in an accelerated nursing program. The pace of the twelve-month accelerated nursing program assisted them in developing critical thinking and prioritization, skills they utilize in their bedside practice. Emma states "Going through the accelerated program and having to learn to manage all of that and like keep myself on a schedule is really helpful with keeping my two patients on a schedule." Marie compared her experience in an accelerated nursing program to working during a pandemic. She states "I think it prepared us pretty well especially because the program was only a year long. And so, we were forced to kind of put our heads down and grind for a year. And that is kind of what it feels like."

*3.8. I Would Still Choose Nursing*

Many participants entered nursing as a second career. They voiced little to no negative feelings about their decision to become a nurse; many felt certain that they would still pursue nursing as a career, even if a global pandemic was in their future. Jane was glad she entered the field, "I love my job and what I do, especially the specialty I'm in." Similarly, Hattie described a passion for nursing, "I absolutely love my job. There is not one aspect of it that I don't like."

There was overwhelming confidence in their role choice and belief that they make a difference in the lives of their patients. Bill stated: "I still would do it all over again. If I knew that this was at the end of the tunnel, I 100% would. I love what I do. I definitely feel that I am helping people each and every day at work." Irena is similarly confident in her decision to become a nurse. She stated:

> I absolutely would do it again, a million times. I love being a nurse. I love helping people. I actually have been nominated twice for Daisy awards at my hospital which is a huge big deal . . . .I don't regret my decision to become a nurse, especially as like a second career.

Though many participants were happy with their decision to be a nurse, many describe a desire to move away from bedside in the future. Several of the participants expressed a need to work in a different (non-inpatient) environment. Irena states: "I definitely have days where I'm like, I need to get out of the hospital. I need to get out of this COVID unit. I don't know how many more times I can double glove and wear masks and, you know, do all this stuff. So always nursing, for sure, just maybe in a different environment." The impact of death has affected Layla and her desire to stay in the inpatient setting. She stated, "I don't think that I'll stay like inpatient forever, or anything like that. I think, I think this experience helped me realize that for some of us, you know, outpatient where you're not dealing with people dying left and right would be nice." Marie expressed a desire to enter a field that focused on research: "... this has all made me want to go back to school, maybe for public health in the future . . . research and epidemiology is cool."

## 4. Discussion

In this study, the experience of being a new nurse during a pandemic left nurses feeling that they were being challenged by the experience and that, at times, they were overwhelmed and struggled to cope with the intensity of the experience. Nurses found that patients were of high acuity and they felt they lacked adequate training to care for them, many patients did not survive despite the best medical and nursing efforts, guidance about PPE was regularly changing, and units were working short-staffed. In a study by Garcia-Martin et al. of novice nurses in the Emergency Department (ED), similar themes emerged from an analysis of 16 semi-structured interviews [16]. One of the themes identified was titled "Fears and concerns" which addressed the nurses caring for highly complex patients with limited training in the ED and fear of becoming ill or taking the illness home to family [16]. A subtheme called "Dealing with new challenges" under a separate theme spoke to the confusion surrounding appropriate PPE to be worn to remain safe and free of illness [16].

In this study, support from colleagues who understood the experiences of caring for these extremely ill patients helped nurses when the process of caring for patients had become difficult for them to handle. While the Garcia-Martin et al. article identified a theme of "Support for novice nurses," the subthemes focused primarily on the need for information and organizing resources to provide care for the patients during a short stay in the ED setting [16].

One of the themes unique to this study was "Everything is not okay" which spoke to the personal coping of nurses who were caring for patients during the pandemic. Some participants described experiencing signs and symptoms such as inability to eat and sleep, nightmares, crying over difficult work situations, reluctance to return to work, and feeling depressed. that are potential evidence of extreme anxiety and stress, depression, or burnout and intention to leave nursing. In an article by Chen et al., the authors looked at predictors for leaving the nursing profession during the pandemic and concluded that clinical stress and frequency of caring for patients with COVID-19 infections impacted the nurses' decision to stay in their career [17].

A systematic review of the literature by Carmassi et al. concludes that post-traumatic stress disorder (PTSD) was present during the first two pandemics and may be present in nurses caring for acutely ill patients during the recent pandemic [18]. An article by d'Ettore et al. also suggests that health care workers have experienced mental health issues during previous epidemics, such as SARS and Middle East respiratory syndrome (MERS) [19]. PTSD is a disorder characterized by recurring symptoms such as bad dreams, flashbacks, avoidance, hyperarousal, difficulty sleeping, and negative thoughts that develops in some people following exposure to a traumatic event [20]. In the Carmassi review, the authors identified exposure level to ill patients, years of work experience, female gender, and a number of other risk and resilience factors as determining if individuals might experience PTSD in the performance of their duties during a pandemic [18]. The International Council of Nurses published a COVID-19 Update suggesting that globally, nurses are experiencing burnout and mental distress associated with extreme pressures of working during the pandemic and number of nurse deaths exceeded 2200 as of January 2021 [21]. In this study, even those nurses without daily direct contact with COVID-19 patients experienced negative psychological effects, such as guilt that they were not doing enough to assist fellow co-workers.

Uncovering the experiences of novice nurses in a pandemic and understanding the unique challenges being faced provides a foundation for educational interventions that have the potential to strengthen and preserve the nursing workforce. In the theme "Nursing school preparation for a pandemic" students described how the demands of nursing school had instilled the ability to plan, organize, think critically, and be flexible in their practice. Clinical rotations and high intensity simulation experiences, post-clinical debriefings, and end-of-life or palliative care discussions were also helpful. In the article by Sparacino, role transition as novice nurses is inevitable but expert, caring, professional experiences with faculty can make a real difference for students in knowing how to engage in a positive way in their professional role especially during stressful times [6]. This education must continue to be enhanced with a focus on self-care and effective team communication.

For nurses in the stressful situation of providing care for patients in a pandemic, hospital management must provide additional support such as counseling sessions at no cost for nurses experiencing symptoms of anxiety, depression, or PTSD, nurse mentoring programs pairing nurses with several years of nursing experience with novice nurses, and providing structured weekly opportunities for debriefing with nursing unit managers, administrators, and colleagues to provide support. Staff educational sessions on the most effective techniques in caring for ill patients and preferred PPE equipment should be conducted.

Participants were asked whether they had used any resilience resources since the pandemic began. Interestingly, only one of 13 participants reported using employer-provided resilience resources, which included support webinars, counseling hotlines, and talking with hospital chaplains. Many sought their own forms of support with physical activity, media vacations, engaging in pleasurable and distracting hobbies, seeking help from their own counselors, or talking with friends and family members. This may point to a lack of understanding on the part of organizations about what resources are most needed by novice frontline nurses, and how best to connect employees to employer-offered resources, which supports findings of the meta-analysis by Pollock and colleagues [9].

*Limitations*

Although the teacher-to-former student relationship of the PI to participants may be a limitation regarding perceptions about nursing school preparation for the pandemic, participants readily responded to calls for participation and shared openly with the PI, perhaps due in part to the established relationship. Additionally, participants noted in a theme that talking with other health care providers who understand was a significant and desirable form of coping with stress during this time, and they may have perceived benefit in sharing this experience with a fellow clinician, and their former teacher.

## 5. Conclusions

Understanding the experiences of novice nurses caring for acutely ill patients during a pandemic and how best to support these nurses was of keen interest to the researchers. The authors believe that this understanding was achieved in the context of this study. Implications of this study include further investigation of the signs and symptoms nurses experienced that were suggestive of anxiety, depression, and PTSD. These nurse participants should be studied longitudinally to uncover the impact on future nursing practice. While nursing education programs provided resources considered helpful for dealing with pandemic-related stressors, programs should build mechanisms into curriculum to focus on crisis management, post-clinical debriefing, strong team communication, and self-care. Employers should build time into the end of shifts for mandatory debriefing to support nurses' mental health.

**Author Contributions:** Conceptualization, H.N.; methodology, C.H. and H.N.; formal analysis, H.N., C.H. and P.T.; investigation, H.N.; resources, H.N.; data curation, H.N.; writing—original draft preparation, H.N., C.H. and P.T.; writing—review and editing, H.N., C.H. and P.T.; visualization, H.N.; supervision, H.N.; project administration, H.N. All authors have read and agreed to the published version of the manuscript.

**Funding:** This research received no external funding.

**Institutional Review Board Statement:** This study was conducted according to the guidelines of the Declaration of Helsinki, and approved by the Institutional Review Board of Creighton University on 22 July 2020 (protocol code 2001237-01).

**Informed Consent Statement:** This project was approved by Creighton University IRB and was determined to be exempt from Federal Policy for Protection of Human Subjects as per 45CFR46.101 (b) 2. Though exemption was received, all participants received information about the study, use of data, confidentiality and privacy, voluntary participation, and IRB contact information. Patient consent was waived due to IRB determination of exempt status. Written informed consent has been obtained from the participant contributing the blog post artifact to publish this paper.

**Data Availability Statement:** The data presented in this study are available on request from the corresponding author. The data are not publicly available due to privacy protection.

**Acknowledgments:** The authors would like to thank Joan M. Lappe, PhD, RN, FAAN, Associate Dean of Research College of Nursing, Creighton University, for her guidance and editorial assistance (https://www.creighton.edu/faculty-directory-profile/340/joan-lappe accessed on 7 May 2021).

**Conflicts of Interest:** The authors declare no conflict of interest.

## References

1. Benner, P.E. *From Novice to Expert: Excellence and Power in Clinical Practice*; Prentice-Hall: Upper Saddle River, NJ, USA, 2001.
2. Washington, G.T. Performance Anxiety in New Graduate Nurses. *Dimens. Crit. Care Nurs.* **2012**, *31*, 295–300. [CrossRef] [PubMed]
3. Hatler, C.; Stoffers, P.; Kelly, L.; Redding, K.; Carr, L.L. Work unit transformation to welcome new graduate nurses: Using nurses' wisdom. *Nurs. Econ.* **2011**, *29*, 88–93. [PubMed]
4. Sledge, J.A.; Potter, P.; Stapleton, P. Participant Voices: Making a Nurse Residency Program Better. *Nurse Lead.* **2016**, *14*, 358–364. [CrossRef]
5. Henderson, A.; Ossenberg, C.; Tyler, S. 'What matters to graduates': An evaluation of a structured clinical support program for newly graduated nurses. *Nurse Educ. Pract.* **2015**, *15*, 225–231. [CrossRef] [PubMed]
6. Sparacino, L.L. Faculty's Role in Assisting New Graduate Nurses' Adjustment to Practice. *SAGE Open Nurs.* **2016**, *2*. [CrossRef]
7. Sandler, M. Why are new graduate nurses leaving the profession in their first year of practice and how does this impact on ED nurse staffing? A rapid review of current literature and recommended reading. *Can. J. Emerg. Nurs.* **2020**, *41*, 23–24. [CrossRef]
8. Sriharan, A.; West, K.J.; Almost, J.; Hamza, J.A.A.A. COVID-19-Related Occupational Burnout and Moral Distress among Nurses: A Rapid Scoping Review. *Can. J. Nurs. Leadersh.* **2021**, *34*, 7–19. [CrossRef] [PubMed]
9. Pollock, A.; Campbell, P.; Cheyne, J.; Cowie, J.; Davis, B.; McCallum, J.; McGill, K.; Elders, A.; Hagen, S.; McClurg, D.; et al. Interventions to support the resilience and mental health of frontline health and social care professionals during and after a disease outbreak, epidemic or pandemic: A mixed methods systematic review. *Cochrane Database Syst. Rev.* **2020**, *11*, CD013779. [CrossRef] [PubMed]
10. Heung, Y.J.; Wong, K.F.; To, S.T.; Wong, H.D. Severe acute respiratory syndrome outbreak promotes a strong sense of professional identity among nursing students. *Nurse Educ. Today* **2005**, *25*, 112–118. [CrossRef] [PubMed]
11. Sun, N.; Wei, L.; Shi, S.; Jiao, D.; Song, R.; Ma, L.; Wang, H.; Wang, C.; Wang, Z.; You, Y.; et al. A qualitative study on the psychological experience of caregivers of COVID-19 patients. *Am. J. Infect. Control.* **2020**, *48*, 592–598. [CrossRef] [PubMed]
12. Neubauer, B.E.; Witkop, C.T.; Varpio, L. How phenomenology can help us learn from the experiences of others. *Perspect. Med. Educ.* **2019**, *8*, 90–97. [CrossRef] [PubMed]
13. Teherani, A.; Martimianakis, T.; Stenfors-Hayes, T.; Wadhwa, A.; Varpio, L. Choosing a Qualitative Research Approach. *J. Grad. Med. Educ.* **2015**, *7*, 669–670. [CrossRef] [PubMed]
14. Tong, A.; Sainsbury, P.; Craig, J. Consolidated criteria for reporting qualitative research (COREQ): A 32-item checklist for interviews and focus groups. *Int. J. Qual. Health Care* **2007**, *19*, 349–357. [CrossRef] [PubMed]
15. Castleberry, A.; Nolen, A. Thematic analysis of qualitative research data: Is it as easy as it sounds? *Curr. Pharm. Teach. Learn.* **2018**, *10*, 807–815. [CrossRef] [PubMed]
16. García-Martín, M.; Roman, P.; Rodriguez-Arrastia, M.; Diaz-Cortes, M.D.M.; Soriano-Martin, P.J.; Ropero-Padilla, C. Novice nurse's transitioning to emergency nurse during COVID-19 pandemic: A qualitative study. *J. Nurs. Manag.* **2021**, *29*, 258–267. [CrossRef] [PubMed]

17. Chen, H.-M.; Liu, C.-C.; Yang, S.-Y.; Wang, Y.-R.; Hsieh, P.-L. Factors Related to Care Competence, Workplace Stress, and Intention to Stay among Novice Nurses during the Coronavirus Disease (COVID-19) Pandemic. *Int. J. Environ. Res. Public Health* **2021**, *18*, 2122. [CrossRef] [PubMed]
18. Carmassi, C.; Foghi, C.; Dell'Oste, V.; Cordone, A.; Bertelloni, C.A.; Bui, E.; Dell'Osso, L. PTSD symptoms in health care workers facing the three coronavirus outbreaks: What can we expect after the COVID-19 pandemic. *Psychiatry Res.* **2020**, *292*, 113312. [CrossRef] [PubMed]
19. D'Ettorre, G.; Ceccarelli, G.; Santinelli, L.; Vassalini, P.; Innocenti, G.P.; Alessandri, F.; Koukopoulos, A.E.; Russo, A.; Tarsitani, L. Post-Traumatic Stress Symptoms in Healthcare Workers Dealing with the COVID-19 Pandemic: A Systematic Review. *Int. J. Environ. Res. Public Health* **2021**, *18*, 601. [CrossRef] [PubMed]
20. National Institute of Mental Health. Post-Traumatic Stress Disorder. 2019. Available online: https://www.nimh.nih.gov/health/topics/post-traumatic-stress-disorder-ptsd/index.shtml (accessed on 27 April 2021).
21. International Council of Nurses. COVID-19 Update. 2021. Available online: https://www.icn.ch/news/covid-19-effect-worlds-nurses-facing-mass-trauma-immediate-danger-profession-and-future-our (accessed on 27 April 2021).

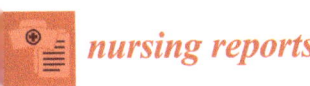 

Article

# Healthcare Provider Attitudes toward the Newly Developed COVID-19 Vaccine: Cross-Sectional Study

Gasmelseed Ahmed [1], Zainab Almoosa [1], Dalia Mohamed [1], Janepple Rapal [1], Ofelia Minguez [1], Issam Abu Khurma [1], Ayman Alnems [1] and Abbas Al Mutair [1,2,3,*]

1. Research Center, Almoosa Specialist Hospital, Al-ahsa 36342, Saudi Arabia; g.yousif@almoosahospital.com.sa (G.A.); z.almoosa@almoosahospital.com.sa (Z.A.); dalia@almoosahospital.com.sa (D.M.); janepple@almoosahospital.com.sa (J.R.); ofelia.minguez@almoosahospital.com.sa (O.M.); issam@almoosahospital.com.sa (I.A.K.); a.alnems@almoosahospital.com.sa (A.A.)
2. School of Mursing, Wollongong University, Wollongong, NSW 2522, Australia
3. Nursing College, Princess Nora University, Riyadh 11564, Saudi Arabia
* Correspondence: abbas.almutair@almoosahospital.com.sa

**Abstract:** Background: During the long wait and the global anxiety for a vaccine against COVID-19, impressively high-safety and effective vaccines were invented by multiple pharmaceutical companies. Aim: We aimed to assess the attitudes of healthcare providers and evaluate their intention to advocate for the vaccine. Methods: This was a cross-sectional study conducted in a tertiary private hospital where an electronic survey was distributed among healthcare providers (HCPs). The survey contained two sections: socio-demographic characteristics and Likert-scale perception, with 72% internal consistency. Results: The response rate to the email survey was 37% (n = 236). In addition, 169 (71.6%) of respondents were women, with more than half (134, 56.8%) aged ≤35 years. A total of 110 (46.6%) had over 10 years of experience, and most of them were nurses (146, 62%). Univariate analysis revealed that older participants significantly accepted and advocated for the new vaccine more than the younger ones. In the multivariate analysis, men were significantly more likely than women to accept and advocate for the new vaccine, as were those with chronic illnesses. Participants with allergy were significantly less likely to accept the vaccine than others. odds ratio (OR) and p-values were 2.5, 0.003; 2.3, 0.04; and 0.4, 0.01, respectively. Conclusion: The acceptance rate for the newly-developed COVID-19 vaccines was average among HCPs. Sex, age, presence of chronic illnesses, and allergy were significant predictors of accepting the vaccine.

**Keywords:** healthcare providers; vaccination; Saudi Arabia; attitudes; acceptance; advocate; COVID-19

Citation: Ahmed, G.; Almoosa, Z.; Mohamed, D.; Rapal, J.; Minguez, O.; Abu Khurma, I.; Alnems, A.; Al Mutair, A. Healthcare Provider Attitudes toward the Newly Developed COVID-19 Vaccine: Cross-Sectional Study. *Nurs. Rep.* **2021**, *11*, 187–194. https://doi.org/10.3390/nursrep11010018

Academic Editor: Richard Gray

Received: 11 February 2021
Accepted: 10 March 2021
Published: 23 March 2021

**Publisher's Note:** MDPI stays neutral with regard to jurisdictional claims in published maps and institutional affiliations.

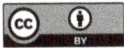

**Copyright:** © 2021 by the authors. Licensee MDPI, Basel, Switzerland. This article is an open access article distributed under the terms and conditions of the Creative Commons Attribution (CC BY) license (https://creativecommons.org/licenses/by/4.0/).

## 1. Background

No specific treatment was available for SARS-CoV-2; therefore, the rapid development of effective vaccines was urgently needed [1,2]. Many patients all over the world used human drugs off-label such as chloroquine, hydroxychloroquine, azithromycin lopinavir-ritonavir, favipiravir, remdesivir, ribavirin, interferon, convalescent plasma, hormones, and anti-IL-6 inhibitors based on either their in vitro antiviral or anti-inflammatory properties [3].

With multiple clinical vaccine studies ongoing, the target time for public distribution of a safe and efficient vaccine was projected as 18 months [4]. Therefore, to avoid the spread of COVID-19, measures to increase the acceptance of COVID-19 vaccines are critical. However, immunization program success depends on high vaccine acceptance versus rejection rates by healthcare providers, who play a crucial role in vaccination [5]. There is a demand to identify factors that may contribute to the acceptance and rejection of the newly-developed COVID-19 vaccine, especially doctors and nurses, who are known for being advocates of patients. Vaccine hesitancy is a global threat, so scientists must focus on understanding the underlying causes of this hesitancy to fight against vaccine misinformation [6]. Vaccine hesitancy is defined by its determinants; confidence, complacency and convenience are on the rise. Exploring the population's concerns through research at the individual and community levels is the best practice to address the trust component of vaccine hesitancy and to promote vaccine acceptance [7] by effectively presenting science-based information, and accordingly presenting immunization as a social norm both in educational materials and in conversations or resilience. However, immunization trust-building and maintaining at the public level will take time [7].

Although immunization has successfully reduced the global burden of illness and deaths, the overall confidence in vaccines among communities can be affected by various concerns. Consequently, vaccine hesitancy can lead to vaccine refusal. Nowadays and due to the massive availability and accessibility of different modes communication media, the intensity, spread, and effects of public opinion on vaccines are speeding up information sharing, contributing to vaccine hesitancy and refusal [8].

While most of the world's countries were in lockdown to limit the spread of COVID-19, scientists from all over the world were racing to provide proven treatment or develop vaccines against COVID-19. Their global access was a priority to end the pandemic [9]. The long-term solution to the COVID-19 pandemic will be a globally implemented and safe vaccination program, which will have both broad clinical and socioeconomic benefits. The vaccine must be delivered to the public as early as it is available to reduce morbidity and mortality from the COVID-19 pandemic. The vaccine must also be accepted by the public as well the healthcare community. Considering vaccine hesitancy as a major barrier to vaccine uptake, a high vaccine refusal rate could significantly affect the preventive goals [10].

In this study, we aimed to assess the attitudes of healthcare providers (HCPs) in a tertiary private hospital toward their acceptance and intention to advocate for the newly developed COVID-19 vaccine amongst patients, friends, and families. The study will identify the possible reasons behind HCP acceptance and rejection of the newly developed vaccines.

## 2. Methods

A cross-sectional study was conducted using a questionnaire. The study was conducted in a tertiary private hospital in the east region of Saudi Arabia, where an electronic survey was distributed to all HCPs. All respondent employees were enrolled consecutively in the study. An ethical approval to conduct the study was obtained from Almoosa Specialist Hospital's Institutional Review Board (IRB) (log No: ARC-20.10.3).

The questionnaire consisted of two sections: the first was socio-demographic characteristics, gathering data on sex, age, educational status, years of experience, nationality, occupation, and marital status; the second used a Likert scale to gather information on perceptions (consisted of twelve items, including medical knowledge, trust in media, trust in manufacturers, and trust in policymakers and leaders). The validation test of the data collection instrument revealed an internal consistency of 72%.

A pre-defined justified sample size for our study was determined in reference to an effect size from similar study by Wang et al., reported 91.3% of participants stated that they would accept COVID-19 vaccination after the vaccine becomes available. Applying the standard categorical variable data sample equation [$(n = z^2 \times PQ/e^2)$, where z is confidence level, p is the reported effect size and e is the margin of error], expecting a 99% confidence level and accepting a narrow margin of error around 0.05, the optimal sample size for this study was calculated as 196 participants [11].

Prior to data collection, IRB approval was sought from the Almoosa Specialist Hospital (ARC-20.10.3). The Almoosa Specialist Hospital is a 220-bed tertiary private care center and the largest in the Al-ahsa region, Saudi Arabia. The study design was cross-sectional, approached using a survey administered to the hospital's employees. The target population for this study was all the people serving in this facility, which has a local catchment population of over two million with all medical specialties including: adult; pediatric; neonatal; cardiology; oncology; internal medicine; infectious diseases; dermatology; gastroenterology; rheumatology; hematology; radiology; geriatrics; obstetrics and gynecology;

neuroscience; nephrology; orthopedics; urology; surgery; ear, nose, and throat care; dental; burn; and intensive care.

## 3. Results

The response rate to the emailed survey was 37% (n = 236). In addition, 169 (71.6%) of respondents were women, with more than half (134, 56.8%) aged ≤35 years. A total of 110 (46.6%) had over 10 years of experience, and most of them were nurses (146, 62%) (Table 1). The common reasons for rejecting the vaccine are outlined in Table 2. Univariate analysis revealed that older respondents significantly accepted and advocated for the new vaccine more than the younger ones (53% vs. 47%, *p*-value = 0.003; Table 3). Multivariate analysis revealed that men were significantly more likely than women to accept and advocate for the new vaccine (OR = 2.5, *p*-value = 0.003), as were those who had chronic illnesses (OR = 2.3, *p*-value = 0.04). Participants with allergy were significantly less than others to accept the vaccine. The results also showed that the trust in healthcare providers is double the trust in other influential people (OR = 2.3, *p*-value = 0.05; Table 4). Healthcare providers' specialties, graduation degree, and years of experience showed no statistically significance differences in the acceptance rate.

Table 1. Socio-demographic characteristics (n = 236).

| Characteristics | N (%) |
|---|---|
| Sex | |
| Female | 169 (71.6%) |
| Male | 67 (28.4%) |
| Age group | |
| ≤35 years | 134 (56.8%) |
| >35 years | 102 (43.3%) |
| Educational degree | |
| Graduate degrees (diploma and bachelor) | 187 (79.2%) |
| Postgraduate degrees (master and Ph.D.) | 49 (20.8%) |
| Country of origin | |
| Indian | 75 (31.8%) |
| Philipino | 73 (30.9%) |
| Saudi | 41 (17.4%) |
| Others (different 11 countries ranging from 1 to 11 nurses) | 47 (19.9%) |
| Do you have a comorbidity (any chronic disease)? | |
| Yes | 032 (13.6%) |
| No | 204 (86.4%) |
| Have allergy to medicine or food? | |
| Yes | 35 (14.8%) |
| No | 201 (85.2%) |
| Years of experience | |
| ≤10 | 126 (53.4%) |
| >10 | 110 (46.6%) |
| Occupation | |
| Nurse | 146 (61.9%) |
| Doctor | 038 (16.1%) |
| Other | 052 (22.0%) |
| Who do you trust the most for information on vaccination? | |
| Healthcare providers (HCPs) | 190 (80.6%) |
| Leaders | 14 (05.9%) |
| Media | 6 (02.5%) |
| Policy makers | 13 (05.5%) |
| None | 13 (05.5%) |

**Table 1.** Cont.

| Characteristics | N (%) |
|---|---|
| Accept the newly developed vaccine? | |
| Yes | 131 (55.5%) |
| No | 105 (44.5%) |
| Advocate for newly developed vaccine | |
| Yes | 142 (60.1%) |
| No | 094 (39.9%) |
| Both accept and advocate for newly developed vaccine | |
| Yes | 121 (51.3%) |
| No | 115 (48.7%) |

**Table 2.** The common reasons for rejection of the vaccines (n = 236).

| Characteristics | N (%) |
|---|---|
| Trust manufacturing country | |
| Agree | 157 (66.5%) |
| Disagree | 079 (33.5%) |
| I trust the manufacturing company of the vaccine | |
| Agree | 159 (67.4%) |
| Disagree | 077 (32.6%) |
| I believe vaccines are tested long enough for safety and efficacy | |
| Agree | 150 (63.6%) |
| Disagree | 086 (36.4%) |
| I think the media have created a negative impression about the vaccine | |
| Agree | 091 (38.6%) |
| Disagree | 145 (61.4%) |
| I think the vaccine's industry is driven by financial motives | |
| Agree | 136 (57.6%) |
| Disagree | 100 (42.4%) |
| I believe forced vaccination by authorities provokes hesitancy | |
| Agree | 172 (72.9%) |
| Disagree | 064 (27.1%) |

**Table 3.** Univariate analysis (n = 236).

| Characteristics | Take and Advocate for Vaccine (%) | Will Not Advocate (%) | $p$-Value |
|---|---|---|---|
| Sex | | | |
| Female | 70 (60.9%) | 99 (81.8%) | |
| Male | 45 (39.1%) | 22 (18.2%) | 0.0001 |
| Age (years) | | | |
| ≤35 | 54 (47.0%) | 80 (66.1%) | |
| >36 | 61 (53.0%) | 41 (33.9%) | 0.003 |
| Occupation | | | |
| Nurse | 69 (60.5%) | 77 (61.7%) | |
| Doctor | 18 (15.4%) | 20 (18.1%) | |
| All other HCPs | 28 (24.1%) | 24 (20.2%) | 0.71 |
| Degree of graduation | | | |
| Graduate degrees | 89 (77.4%) | 98 (81.0%) | |
| Postgraduate | 26 (22.6%) | 23 (19.0%) | 0.49 |

**Table 3.** *Cont.*

| Characteristics | Take and Advocate for Vaccine (%) | Will Not Advocate (%) | p-Value |
|---|---|---|---|
| Years of experience | | | |
| 10 years or more | 59 (51.3%) | 51 (42.1%) | |
| Less than 10 years | 56 (48.7%) | 70 (57.9%) | 0.16 |
| Do you have any chronic disease? | | | |
| Yes | 22 (19.1%) | 10 (08.3%) | |
| No | 94 (80.9%) | 110 (91.7%) | 0.02 |
| Have allergy to medicine or food | | | |
| Yes | 009 (07.8%) | 26 (21.5%) | |
| No | 106 (92.2%) | 95 (78.5%) | 0.003 |
| Who do you trust the most for information on vaccination | | | |
| Health policymakers and leaders | 18 (15.7%) | 009 (07.4%) | |
| Others | 97 (84.3%) | 112 (92.6%) | 0.048 |

**Table 4.** Multivariate analysis (n = 236). OR, odds ratio.

| Characteristics | OR | 95% CI | p-Value |
|---|---|---|---|
| Sex | | | |
| Male vs. female | 2.5 | (1.35–4.56) | 0.003 |
| Having allergy to medicine or food | | | |
| Those with allergy vs. others | 0.4 | (0.16–0.83) | 0.02 |
| Presence of chronic disease? | | | |
| Those with chronic disease vs. others | 2.3 | (1.02–5.39) | 0.04 |
| Who do you trust the most for information on vaccination | | | |
| Health policy makers and leaders vs. others | 2.3 | (0.99–5.37) | 0.05 |

## 4. Discussion

In this study, we assessed the attitudes of healthcare providers toward the newly developed vaccine and evaluated their intention to advocate for it. The literature shows that several studies have been conducted on factors associated with the acceptance of vaccines among healthcare workers [12–14]. A cross-sectional study examining healthcare workers' knowledge, attitude, and acceptance of influenza vaccination in Saudi Arabia has found that the acceptance and participation in influenza vaccination have markedly increased in the 2016 season compared with previous years, indicating highly motivated practitioners who seem prepared to encourage the adoption of influenza vaccination [15]. A systematic review focused on the factors influencing pandemic influenza vaccination among healthcare providers found that the H1N1 vaccine was likely to be accepted by healthcare workers if they perceived the vaccine as safe. Immunization effectively prevents infection of self and others and H1N1 is perceived as a serious and severe infection [16].

In the current study, we found above-average rates of acceptance and intention for advocating for the vaccine (56% and 60%, respectively). However, both accepting and advocating were reported by half of the study group (51.3%). The average rate of acceptance in our results is higher than for an online survey conducted in France in late March 2020 in a population aged 18 years: only 26% of participants agreed that they will use the vaccine against COVID-19 if it becomes available [17]. A survey conducted in 19 countries, which aimed to determine potential acceptance rates and factors influencing the acceptance of a COVID-19 vaccine, revealed differences in acceptance rates among participants ranging from almost 90% in China to less than 55% in Russia [18].

Despite the low rate of acceptance and the low trust caused by different factors, participants in this study mostly trust health policymakers and health leaders. Another study in India reported that vaccination decision-makers had different perceptions about building trust with the communities and foster engagement to function optimally toward achieving national vaccination goals [19].

A survey study on Israeli populations, which included both medical and non-medical staff, evaluated the current vaccination compliance rates and assessed whether participants would agree to receive a COVID-19 vaccine once available. The study results indicated that the rate of vaccine suspicion was high among medical professionals, which depended on the personal risk–benefit perception, which may be affected by misinformation about vaccine safety and efficacy. Due to the rapidly developed vaccine, many of the study respondents were non-compliant and raised fears about the safety of the vaccine. However, individuals who believe that they are at a higher risk of illness displayed greater vaccine acquiescence [20]. This finding agrees with our findings for our participants with chronic illnesses, where 22 of 32, (69%) of them reported to be willing to accept the newly developed vaccine. In a different study conducted in Hong Kong, a low rate of intention to accept COVID-19 vaccination and a high proportion of hesitation were found despite the evolution of the pandemic. As indicated by the authors, the reasons for this finding are related to suspicion regarding the safety and efficacy of the new vaccine [21].

Misinformation and conspiracy theories may decrease vaccine uptake, so the key to overcoming the anti-vaccination movement is establishing a consensus on how groups of the population will obtain access to the vaccine and mitigate any doubts and concerns that exist to generate demand for vaccinations. [22]. The threshold for COVID-19 herd immunity, as previously reported, was estimated to be between 55% and 82% of the total population. This could be significantly affected by a vaccine refusal rate of more than 10% to 15%, as reported in countries such as Australia [23]. An influential call to promote and advocate for the broader continuum of health and critical thinking is needed for preparing healthcare workers to meet the expected challenges of healthcare equity, environmental justice, and economic recovery [24]. Some health belief model (HBM) studies reported that a person will take health-related actions if they feel that a negative condition or side effects can be avoided, or if they have a positive expectation of taking a recommended action [25]. One of our concerns in the findings of our study is low level of acceptance and low trust in the newly produced vaccine. Similar findings were reported in study by Ozawa and Stack, revealing a wide vaccine confidence gap due to different factors, which necessitate building public trust by engaging all stakeholders including parents, healthcare providers, community leaders, policy makers, and the media [26].

## 5. Conclusions

The overall rate of acceptance for a newly developed COVID-19 vaccine among healthcare providers was average in this study. The results also demonstrated that sex, age, presence of chronic illnesses, and allergy are significant predictors for accepting the vaccine. It is strongly recommended that healthcare providers are prepared for a science- and evidence-based approach that addresses the safety and efficacy of the vaccines in the community to build and maintain public trust in the vaccine. Well-planned media and a positive influential campaign led by HCPs can be used to share transparent and scientific information with the community in terms of epidemiological details, scientific facts, and methodological process of the vaccine to promote critical thinking, which could result in increased confidence to optimize the uptake of the vaccine. Senior health are policy makers and leaders in public taking the vaccine will encourage more people to accept vaccination. The findings of the current study should be interpreted considering its several limitations: the cross-sectional approach of the study and using a survey tool with the lowest margin of internal consistency. Additionally, the survey was a self-administered questionnaire. Other limitations were the small sample taken from a single center, and the limited number of men and physicians participated in the survey. We acknowledge these limitations might potentially impact the study and limit generalizability of the findings. Hence, we recommend a future multicenter national study. Surveying a larger population by applying highly validated tool will rely on subjective rather than objective methods for increased understanding of valid perception and acceptance of the newly developed vaccine among healthcare providers.

**Author Contributions:** Conceptualization, G.A, Z.A., D.M. and A.A.M.; methodology, G.A.; validation and formal analysis, J.R., O.M., I.A.K. and A.A. data curation, Z.A., A.A.M. and G.A.; original draft preparation, writing, review and editing. All authors have read and agreed to the published version of the manuscript.

**Funding:** This research received no external funding.

**Institutional Review Board Statement:** The study was conducted according to the guidelines of the Declaration of Helsinki, and approved by the Institutional Review Board of Almoosa Specialist Hospital.

**Informed Consent Statement:** Informed consent was obtained from all subjects involved in the study.

**Data Availability Statement:** Data used and analyzed in this study will be promptly available for the publisher upon request.

**Conflicts of Interest:** The authors declare no conflict of interest.

# References

1. World Health Organization. WHO Coronavirus Disease (COVID-19) Dashboard. Available online: https://covid19.WHO.int/ (accessed on 7 November 2020).
2. Gao, Q.; Bao, L.; Mao, H.; Wang, L.; Xu, K.; Li, Y.; Zhu, L.; Wang, N.; Lv, Z.; Gao, H.; et al. Rapid development of an inactivated vaccine for SARS-CoV-2. *bioRxiv* **2020**, in press.
3. Kalil, A.C. Treating COVID-19—Off-label drug use, compassionate use, and randomized clinical trials during pandemics. *JAMA* **2020**, *323*, 1897–1898. [CrossRef] [PubMed]
4. Callaway, E. The race for coronavirus vaccines: A graphical guide. *Nature* **2020**, *580*, 576. [CrossRef]
5. Omer, S.B.; Salmon, D.A.; Orenstein, W.A.; Dehart, M.P.; Halsey, N. Vaccine refusal, mandatory immunization, and the risks of vaccine-preventable diseases. *N. Engl. J. Med.* **2009**, *360*, 1981–1988. [CrossRef] [PubMed]
6. McAteer, J.; Yildirim, I.; Chahroudi, A. The VACCINES Act: Deciphering Vaccine Hesitancy in the Time of COVID-19. *Clin. Infect. Dis.* **2020**, *71*, 703–705. [CrossRef]
7. Sondagar, C.; Xu, R.; MacDonald, N.E.; Dubé, E. Vaccine acceptance: How to build and maintain trust in immunization. *Eur. PMC* **2020**, *46*, 155–159. [CrossRef]
8. Larson, H.J.; Smith, D.M.D.; Paterson, P.; Cumming, M.; Eckersberger, E.; Freifeld, C.C.; Ghinai, I.; Jarrett, C.; Paushter, L.; Brownstein, J.S.; et al. Measuring vaccine confidence: Analysis of data obtained by a media surveillance system used to analyse public concerns about vaccines. *Lancet Infect Dis.* **2013**, *13*, 606–613. [CrossRef]
9. Yamey, G.; Schäferhoff, M.; Hatchett, R.; Pate, M.; Zhao, F.; McDade, K.K. Ensuring global access to COVID-19 vaccines. *Lancet* **2020**, *395*, 1405–1406. [CrossRef]
10. DeRoo, S.S.; Pudalov, N.J.; Fu, L.Y. Planning for a COVID-19 Vaccination Program. *JAMA* **2020**, *323*, 2458–2459. [CrossRef]
11. Wang, J.; Jing, R.; Lai, X.; Zhang, H.; Lyu, Y.; Knoll, M.D.; Fang, H. Acceptance of COVID-19 Vaccination during the COVID-19 Pandemic in China. *Vaccines (Basel)* **2020**, *8*, 482.
12. Asghar, M.S.; Kazmi, S.J.H.; Khan, N.A.; Akram, M.; Khan, S.A.; Rasheed, U.; Hassan, M.; Memon, G.M. Clinical Profiles, Characteristics, and Outcomes of the First 100 Admitted COVID-19 Patients in Pakistan: A Single-Center Retrospective Study in a Tertiary Care Hospital of Karachi. *Cureus* **2020**, *12*, e8712. [PubMed]
13. Bhagavathula, A.S.; Aldhaleei, W.A.; Rahmani, J.; Mahabadi, M.A.; Bandari, D.K. Knowledge and Perceptions of COVID-19 among Health Care Workers: Cross-Sectional Study. *JMIR Public Health Surveill.* **2020**, *6*, e19160. [CrossRef] [PubMed]
14. Available online: https://www.moh.gov.sa/en/Ministry/MediaCenter/News/Pages/News-2020-03-02-002.aspx (accessed on 3 March 2020).
15. Alshammari, T.M.; Yusuff, K.B.; Aziz, M.M.; Subaie, G.M. Healthcare professionals' knowledge, attitude and acceptance of influenza vaccination in Saudi Arabia: A multicenter cross-sectional study. *BMC Health Serv. Res.* **2019**, *19*, 229. [CrossRef] [PubMed]
16. Prematunge, C.; Corace, K.; McCarthy, A.; Nair, R.C.; Pugsley, R.; Garber, G. Factors influencing pandemic influenza vaccination of healthcare workers—A systematic review. *Vaccine* **2012**, *30*, 4733–4743. [CrossRef] [PubMed]
17. COCONEL Group. A future vaccination campaign against COVID-19 at risk of vaccine hesitancy and politicisation. *Lancet Infect. Dis.* **2020**, *20*, 769. [CrossRef]
18. Lazarus, J.V.; Ratzan, S.C.; Palayew, A.; Gostin, L.O.; Larson, H.J.; Rabin, K.; Kimball, S.; El-Mohandes, A. A global survey of potential acceptance of a COVID-19 vaccine. *Nat. Med.* **2020**, *27*, 225–228. [CrossRef]

19. Dutta, T.; Meyerson, B.E.; Agley, J.; Barnes, P.A.; Sherwood-Laughlin, C.; Nicholson-Crotty, J. A qualitative analysis of vaccine decision makers' conceptualization and fostering of 'community engagement' in India. *Int. J. Equity Health* **2020**, *19*, 185. [CrossRef]
20. Dror, A.A.; Eisenbach, N.; Taiber, S.; Morozov, N.G.; Mizrachi, M.; Zigron, A.; Srouji, S.; Sela, E. Vaccine hesitancy: The next challenge in the fight against COVID-19. *Eur. J. Epidemiol.* **2020**, *35*, 775–779. [CrossRef]
21. Wang, K.; Wong, E.L.; Ho, K.F.; Cheung, A.W.; Chan, E.Y.; Yeoh, E.K.; Wong, S.Y. Intention of nurses to accept coronavirus disease 2019 vaccination and change of intention to accept seasonal influenza vaccination during the coronavirus disease 2019 pandemic: A cross-sectional survey. *Vaccine* **2020**, *38*, 7049–7056. [CrossRef] [PubMed]
22. French, J.; Deshpande, S.; Evans, W.; Obregon, R. Key Guidelines in Developing a Pre-Emptive COVID-19 Vaccination Uptake Promotion Strategy. *Int. J. Environ. Res. Public Health* **2020**, *17*, 5893. [CrossRef]
23. Danchin, M.; Biezen, R.; Manski-Nankervis, J.A.; Kaufman, J.; Leask, J. Preparing the public for COVID-19 vaccines: How can general practitioners build vaccine confidence and optimize uptake for themselves and their patients? *Aust. J. Gen. Pract.* **2020**, *49*, 625. [CrossRef] [PubMed]
24. Watson, M.F.; Bacigalupe, G.; Daneshpour, M.; Han, W.J. Parra-Cardona R. COVID-19 interconnectedness: Health inequity, the climate crisis, and collective trauma. *Fam. Process* **2020**, *59*, 832–846. [CrossRef] [PubMed]
25. Albashtawy, M.; Gharaibeh, H.; Alhalaiqa, F.; Batiha, A.; Freij, M.; Saifan, A.; L-Awamreh, K.A.; Hamadneh, S.; L-Kloub, M.A.; Khamaiseh, A. The Health Belief Model's Impacts on the Use of Complementary and Alternative Medicine by Parents or Guardians of Children with Cancer. *Iran J. Public Health* **2016**, *45*, 708–709. [PubMed]
26. Ozawa, S.; Stack, M.L. Public trust and vaccine acceptance-international perspectives. *Hum. Vaccines Immunother.* **2013**, *9*, 1774–1778. [CrossRef]

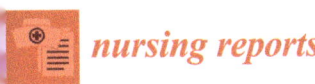 

Article

# Impacts of Coping Mechanisms on Nursing Students' Mental Health during COVID-19 Lockdown: A Cross-Sectional Survey

Son Chae Kim *, Christine Sloan, Anna Montejano and Carlota Quiban

School of Nursing, Point Loma Nazarene University, 2600 Laning Road, San Diego, CA 92106, USA; christinesloan@pointloma.edu (C.S.); amonteja@pointloma.edu (A.M.); carlotaquiban@pointloma.edu (C.Q.)
* Correspondence: skim@pointloma.edu

**Citation:** Kim, S.C.; Sloan, C.; Montejano, A.; Quiban, C. Impacts of Coping Mechanisms on Nursing Students' Mental Health during COVID-19 Lockdown: A Cross-Sectional Survey. *Nurs. Rep.* 2021, *11*, 36–44. https://doi.org/10.3390/nursrep11010004

Received: 30 November 2020
Accepted: 5 January 2021
Published: 12 January 2021

**Publisher's Note:** MDPI stays neutral with regard to jurisdictional claims in published maps and institutional affiliations.

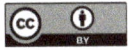

**Copyright:** © 2021 by the authors. Licensee MDPI, Basel, Switzerland. This article is an open access article distributed under the terms and conditions of the Creative Commons Attribution (CC BY) license (https://creativecommons.org/licenses/by/4.0/).

**Abstract:** The COVID-19 pandemic and consequent lockdown have precipitated significant disruption in the educational system. Nursing students are known to have higher levels of stress and anxiety than other non-nursing students, but there is a dearth of evidence regarding the impacts of the COVID-19 lockdown on their mental health and coping mechanisms. Purpose: The aim of this study was to explore the influence of coping mechanisms as predictors of stress, anxiety, and depression among nursing students during the COVID-19 lockdown. Methods: A cross-sectional online survey was conducted from 20 April to 10 May 2020 among 173 nursing students at a private university in Southern California, USA. Results: Self-reported stress, anxiety, and depression were significantly higher during the lockdown compared to the pre-lockdown period ($p < 0.001$). Almost a quarter of participants reported high stress, while more than half reported moderate-to-severe symptoms of anxiety and depression. High resilience was negatively associated with high stress (Odds Ratio (OR) = 0.46; 95% Confidence Interval (CI) = 0.22–0.98; $p = 0.045$), moderate-to-severe anxiety (OR = 0.47; 95%CI = 0.25–0.90; $p = 0.022$), and moderate-to-severe depression (OR = 0.50; 95%CI = 0.26–0.95; $p = 0.036$). Similarly, high family functioning was negatively associated with high stress (OR = 0.41; 95%CI = 0.20–0.86; $p = 0.018$), moderate-to-severe anxiety (OR = 0.41; 95%CI = 0.21–0.80; $p = 0.009$), and moderate-to-severe depression (OR = 0.41; 95%CI = 0.20–0.81; $p = 0.011$). High spiritual support was negatively associated with moderate-to-severe depression (OR = 0.48; 95%CI = 0.24–0.95; $p = 0.035$). Conclusions: During the COVID-19 lockdown, nursing students experienced remarkable levels of poor mental health. High levels of resilience and family functioning were associated with 2- to 2.4-fold lower risk of stress, anxiety, and depression, whereas high spiritual support was associated with 2-fold lower risk of depression. As the pandemic evolves, fostering these coping mechanisms may help students to maintain their psychological wellbeing.

**Keywords:** COVID-19; anxiety; stress; depression; coping mechanism; resilience; spirituality; family functioning

## 1. Introduction

The COVID-19 pandemic and subsequent mandatory lockdown to suppress transmission of the SARS-CoV-2 virus have caused significant global disruption of the educational system. According to the United Nations Educational, Scientific and Cultural Organization (UNESCO), more than a billion students globally have experienced closures of educational institutions during the pandemic [1]. In California, USA, the state governor issued a statewide mandatory stay-at-home order on 19 March 2020, resulting in the shutdown of face-to-face education for students [2]. For college students, the rapid shift from in-person to online learning, as well as concerns over educational progress and future job opportunities, contributed greatly to increased levels of stress and anxiety [3,4].

Before the pandemic, a national survey of 26,181 college students in USA reported that about a half were either diagnosed or treated for anxiety, depression, or panic attacks within the past year [5]. Nursing students experienced even higher levels of stress as they adjust to challenges of rigorous academic requirements as well as clinical demands, resulting in stress-related illnesses, depression, and sleep disturbances [6,7]. In China, the arrival of the COVID-19 pandemic has resulted in even higher levels of stress, anxiety, and depression among college students [8,9]. A study from Israel demonstrated that during the third week of COVID-19 lockdown, more than half of nursing students reported moderate-to-severe anxiety symptoms [10]. The study findings showed that female gender, concerns of academic progress, and fear of infection correlated with higher anxiety.

In addition to the immediate impact of the pandemic, previous studies of earlier coronavirus outbreaks have indicated that quarantine or lockdown can result in long-term psychological consequences [11]. Anxiety symptoms and feelings of anger remained present four to six months following quarantine during the Middle East Respiratory Syndrome (MERS) outbreak in Korea [12]. Furthermore, long-term consequences of psychological distress and burnout among nurses persisted nearly two years after the original Severe Acute Respiratory Syndrome (SARS) outbreak in Canada [13].

In managing psychological distress during epidemics, various coping mechanisms appear to be effective [14]. For example, having a support group for college students quarantined at home during the earlier SARS outbreak was found to be helpful [15]. Similarly, the presence of parental support was associated with lower anxiety among college students during the COVID-19 outbreak [16]. Spiritual support also seems to be an effective coping mechanism. College students with high spiritual support had greater personal happiness and satisfaction with life, as well as better adjustment to college life [17–19]. Minority college students with high spiritual support employed more problem-oriented coping behaviors, such as positive reinterpretation of adverse events, resulting in lower stress and better academic performance [20]. Resilience, another coping mechanism, refers to an individual's ability to bounce back from adversity and effectively respond to challenges [21]. Postgraduate nursing students exhibited a higher level of resilience than undergraduate nursing students, and the resilience was a positive predictor of perceived wellbeing [22]. Resilience was also positively associated with clinical communication ability and academic success [23,24]. During the COVID-19 pandemic, high resilience among nursing students was negatively associated with anxiety [10].

The psychological wellbeing of nursing students during the pandemic is critical for their academic success, and assessment of various coping mechanisms is necessary. However, there are limited studies on various coping mechanisms that enhance overall mental health of nursing students during the pandemic [10]. The aim of this study was to explore the influence of coping mechanisms as predictors of stress, anxiety, and depression among nursing students during the COVID-19 pandemic and subsequent lockdown.

## 2. Methods

### 2.1. Design and Sample

This cross-sectional study was conducted using an online survey platform Qualtrics XM (Provo, UT, USA) during the COVID-19 pandemic lockdown. All undergraduate and graduate nursing students enrolled in the spring semester 2020 at a private university in Southern California, USA were eligible to participate in the study.

### 2.2. Study Questionnaire

The study survey included valid and reliable instruments that measure resilience, spiritual support, family functioning, stress, anxiety, and depression. The respondents were asked to assess their current mental health status as well as to estimate their pre-lockdown mental health. Demographic information, including age, gender, ethnicity, and nursing program enrollment, was also collected.

The Connor–Davidson Resilience Scale (CD-RISC)-10 asks respondents to assess their adaptability in challenging situations and the ability to bounce back [25]. The response options on a 5-point Likert scale range from 0 (not true at all) to 4 (true all the time).

The possible maximal score is 40, with a higher score indicating higher resilience. The Cronbach's alpha was previously reported as 0.92 and was 0.83 in this study.

The 12-item Spirituality Support Scale evaluates respondents' perceived spiritual support from a higher power, religious faith, or beliefs on a 4-point Likert scale ranging from 1 (strongly disagree) to 4 (strongly agree) [26]. The summation scores range from 12 to 48, with a higher score indicating higher spiritual support. The Cronbach's alpha was previously reported as 0.97 and was 0.96 in this study.

The Family APGAR questionnaire measures satisfaction with support from family members [27]. It includes five indicators of family functioning: adaptation, partnership, growth, affection, and resolve, on a 3-point Likert scale ranging from 0 (hardly ever) to 2 (almost always). Scores of 8–10 indicate a highly functional family, while scores of 4–7 and 0–3 indicate moderate and severely dysfunctional families, respectively. The inter-item correlation coefficients were reported to be 0.63 to 0.71.

The Perceived Stress Scale (PSS) assesses respondents' perception of stress by eliciting thoughts and feelings during the past month [28]. It consists of 10 items in two subscales, including 6-item positive and 4-item negative factors on a 5-point Likert scale ranging from 0 (never) to 4 (very often). The responses of four items in the negative factor were reversed with possible total scores ranging from 0 to 40. Scores of 0–13, 14–26, and 27–40 were assessed as low, moderate, and high stress, respectively. Cronbach's alpha was previously reported as 0.83, and was 0.85 in this study.

The General Anxiety Disorder-7 (GAD-7) and Patient Health Questionnaire-9 (PHQ-9) are widely used tools that assess the symptoms of anxiety and depression, respectively [29]. The response options range from 0 (not at all) to 3 (nearly every day). Scores $\geq 10$ are considered moderate-to-severe anxiety or depression that potentially warrant further follow-up. The sensitivity and specificity of the GAD-7 for anxiety disorder were 72% and 80%, respectively. Similarly, the sensitivity and specificity of the PHQ-9 for the major depressive disorder were 88% and 88%, respectively.

### 2.3. Data Collection Procedures

The Institutional Review Board of the university approved this study (PLNU IRB ID#17877). Recruitment emails containing a hyperlink to the online survey were sent to all nursing students enrolled in the spring semester 2020. Written informed consent was waived due to minimal risk associated with participation. Students were assured that their participation in the study was confidential and voluntary. They were also reminded that participation or lack thereof would not affect their course grades or relationship with the school. Completion of the online survey indicated their consent to the study. Data were collected from 20 April to 10 May 2020, and at study closure, a $10 gift card was given to 10 randomly selected students. This study was carried out following the rules of the Declaration of Helsinki.

### 2.4. Data Analysis

In this study, poor mental health was defined using the symptom severity cutoff scores for high stress (PSS scores $\geq 27$), moderate-to-severe anxiety (GAD-7 scores $\geq 10$), and moderate-to-severe depression (PHQ-9 scores $\geq 10$). Coping mechanisms were categorized into dichotomous variables using the following cutoff scores: CD-RISC-10 scores $\geq$ median of 29 (high resilience); Spirituality Support Scale scores $\geq$ median of 36 (high spiritual support); and family APGAR scores $\geq 8$ (high family functioning).

Descriptive statistics summarized sample characteristics and key study variables. Wilcoxon signed-rank tests were performed to compare the median scores of high stress, moderate-to-severe anxiety, and moderate-to-severe depression before and during the lockdown. Kendall's tau correlation procedures were performed to explore potential correlations between the dichotomous variables of poor mental health, coping mechanisms, and demographic variables. Statistically significant demographic variables and coping mechanisms were entered into multivariate logistic regression models to explore the influence of coping mechanisms as predictors of poor mental health. All statistical analyses were performed using SPSS software, version 26.0 (IBM Corporation, Armonk, NY, USA). The level of significance level was set at $p$-value < 0.05, and all tests were two-tailed.

## 3. Results

### 3.1. Sample Characteristics

Of 447 students invited, 173 completed the survey and were included in the statistical analysis (38.7% participation rate). The average age was 25 years old, and most were female (93.1%). More than half were white (57.8%) and pre-licensure undergraduate students (76.8%). Almost a quarter (23.1%) were registered nurses enrolled in graduate programs or a baccalaureate degree completion program. About 14 percent had worked with COVID-19 patients, while three quarters had experienced quarantine or self-isolation during the pandemic (75.7%). For coping mechanisms, the median (IQR) scores of resilience, spiritual support, and family functioning were 29 (25, 32), 36 (33, 43), and 9 (6.5, 10), respectively.

### 3.2. Mental Health before and during COVID-19 Lockdown

Compared with the pre-lockdown period, students reported higher stress (median [IQR]; 16 [13, 18] vs. 23 [18, 26.3]; $p < 0.001$), moderate-to-severe anxiety (median [IQR]; 4 [2, 8.3] vs. 10 [5, 15]; $p < 0.001$), and moderate-to-severe depression (median [IQR]; 3 [1, 6] vs. 10 [4, 15]; $p < 0.001$) during the lockdown. Similarly, more students experienced high stress (4.1% vs. 24.7%), moderate-to-severe anxiety (19.4% vs. 55.2%), and moderate-to-severe depression (12.9% vs. 51.5%) during the lockdown (Figure 1).

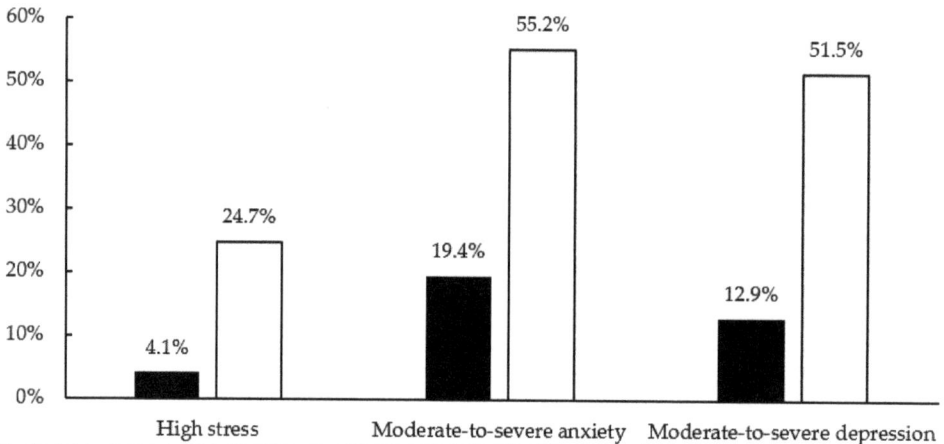

**Figure 1.** Poor mental health status before and during COVID-19 lockdown ($N$ = 173). Black bars and white bars represent the poor mental health status before and during the COVID-19 lockdown, respectively. High stress = Perceived Stress Scale scores $\geq$ 27; moderate-to-severe anxiety = GAD-7 scores $\geq$ 10; moderate-to-severe depression = PHQ-9 scores $\geq$ 10.

### 3.3. Predictors of Poor Mental Health

Table 1 shows bivariate Kendall's tau correlations between coping mechanisms and poor mental health. High resilience and high family functioning were negatively correlated with high stress, moderate-to-severe anxiety, and moderate-to-severe depression ($p < 0.05$). Similarly, there were significant negative correlations between high spiritual support and anxiety and depression. By contrast, none of the demographic variables correlated significantly with high stress, moderate-to-severe anxiety, or moderate-to-severe depression.

**Table 1.** Correlations with poor mental health during COVID-19 lockdown (N = 173).

|  | High Stress (r) | Moderate-to-Severe Anxiety (r) | Moderate-to-Severe Depression (r) |
|---|---|---|---|
| Age | −0.07 | −0.14 | −0.09 |
| Female | 0.09 | 0.01 | 0.03 |
| Pre-licensure undergraduate students | 0.11 | 0.02 | 0.06 |
| Quarantine or self-isolation experience | 0.10 | 0.06 | −0.03 |
| High resilience [a] | −0.20 * | −0.22 ** | −0.23 ** |
| High family functioning [b] | −0.22 ** | −0.24 ** | −0.28 *** |
| High spiritual support [c] | −0.08 | −0.21 * | −0.24 ** |

* $p < 0.05$; ** $p < 0.01$; *** $p < 0.001$ by Kendall's Tau test. High stress = Perceived Stress Scale scores $\geq 27$; moderate-to-severe anxiety = GAD-7 scores $\geq 10$; moderate-to-severe depression = PHQ-9 scores $\geq 10$. [a] CD-RISC-10 scores $\geq 29$; [b] Family APGAR scores $\geq 8$; [c] Spirituality Support Scale scores $\geq 36$.

The results of multivariate logistic regression procedures are shown in Table 2. High resilience was a significant predictor of lower risks of high stress (Odds Ratios (OR) = 0.46; 95% Confidence Interval (CI) = 0.22–0.98; $p = 0.045$), moderate-to-severe anxiety (OR = 0.47; 95%CI = 0.25–0.90; $p = 0.022$), and moderate-to-severe depression (OR = 0.50; 95%CI = 0.26–0.95; $p = 0.036$). Similarly, high family functioning was also a significant predictor of lower risks of high stress (OR = 0.41; 95%CI = 0.20–0.86; $p = 0.018$), moderate-to-severe anxiety (OR = 0.41; 95%CI = 0.21–0.80; $p = 0.009$), and moderate-to-severe depression (OR = 0.41; 95%CI = 0.20–0.81; $p = 0.011$). In addition, high spiritual support was a significant predictor of lower risk of depression (OR = 0.48; 95%CI = 0.24–0.95; $p = 0.035$).

**Table 2.** Predictors of poor mental health during COVID-19 lockdown (N = 173).

|  | OR | 95%CI | p-Value |
|---|---|---|---|
| **High stress** |  |  |  |
| High resilience [a] | 0.46 | 0.22–0.98 | 0.045 |
| High family functioning [b] | 0.41 | 0.20–0.86 | 0.018 |
| **Moderate-to-severe anxiety** |  |  |  |
| High resilience [a] | 0.47 | 0.25–0.90 | 0.022 |
| High family functioning [b] | 0.41 | 0.21–0.80 | 0.009 |
| **Moderate-to-severe depression** |  |  |  |
| High resilience [a] | 0.50 | 0.26–0.95 | 0.036 |
| High family functioning [b] | 0.41 | 0.20–0.81 | 0.011 |
| High spiritual support [c] | 0.48 | 0.24–0.95 | 0.035 |

OR = odds ratio; CI = confidence interval. High stress = Perceived Stress Scale scores $\geq 27$; moderate-to-severe anxiety = GAD-7 scores $\geq 10$; moderate-to-severe depression = PHQ-9 scores $\geq 10$; [a] CD-RISC-10 scores $\geq 29$; [b] Family APGAR scores $\geq 8$; [c] Spirituality Support Scale scores $\geq 36$.

## 4. Discussion

It is remarkable how much the COVID-19 lockdown has impacted the psychological wellbeing of nursing students. The proportion of students with high stress level during the lockdown jumped 6-fold compared to the pre-lockdown period, while moderate-to-severe anxiety and depression increased nearly 3–4-fold. Interestingly, psychological distress appears to be ameliorated by potentially modifiable factors, such as resilience, family functioning, and spiritual support. In multivariate analyses, high resilience and family functioning were independently associated with a 2- to 2.4-fold lower risk of high stress, moderate-to-severe anxiety, and moderate-to-severe depression. In addition, high spiritual support was also independently associated with 2-fold lower risk of moderate-to-severe depression. By contrast, demographic variables, such as age, educational background, or ethnicity, showed no correlation with poor mental health during the lockdown.

It is plausible that resilience, family functioning, and spiritual support among nursing students can be nurtured so that they can better manage unexpected challenges impacting psychological equilibrium. For example, a randomized controlled trial (RCT) of resilience training based on cognitive behavior therapy among newly licensed registered nurses showed significant decreases in stress, anxiety, and depression [30,31]. Perhaps, resilience and spiritual support are complimentary coping mechanisms. Spiritual support arises from a sense of connection to an external higher power, whereas resilience is one's internal capacity to bounce back and adapt to stressful circumstances [32–35]. In our study, about half of the students reported moderate-to-severe anxiety and depression during the lockdown, which is consistent with a study of nursing students in Israel that reported more than half with anxiety [10]. However, other dimensions of psychological distress, such as perceived stress and depression, were not assessed in this previous study. Another study among university students and associates in Germany also showed higher levels of health anxiety during the COVID-19 pandemic compared to pre-pandemic [36]. High family function as a protective factor against poor mental health is consistent with another previous study. Among college students in China, lower anxiety symptoms were associated with living with parents during the COVID-19 pandemic [16]. Although these authors did not assess family functioning as a coping mechanism, it is likely that simply living with parents during isolation reduces symptoms of anxiety and depression among college students.

*4.1. Implications for Nursing Education*

The COVID-19 pandemic has caused significant disruption in education worldwide. Although most colleges have shifted to online learning, nursing schools must continue to have clinical practicums, which require students to work in close contact with patients. The concern of viral transmission and the unpredictable progression of the COVID-19 pandemic may further increase students' uncertainty of academic advancement and affect their mental health negatively. Therefore, it is imperative for nurse educators to help students to identify and develop optimal coping strategies to minimize anxiety due to the pandemic. Providing clear guidelines for infection control will help students to feel confident about their safety and minimize stress as they work with patients. Furthermore, it is critical to provide a supportive learning environment that helps students to develop effective coping strategies [32]. For example, nursing school can develop and integrate a resilience-building program throughout the nursing curriculum to assist students in managing stress associated with academic, social, and personal challenges. Such a resilience-building program may include mindfulness-based stress reduction strategies, muscle relaxation exercise, self-care, communication skills, problem-solving skills, or study skills. These activities may be implemented via lectures, reflective journaling, experience sharing, role-playing, or homework assignments [33]. Studies have shown that such programs can help students to utilize effective coping strategies and time management, which improves mental health and academic success [33–35,37]. In addition, tailored resilience interventions based on needs assessment and skill-building activities may be helpful [36]. Given the need for social distancing, online platforms may also be useful for spiritual and peer support, as well as resilience training to enhance psychological wellbeing [15,38,39].

*4.2. Limitations*

There are several limitations to this study. Because this was a cross-sectional study, the resilience, family functioning, and spiritual support as predictors of mental health should not be taken as a cause-and-effect relationship. Such a causal relationship can be determined only through interventional studies. Second, less than 40% of the enrolled students completed the survey, which is not unusual for an online survey. However, this may have introduced a selection bias. Third, the self-reported data collection method could have over- or underestimated the symptoms of stress, anxiety, and depression. Fourth, pre-lockdown data were collected retrospectively, which may have introduced recall bias. Fifth, this study was conducted in spring 2020 during the initial wave of the COVID-19 pandemic in the US. Thereafter, the pandemic has evolved rapidly with subsequent case spikes, as well as the advent of improved treatments and vaccines. Therefore, the study findings may be most applicable to the initial phase of such pandemics. Finally, the study findings are based on a relatively small sample size from a single institution and may not be broadly generalizable. Future interventional studies are needed to confirm these study findings as well as to determine the effectiveness of fostering coping mechanisms among nursing students.

## 5. Conclusions

During the COVID-19 lockdown, nursing students experienced remarkable levels of poor mental health. This study showed that high resilience, family functioning, and spiritual support were predictors of lower stress, anxiety, and depression. As the pandemic evolves, fostering these coping mechanisms may help students to maintain their psychological wellbeing.

**Author Contributions:** Conceptualization, S.C.K., C.S., A.M., and C.Q.; methodology, S.C.K., C.S., A.M., and C.Q.; software, C.S.; validation, S.C.K.; formal analysis, S.C.K.; investigation, S.C.K., C.S., A.M., and C.Q.; resources, S.C.K.; data curation, C.S.; writing—original draft preparation, S.C.K., C.S., and A.M.; writing—review and editing, S.C.K., C.S., A.M., and C.Q.; visualization, S.C.K.; supervision, S.C.K.; project administration, S.C.K.; All authors have read and agreed to the published version of the manuscript.

**Funding:** This research received no external funding.

**Institutional Review Board Statement:** The study was conducted according to the guidelines of the Declaration of Helsinki, and approved by the Institutional Review Board of Point Loma Nazarene University (IRB ID# 17877, 20 April 2020).

**Informed Consent Statement:** Subject consent was waived due to no more than minimal risks involved in this online survey study.

**Data Availability Statement:** The data presented in this study are available on request from the corresponding author. The data are not publically available due to ethical considerations.

**Conflicts of Interest:** The authors declare no conflict of interest.

## References

1. United Nations Educational, Scientific and Cultural Organization (UNESCO). COVID-19 Educational Disruption and Response. 2020. Available online: https://en.unesco.org/covid19/educationresponse (accessed on 10 July 2020).
2. Executive Department, State of California. Executive Order N-33-20. 2020. Available online: https://www.politico.com/states/f/?id=00000170-f5a4-d209-af70-fdae4c930000 (accessed on 22 June 2020).
3. Dewart, G.; Corcoran, L.; Thirsk, L.; Petrovic, K. Nursing education in a pandemic: Academic challenges in response to COVID-19. *Nurse Educ. Today* **2020**, *92*, 104471. [CrossRef]
4. Elmer, T.; Mepham, K.; Stadtfeld, C. Students under lockdown: Comparisons of students' social networks and mental health before and during the COVID-19 crisis in Switzerland. *PLoS ONE* **2020**, *15*, e0236337. [CrossRef]
5. American College Health Association. National College Health Assessment: Reference Group Executive Summary. 2018. Available online: https://www.acha.org/documents/ncha/NCHA-II_Fall_2018_Reference_Group_Executive_Summary.pdf (accessed on 7 July 2020).
6. Bartlett, M.L.; Taylor, H.; Nelson, J.D. Comparison of mental health characteristics and stress between baccalaureate nursing students and non-nursing students. *J. Nurs. Educ.* **2016**, *55*, 87–90. [CrossRef]
7. Chen, C.J.; Chen, Y.C.; Sung, H.C.; Hsieh, T.C.; Lee, M.S.; Chang, C.Y. The prevalence and related factors of depressive symptoms among junior college nursing students: A cross-sectional study. *J. Psychiatr. Ment. Health Nurs.* **2015**, *22*, 590–598. [CrossRef] [PubMed]
8. Wang, C.; Pan, R.; Wan, X.; Tan, Y.; Xu, L.; Ho, C.S.; Ho, R.C. Immediate psychological responses and associated factors during the initial stage of the 2019 coronavirus disease (COVID-19) epidemic among the general population in China. *Int. J. Environ. Res. Public Health.* **2020**, *17*, 1729. [CrossRef] [PubMed]
9. Wang, C.; Zhao, H. The impact of COVID-19 on anxiety in Chinese university students. *Front. Psychol.* **2020**, *11*, 1168. [CrossRef] [PubMed]
10. Savitsky, B.; Findling, Y.; Ereli, A.; Hendel, T. Anxiety and coping strategies among nursing students during the COVID-19 pandemic. *Nurse Educ. Pract.* **2020**, *46*, 102809. [CrossRef] [PubMed]

11. Brooks, S.K.; Webster, R.K.; Smith, L.E.; Woodland, L.; Wessely, S.; Greenberg, N.; Rubin, G.J. The psychological impact of quarantine and how to reduce it: Rapid review of the evidence. *Lancet* **2020**, *395*, 912–920. [CrossRef]
12. Jeong, H.; Yim, H.W.; Song, Y.J.; Ki, M.; Min, J.A.; Cho, J.; Chae, J.H. Mental health status of people isolated due to Middle East Respiratory Syndrome. *Epidemiol. Health* **2016**, *38*, e2016048. [CrossRef]
13. Maunder, R.G.; Lancee, W.J.; Balderson, K.E.; Bennett, J.P.; Borgundvaag, B.; Evans, S.; Fernandes, C.M.; Goldbloom, D.S.; Gupta, M.; Hunter, J.J.; et al. Long-term psychological and occupational effects of providing hospital healthcare during SARS outbreak. *Emerg. Infect. Dis.* **2006**, *12*, 1924–1932. [CrossRef]
14. Brooks, S.K.; Dunn, R.; Amlot, R.; Rubin, G.J.; Greenberg, N. A systematic, thematic review of social and occupational factors associated with psychological outcomes in healthcare employees during an infectious disease outbreak. *J. Occup. Environ. Med.* **2018**, *60*, 248–257. [CrossRef] [PubMed]
15. Pan, P.; Chang, S.; Yu, Y. A support group for home-quarantined college students exposed to SARS: Learning from practice. *J. Spec. Group Work* **2006**, *30*, 363–374. [CrossRef]
16. Cao, W.; Fang, Z.; Hou, G.; Han, M.; Xu, X.; Dong, J.; Zheng, J. The psychological impact of the COVID-19 epidemic on college students in China. *Psychiatry Res.* **2020**, *287*, 112934. [CrossRef] [PubMed]
17. Francis, L.J.; Ok, U.; Robbins, M. Religion and happiness: A study among university students in Turkey. *J. Relig. Health* **2017**, *56*, 1335–1347. [CrossRef] [PubMed]
18. Ross, K.; Handal, P.J.; Clark, E.M.; Vander Wal, J.S. The relationship between religion and religious coping: Religious coping as a moderator between religion and adjustment. *J. Relig. Health* **2009**, *48*, 454–467. [CrossRef] [PubMed]
19. Bryan, J.L.; Lucas, S.; Quist, M.C.; Steers, M.N.; Foster, D.W.; Young, C.M.; Lu, Q. God, can I tell you something? The effect of religious coping on the relationship between anxiety over emotional expression, anxiety, and depressive symptoms. *Psychol. Relig. Spirit.* **2016**, *8*, 46–53. [CrossRef]
20. Greer, T.M.; Brown, P. Minority status and coping processes among African American college students. *J. Divers. High. Educ.* **2011**, *4*, 26–38. [CrossRef]
21. Cleary, M.; Visentin, D.; West, S.; Lopez, V.; Kornhaber, R. Promoting emotional intelligence and resilience in undergraduate nursing students: An integrative review. *Nurse Educ. Today* **2018**, *68*, 112–120. [CrossRef]
22. Chow, K.M.; Tang, W.K.F.; Chan, W.H.C.; Sit, W.H.J.; Choi, K.C.; Chan, S. Resilience and well-being of university nursing students in Hong Kong: A cross-sectional study. *BMC Med. Educ.* **2018**, *18*, 13. [CrossRef]
23. Kong, L.; Liu, Y.; Li, G.; Fang, Y.; Kang, X.; Li, P. Resilience moderates the relationship between emotional intelligence and clinical communication ability among Chinese practice nursing students: A structural equation model analysis. *Nurse Educ. Today* **2016**, *46*, 64–68. [CrossRef]
24. Slatyer, S.; Cramer, J.; Pugh, J.D.; Twigg, D.E. Barriers and enablers to retention of Aboriginal diploma of nursing students in Western Australia: An exploratory descriptive study. *Nurse Educ. Today* **2016**, *42*, 17–22. [CrossRef] [PubMed]
25. Connor, K.M.; Davidson, J.R.T. Development of a new resilience scale: The Connor-Davidson Resilience Scale (CD-RISC). *Depress. Anxiety* **2003**, *18*, 76–82. [CrossRef] [PubMed]
26. Ai, A.L.; Tice, T.N.; Peterson, C.; Huang, B. Prayers, spiritual support, and positive attitudes in coping with the September 11 national crisis. *J. Personal.* **2005**, *73*, 763–791. [CrossRef] [PubMed]
27. Smilkstein, G.; Ashworth, C.; Montano, D. Validity and reliability of the family APGAR as a test of family function. *J. Fam. Pract.* **1982**, *15*, 303–311. [PubMed]
28. Cohen, S.; Kamarck, T.; Mermelstein, R. A global measure of perceived stress. *J. Health Soc. Behav.* **1983**, *24*, 385–396. [CrossRef]
29. Spitzer, R.L.; Kroenke, K.; Williams, J.B.; Lowe, B. A brief measure for assessing generalized anxiety disorder: The GAD-7. *Arch. Intern. Med.* **2006**, *166*, 1092–1097. [CrossRef]
30. Sampson, M.; Melnyk, B.M.; Hoying, J. Intervention effects of the MINDBODYSTRONG cognitive behavioral skills building program on newly licensed registered nurses' mental health, healthy lifestyle behaviors, and job satisfaction. *J. Nurs. Adm.* **2019**, *49*, 487–495. [CrossRef]
31. Sampson, M.; Melnyk, B.M.; Hoying, J. The MINDBODYSTRONG intervention for new nurse residents: 6-month effects on mental health outcomes, healthy lifestyle behaviors, and job satisfaction. *Worldviews Evid. Based Nurs.* **2020**, *17*, 16–23. [CrossRef]
32. Huang, L.; Xu, F.; Liu, H. Emotional responses and coping strategies of nurses and nursing college students during COVID-19 outbreak. *MedRxiv* **2020**. [CrossRef]
33. Boardman, L. Building resilience in nursing students: Implementing techniques to foster success. *Int. J. Emerg. Ment. Health Hum. Resil.* **2016**, *18*, 1–5.
34. Rios-Risquez, M.I.; Garcia-Izquierdo, M.; Sabuco-Tebar, E.L.; Carrillo-Garcia, C.; Martinez-Roche, M.E. An exploratory study of the relationship between resilience, academic burnout and psychological health in nursing students. *Contemp. Nurse* **2016**, *52*, 430–439. [CrossRef]
35. Onan, N.; Karaca, S.; Unsal Barlas, G. Evaluation of a stress coping course for psychological resilience among a group of university nursing students. *Perspect. Psychiatr. Care* **2019**, *55*, 233–238. [CrossRef] [PubMed]
36. Sauer, K.S.; Jungmann, S.M.; Witthöft, M. Emotional and behavioral consequences of the COVID-19 pandemic: The role of health anxiety, intolerance of uncertainty, and distress (in)tolerance. *Int. J. Environ. Res. Public Health* **2020**, *17*, 7241. [CrossRef] [PubMed]
37. Lanz, J.J. Evidence-based resilience interventions for nursing students: A randomized controlled pilot trial. *Int. J. Appl. Posit. Psychol.* **2020**, *5*, 217–230. [CrossRef]

38. Ho, C.S.; Chee, C.Y.; Ho, R.C. Mental health strategies to combat the psychological impact of COVID-19 beyond paranoia and panic. *Ann. Acad. Med. Singap.* **2020**, *49*, 155–160. [CrossRef] [PubMed]
39. Joyce, S.; Shand, F.; Lal, T.J.; Mott, B.; Bryant, R.A.; Harvey, S.B. Resilience@Work mindfulness program: Results from a cluster randomized controlled trial with first responders. *J. Med. Internet Res.* **2019**, *21*, e12894. [CrossRef]

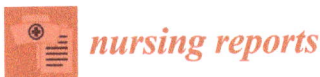 

Article

# Blessings and Curses: Exploring the Experiences of New Mothers during the COVID-19 Pandemic

Phillip Joy [1,*], Megan Aston [2], Sheri Price [2], Meaghan Sim [2], Rachel Ollivier [2], Britney Benoit [3], Neda Akbari-Nassaji [4] and Damilola Iduye [2]

1. Department of Applied Human Nutrition, Mount Saint Vincent University, Halifax, NS B3M 2J6, Canada
2. School of Nursing, Dalhousie University, Halifax, NS B3H 4R2, Canada; megan.aston@dal.ca (M.A.); sheri.price@iwk.nshealth.ca (S.P.); meaghan.sim@dal.ca (M.S.); rachel.ollivier@dal.ca (R.O.); damilola.iduye@dal.ca (D.I.)
3. Rankin School of Nursing, St. Francis Xavier University, Antigonish, NS B2G 2W5, Canada; bbenoit@stfx.ca
4. School of Nursing, Abadan Faculty of Medical Sciences, Abadan, Iran; neda.akbari@dal.ca
* Correspondence: phillip.joy@msvu.ca

Received: 25 November 2020; Accepted: 15 December 2020; Published: 21 December 2020

**Abstract:** The aim of this study was to explore the postpartum experiences of new parents during the COVID-19 pandemic. The postpartum period can be a time of significant transition, both positive and negative, for parents as they navigate new relationships with their babies and shifts in family dynamics. Physical distancing requirements mandated by public health orders during the COVID-19 pandemic had the potential to create even more stress for parents with a newborn. Examining personal experiences would provide health care professionals with information to help guide support during significant isolation. Feminist poststructuralism guided the qualitative research process. Sixty-eight new mothers completed an open-ended on-line survey. Responses were analyzed using discourse analysis to examine the beliefs, values, and practices of the participants relating to their family experiences during the pandemic period. It was found that pandemic isolation was a time of complexity with both 'blessings and curses'. Participants reported that it was a time for family bonding and enjoyment of being a new parent without the usual expectations. It was also a time of missed opportunities as they were not able to share milestones and memories with extended family. Caring for a newborn during the COVID-19 pandemic where complex contradictions were constructed by competing social discourses created difficult dichotomies for families. In acknowledging the complex experiences of mothers during COVID-19 isolation, nurses and midwives can come to understand and help new parents to focus on the blessings of this time while acknowledging the curses.

**Keywords:** family; bonding; COVID-19; mother; post-partum

## 1. Introduction

The postpartum period is often a complex time for new parents. Social, cultural, and medical discourses have created norms and shaped the beliefs, values, and practices of new parents during this time. These discourses position the postpartum period as a time for new parents to bond and form connections not only with their baby but within their larger family. Postpartum is well acknowledged as an opportunity for family-forming [1]. Social, health, and nursing discourses of mother-child bonding are dominant during this period and positions such bonding as critical for the development of healthy relationships, positive mental health and confident parents [2,3].

Family health nursing is a specialty clinical practice that focuses on understanding how relations within the family impact their health [4,5]. Decades of research have demonstrated the need to understand the family as a unit where " ... family has a significant impact on the health and well-being of individual members (p. 1)" [6]. However, the family does not operate in isolation and supportive relations with extended family, friends, health care professionals, and others are extremely important [6,7].

The postpartum period is also a time for much needed social support [2]. New parents often seek and need social support for a variety of reasons from extended family members, friends, other parents outside their immediate social networks, nurses, midwives, lactation consultants, and other health care professionals. It is a time when new parents learn about their babies and when new families adapt to their changing experiences and the expectations placed upon them. Social discourses about the role of mothers perpetuates knowledge about what it means to be a mother and (re)creates many expectations for them [8,9]. New parents are challenged to balance new parental roles, work, extended family relations, and a myriad of other responsibilities while also attempting to enjoy these early moments with their baby [10].

Postpartum is also a period of time in which new parents are tasked to ensure they start their babies off onto the "right" path to be successful, whether this involves creating loving moments of family bonding, socialization with their babies, or ensuring proper nutrition [9]. Emotional and social well-being of infants and children are significant parts of these expectations. In the field of psychology, research continues to examine the emotional and psychological development of children and correlations with socialization and behaviour. Brownell [11] states: " ... socialization of prosocial behavior occurs continuously via social engagement beginning at birth. Because the infant participates actively and eagerly in social and emotional exchanges, socialization encompasses more than top-down teaching or shaping processes and selected social-learning processes such as imitation. Instead, socialization includes many bidirectional social processes, some of which are quite subtle (p. 223)".

Furthermore, social networking for new parents is one way to seek out relationships with other parents to share information, experience support and gain confidence in their parenting abilities with their newborns [12–17]. Social networking occurs both online and offline with the purpose of facilitating supportive meeting spaces for babies and parents. Research has identified that peer and social supports are essential in the postpartum period to improve outcomes such as breastfeeding or maternal mental health, including postpartum depression [18–21].

Isolation can put parents at risk for mental health issues; therefore, connections between people can help to alleviate some of the risks. Postpartum programs and services offered by health care professional and community groups all focus on supporting the physical, emotional, and social well-being of parents. Our research to date has demonstrated that social networking is an essential part of the postpartum period [22,23] and is important for both parents and babies to ensure healthy short term and long term mental and emotional health. The COVID-19 pandemic has significantly reduced opportunities for parents to gather or meet with family, friends, other parents and health care professionals [16,24–26]. Therefore, examining the postpartum experiences of parents during the COVID-19 pandemic and required self-isolation, enabled us to examine how parents in Nova Scotia coped with the social and relational aspects of postpartum.

The overarching aim of this study was to examine parents' experiences of the postpartum period during the mandated health protection orders in response to the COVID-19 pandemic. The research also explored how various social and institutional discourses shaped their experiences. The research question was 'How do parents experience the postpartum period during COVID-19'?

## 2. Experimental Section

### 2.1. Theoretical Framework

Feminist poststructuralism was used as the guiding methodology [27–32] as it provided a way to understand how experiences were personally, socially and institutionally constructed through different subject positions. A feminist poststructuralist methodology allowed us to look for moments of negotiation to understand how different beliefs, values, and practices were constructed through relations of power between people [27–32]. The concept of subjectivity enabled us to examine how participants felt in relation to others (health professionals, family or peers). The concept of agency guided our analysis to consider how all individuals have power and therefore the potential to control their lives and make change [27–32]. Feminist poststructuralist methodology is based on the belief that participants are the primary experts of their experiences, and therefore are credible sources of data who are self-reflexive, conscious of their own locations (social, historical, gendered, cultural, racial, sexual), able to question, challenge, and possibly change their own circumstances. They also have the potential to recognize the oppressive nature of social structures, stereotypes, and ideologies. The study employed the Standards for Reporting Qualitative Research (SRQR) [33].

## 2.2. The Researchers

The team consists of nursing and health experts in the area of maternal child and infant health, public health nursing, women's, family, and community health. Members of the team use qualitative methodologies, in particular feminist poststructuralism to explore how the health practices of individuals and families in modern society are shaped by historical contexts. Several members are registered nurses within Canada.

## 2.3. Context of the Study

The study took place in Nova Scotia, Canada. Approval for the study was received through the IWK Health Centre's Research Ethics Board (#1025663). Data was collected from May to June 2020, which represented the emergence of the recovery period of the COVID-19 pandemic in Nova Scotia, Canada. The peak COVID-19 or first wave of the COV-19 pandemic period was March and April 2020. During this time, the provincial public health measures were implemented within the province. The public health order was for households to stay physically distanced from one another. This requirement was from March to May, at which point the bubble family was introduced (early May), followed by small groups of less than 10 outdoors. Self-isolation (or isolation/quarantine) was much more restrictive and for certain persons/families, such as those that travelled outside the province. Following the public health orders, travel was restricted, and many workplaces were either closed or employees were instructed to work from home, if possible. Many retail stores and resources for new mothers, such as daycares, family resource centres, and public libraries, were also closed, although grocery stores remained open. Hospital services were restricted, and many consultations were done virtually (via phone or through the use of other technologies) rather than in person [34]. All of these factors led to periods of isolation experienced by the parents/families in this study and the inability to access their usual support networks.

## 2.4. The Qualitative Survey and Participants

Parents (biological, adoptive, foster, kin) who self-identified as the primary caretakers of a newborn baby aged 0–12 months during the time of the COVID-19 pandemic (beginning March 2020) were recruited through social media recruitment to participate in an on-line open ended survey. Participants were encouraged to write as much as they wanted to describe their experiences within their families, as well as any supports they may have had during this period. Specifically, three opened ended questions were asked. These questions were (1) Tell us about your experience at home with your new baby and how the situation created by the COVID-19 pandemic affected you and your family; (2) Tell us about your experience of support (from friends, family, healthcare professionals) during the COVID-19 pandemic; and (3) Tell us about your experience of searching for and receiving information about caring for yourself, your baby, and your family during the COVID-19 pandemic. Responses varied in length.

We recruited 68 participants to complete the qualitative survey. All participants lived in the province of Nova Scotia in Canada, with over two thirds of them living in cities or towns in the province. Although we purposefully put out a call to include a variety of parents/guardians, all participants self-identified as mothers who gave birth within the last year and predominantly identified as heterosexual, white women. Most participants were living with their partners, with only a few identifying as a single parent. Approximately half of the participants reported having other children in their care during this time.

*2.5. Data Analysis*

Discourse analysis was used to analyze the data. Consistent with the feminist poststructuralist approach of the research, the use of discourse analysis [29] enabled the meaning of personal experiences to be deconstructed as a means of exploring how they related to social and institutional beliefs, values and practices. Discourse analysis is a non-linear process that attempts to look beyond the surface meanings of text to situate them within historical, political, social, and cultural contexts [29]. For this process, we paid close attention to language, meaning and relationships between participants, others and the health care system. All researchers independently reviewed the participants' responses and noted the beliefs, values, and practices of the participants relating to their family experiences during the pandemic period, the language of the participants, as well as any tensions expressed. The team met as a whole to discuss the independent analysis and came to a consensus on the final discursive considerations.

Several key characteristics, such as rigor, trustworthiness, and credibility were attained through various processes. For example, the maintenance of accurate documentation, an audit trail that included detailed notes on the way responses were analyzed by each team member, positionality and reflections of researchers, and notes that recorded the ongoing discussions between the team during the analysis ensured rigor, trustworthiness, and creditability [35].

## 3. Results

This research revealed that public health orders due to COVID-19 pandemic created situations where the majority of parents had to negotiate complex family relationships that were often expressed as a duality between positive (blessings) and negative (curses) experiences. The period of isolation during COVID-19 was seen as both emotionally stressful and emotionally rewarding for many of the participants. Most participants responded with personal examples of the complexity of experiences, their comments discussing what they enjoyed during the postpartum period, while also moving on to discuss the tensions and stresses of their experiences.

The nature of qualitative analysis is often complex and not easily separated into distinct sections. As such, we present in this section not only the results but also the analysis of the associated social discourses. The first Section 3.1 examines the construction of positive experiences/ "blessings" through discourses and the second Section 3.2 examines the construction of challenges/ "curses" through discourses. Participants' quotes are used throughout to represent the discursive considerations.

*3.1. The Blessings*

In this study, we define blessings as a beneficial thing for which one is grateful and something that brings well-being. The following section explores the various positive blessings that the participants perceived from their experiences during COVID-19. The described blessings that resulted from following public health orders were multi-faceted and took many forms in the data.

*3.2. The Blessings of Freedom*

One such blessing was participants' freedom to enjoy their babies. A common experience for many mothers was the feeling of freedom from social expectations, including fulfilling the dominant socially constructed roles and identities set before many new moms, as illustrated in the following quote.

> COVID has been a blessing and a nightmare for our new family ... [our baby] gets a lot more daddy time every day and I get help during the day if I need it ... I now feel no pressure

to be a "super mom". I just focus on spending time with her [baby] and enjoying her baby days. I know if the pandemic hadn't happened, I'd be out doing "mommy and me" classes, doing visits, and generally trying to be more productive.

The requirement for families to stay within their own household was seen as a blessing for many of the participants because it created a sense of freedom from the social expectations placed upon new mothers to engage in "productive", externally-focused activities, like mommy classes, visits from family members and friends, and other activities. Instead of feeling obligated by societal pressures and a cultural discourse of productivity to participate in new mother activities and obligations, several participants were able to find a relief from these pressures.

It is interesting to look at how the participant in the quote above constructed the word 'productivity' outside of the home. This dichotomy has been created through a cultural discourse of productivity that gives more respect to work outside the family or household unit [36]. Parenting has been socially constructed to be less visible and less respected compared to work outside the home, an issue that is highly influenced by the gendered norms within society that also work to devalue emotional labour [36]. This socially constructed meaning about caring for a new baby often leads to unrealistic expectations for mothers to 'do it all' while caring for their children [36]. Previous research has shown that pressures to do the right things, and to be a "super mommy" can add a lot of pressure and stress to the experiences of new motherhood [8,9]. Many of the participants in our study expressed similar experiences of feeling less pressure to have to do it all. One participant said, "I found it great to bond as a family" and another stated "spending a lot of time doing things together ... relaxed and no pressure to go anywhere".

### 3.3. The Blessings of Quiet Enjoyment

Similar to the participants above, many of the participants in this study, found the period during the COVID-19 pandemic to be a time for quiet enjoyment of their baby and their new family as they were required to stay at home. Using the lens of feminist poststructuralism, we can see how these mothers were challenging social norms and expectations of new mothers. Challenging social ideals was a way of using their agency as they clearly articulated their beliefs about how being at home with their babies was very positive and for some a 'blessing'. Many participants believed that this was a time for more personal and intimate family enjoyment. A time where the immediate family could not only enjoy each other but also their new baby.

> It's been great ... we have this opportunity to bond as a family and he [partner] is here for every moment during the newborn stage! It has been amazing not having to worry about visitors coming and going and cleaning out home and me worrying about breastfeeding in front of others - instead we have a very relaxed atmosphere for everything!

As the above quote reveals, the participant believed that this was an opportunity to connect with her son in a way that would not have been possible outside of the COVID-19 pandemic. It was a time without the worry about visitors and the social expectations that are often placed upon new parents to be perfect and have everything altogether, such as keeping a clean and immaculate house, while tending to the needs of their new baby. It was a time to let go of the many worries of being a new mother that stem from social and cultural discourses of new motherhood, such as breastfeeding discourses. Social breastfeeding discourse often positions public displays of breastfeeding to be inappropriate and can create feelings of discomfort for the general public as well as mothers who are breastfeeding [37]. The participant revealed that isolation during COVID-19 allowed her to put aside such worries and pressures relating to breastfeeding so that she could relax. For many participants, as exemplified here, isolation was constructed as a time to be removed from societal pressures and to bond as a family.

## 3.4. The Blessings of Learning

The COVID-19 pandemic not only provided an opportunity for intimate family bonding and freedom from the social pressures of new parenthood, but it also provided time for many participants to learn. Their learning was focused on their new baby as well as learning about themselves as new parents. For example, one participant believed that they [parents] "had this time to support each other and see each other grow as parents". This time was valued as a time in which they could come to understand their new identities as parents - a time for her and her partner to grow together in these new roles and identities. Other participants also noted similar experiences, as illustrated in the quote below:

> We were able to spend so much time alone as a family, and constantly being with our new baby has made us able to learn so much about her and enjoy spending our time with her without any distractions.

The time without distractions was seen as a benefit of being a new family. For participants, isolation during COVID-19 gave their families the opportunity to learn about their new baby and each other. It was a time for enjoyment and coming to know and understand their baby without the interference of others.

## 3.5. The Blessings of Bonding and Snuggles

Participants noted how the experience of COVID-19 created time for their family to bond and learn about each other. "I found it great to bond as a family. I've really learned what works and doesn't work for us". This participant believed that this period facilitated greater understanding of their family dynamics and individual roles. Time and space had been created so that they could figure out family strategies that worked and that did not work for them, without interference, judgement, or input from others.

COVID-19 was also a time for the enjoyment of the simple pleasures of having a new baby that many times can often be overlooked in the attempt to be "super moms". For example, another participant recognized that although following the requirements to stay at home was "extremely hard" it was also enjoyable, noting that she has "been loving all of the one-on-one time with my son, the snuggles, and the fact that there have been limited distractions". During isolation, distractions from others was limited and in this less hectic space, some participants were also able to find time to touch, bond, and snuggle more than they would have otherwise. They were able to experience the blessing of snuggles and connections with their babies even within the difficult times of the pandemic. Snuggling, touching, holding, kissing, and hugging are all noted to be deeply involved with bonding and mothers are told through social discourse that such bonding is critical to experience as a 'good mother' [38].

However, the social construction of mothering and parenting in Western societies often produce knowledge and competing discourses about how to hold, touch, and be with one's newborn, especially in public spaces amid the distractions of daily life and other people. Being out in public can interfere with the way parents interact with their newborn. Often within public spaces, certain types of bonding and touching are positioned as too intimate and inappropriate for others. This can create experiences of tension for some mothers as they try to bond with their babies in publicly appropriate ways [39]. For example, as previously described, it has been noted that some mothers experience feelings of embarrassment while breastfeeding in public places [37]. Parents continue to struggle with these competing discourses when making decisions about how to interact and bond with their babies and figure out what is right for themselves and their babies. Participants, however, found that during COVID-19 they were able to better navigate these competing discourses to experience intimate bonding with their babies. As highlighted, in the previous quote, the mother's focus on the joy of snuggling is not just a simple act; her emotional connection and her desire to bond in the best way for her baby was evident in her experience. This demonstrated the participant's value of shared, dedicated, and intimate time with her baby, physical connection and bonding, and respect for the sacred space that is shared between parent and baby. In their bonding, participants challenged public norms of distancing, as well as mainstream judgements and 'distractions'. Such participants enacted their own agency and chose to enjoy their family space during COVID-19 for important snuggling.

*3.6. The Curses*

In this study, we define curses as a challenge, a cause of harm or misery, or something that negatively influences well-being. In addition to identifying many unexpected rewards and positive outcomes during this period of public health measures, new parents also identified many challenges. The majority of mothers in our study revealed that they experienced complex contradictions during this time. In contrast to the 'Blessings' there were many 'Curses'.

*3.7. The Curses of Isolation*

Many participants believed COVID-19 had been a blessing but also a nightmare for their family. As noted in the preceding section, the first participant contrasted being free from the pressure to be a "super mom" against feeling as if she was living a nightmare. Using strong sentiments, she said, "In bad moments I just want to cry because of the pandemic. I am so sad that I can't share her [the baby] with anyone". This mother believed that sharing the experiences of having a new baby was important and felt sadness that she was not able to do this on account of the public health orders in place. Feeling 'so sad' revealed the meaning this experience held for this mother and that it was very significant. This was further emphasized as the participant gave more context to her experiences.

> We were supposed to fly to Alberta to see my family at the end of March but had to cancel the trip. This is my family's first grandchild so it just breaks my heart they will miss her whole babyhood. I also feel so alone with the baby. I have nobody here to help me figure out what is normal or how to progress through these early days. Although people can video chat it isn't the same. I just want somebody to be in the room with me and the baby to see the things she can do and help me with things.

While isolation created the opportunity to bond together and feel free from outside pressures, it also created concerns. This participant expressed that she felt like she was missing opportunities to share the joy of her baby with others, which also resulted in lost moments for her and her baby. In the above quote, the mother also expressed feeling a lack of support and that although there were other options, like video chat, they were not the same. It was important to have others physically in the room to help which was not possible during this time. Without such in person support she felt loss on what was normal or how to progress as a new mother. New mothers are often faced with many contradictory social discourses on how to be mothers and what is best for their babies. Many participants felt that if public health measures requiring that people stay within their household were not in place than they would be better able to access support from others to help them figure out what was "normal" for new babies (discourses of normalcy). Previous research has explored how mothers navigate the discourses of normalcy through networks and connections with other new parents [22,23]. However, these usual networks were generally not accessible during the COVID-19 pandemic.

*3.8. The Curses of Robbed Momemts*

Welcoming an infant into a family is not only an experience for the new parents but is also a significant experience for extended family and friends. Feelings of loss as a result of not being able to be around other people during this time was shared by many of the participants. One significant finding was that parents felt "robbed" of the ability to share their baby with their extended family and close network. One participant noted that, although the peak period of the COVID-19 pandemic was a time for family learning and creating connections between herself, her partner, and her baby, it was also a time of negativity for her and her family. She stated that the pandemic "affected us negatively because as much as we love having our new baby all to ourselves, we are also longing to show off our new baby to our family and friends". She had the desire to share her new baby with others outside of her immediate partner. She further clarified what missing the shared experiences with her friends and family meant to her.

> This pandemic has robbed us of so many other things, things that may not seem important to others. We had a photo shoot booked to capture pictures of her as a newborn, which was also cancelled due to the pandemic. I know in the grand scheme of things that is not a huge deal, but it does take a toll when it's something you were looking forward to.

She believed that many of the typical experiences of new motherhood, experiences she was looking forward to, had been robbed from her and it had "taken a toll". Although she recognized that these may be little moments in the "grand scheme of things" they were nevertheless moments or experiences that she valued as being an integral part of being a new mother and changing family. For example, the act of creating a family portrait through a professional photographer was lost to her and could not be recaptured. Although future photographs will happen, the opportunity to have photographs of her, her baby, and her family captured at that specific time is forever gone. Her baby will never be at this stage of life again.

### 3.9. The Curses of Limited Socialiation and Bonding

Many of the participants said they were concerned that their babies would not be socialized properly. It was felt by many that the COVID-19 pandemic limited their ability to socialize their babies with people, including family, friends, and other babies. One participant said,

> I am home with a now six-month-old. She is missing out on social interaction with family, friends, and other babies. I can't take my child shopping or to meet with other moms for coffee. I worry she will be overly attached to myself and husband, as we are who she sees outside of driveway visits from grandparents.

Another participant also spoke about the dichotomy created by staying home. On one hand, she expressed that "It was much easier to get into a routine. Without the constant onslaught of visitors..". However, she was also negatively affected, evidenced with the following statement, "With that being said, it was VERY hard to not have the grandparents over to hold their new granddaughter. Many tears were shed behind panes of glass".

In addition to the little moments that were lost and lack of socializing, another participant also believed she lost precious alone time with her baby, stating that although her family grew closer together she was also "sad that (she) was missing that alone time with my daughter". Time to be alone with her baby, without her partner or others, was valued by this participant. She believed that as a new mother it is necessary to bond with your baby alone. The public health orders for family members of the same households to stay together prevented this participant from experiencing alone time with her child. The participant mourned this missed alone time to bond with her child.

To understand this mother's experience, we need to look more closely at the meaning of alone time with her daughter. How had this ideal been constructed for this mother? Did she believe that she should be the main caretaker of her baby with the co-parent/father not so close? This can be viewed as a socially constructed discourse informed by heteronormative stereotypes of the roles of mothers and fathers [40]. Such discourse, also rooted in hegemonic gender binaries, often position women in the primary role of nurturer and the parent to bond with newborns. However, it is also possible that this mother valued time alone because it allowed her to more fully, holistically connect with her baby in a way that was unique to her and honoured her identity as a new mother. Following public health orders of staying at home brought out unique feelings about bonding and spending special time with one's baby. In contrast, other mothers spoke about the importance of their partners being able to spend time with their babies. Time that otherwise may not have happened without the isolation measures put in place as a result of the pandemic.

*3.10. The Blessing and Curses of Partners*

Experiences with partners was also discussed by many participants as a result of changing work habits and family circumstances, as exemplified by one participant's comment, "since COVID-19 occurred, my husband has been working from home. While I continue to be on my maternity leave, balancing his work at home has been a little bit of an adjustment". Experiences with partners were often viewed by many participants as both blessings and curses. This was reflected in the words of one participant, "my husband is home constantly which is positive and negative". The blessing of partners included more support and help with the daily activities of their homes, including cooking and cleaning, as well as baby duties, such as changing diapers and holding. As another participant clarified this sentiment, saying, "he is available to help with diaper changes and to hold the baby when I need a quick break, but it isn't what I pictured for my maternity leave". The curse side of having partners home often took the form of more chores and mess relating to them being constantly at home. As another participant discussed, "my husband has been more supportive as he's home more but there is also more to do since there are more meals to cook and more messes to clean and more activities to plan". More chores, more messes, and more planning of activities were created for many participants as a result of their partners always being home during the pandemic. It was noted by several participants that the constant nearness of partners sometimes created certain tensions in their relationship. For example, one participant noted that "although having my husband home allowed him to spend more time with the kids, it increased stress between us we argued more". This quote emphasized the experiences of participants who believed that the pandemic heightened stress and created strains within their personal relationships. Social and medical discourses often position family togetherness as critical during this time [6].

## 4. Discussion

According to Foucault [41], language, discourse, and knowledge are concepts that are interconnected to (re)produce social meanings and practices. Feminist poststructuralism positions language as structuring the way things are thought, and the way people act on the basis of those thoughts. Language is, however, set within historical contexts and as a result, is not stable nor does language represent a truth or one meaning. Language has multiple meanings that change depending on the social and political circumstances in which people live [32,41,42]. Discourse, however, moves beyond language to represent the interrelated systems of social meanings and practices "that systematically form the objects of which they speak" ([41], p. 49). Discourses are constantly being re-created as people collectively think and talk in different ways about the world. Language and discourses, therefore, (re)create knowledge and knowledge (re)creates the way people speak, come to know themselves, and shapes their values, beliefs, and practices. In other words, the subject. We can never fully understand all the influences that affect our subjectivity [42]. The subject is "written and overwritten through multiple and contradictory discourses" ([43], p. 275). The subject can be thought of as a palimpsest, a manuscript on which the writing has been partially erased to make room for other writings but with traces of the original remaining [43]. This metaphor illustrates how a subject is constantly in process and being shaped; written through multiple discourses layered upon and affecting each other. The subject is not ever blank. There is no pre-discursive self as one is never outside the influence of discourses [43].

This research revealed that there were many social discourses that shaped how the mothers experienced their babies and their wellbeing during the self-isolation period of the COVID-19 pandemic. Discourses of productivity for new mothers, discourses of bonding and connections during the postpartum period, discourse of touching, snuggling, and breastfeeding, discourses of normalcy, as well as heteronormative discourses of gender were all revealed through the analysis of participants' responses. These discourses (re)shaped the experiences of the mothers reported in this study. The mothers' experiences were seen as either positive blessings, negative curses, or, more often, seen as a complex interplay of blessings and curses, as highlighted in the results. Discourses of productivity, for example, created experiences for some mothers of freedom from the pressures associated with being a productive new mom, or as some participants said a supermom. This allowed them time to get to know their baby and time to enjoy living in the moment with them, a blessing of freedom. Discourses also created experiences that were negative or curses. For example, discourses of normalcy allow mothers to know and understand what is "normal" for their babies. Since the COVID-19 pandemic resulted in isolation many mothers felt that they were not able to connect with others to understand what is normal for babies. Participants also described the importance of special moments with babies, partners, and extended family. It is known that sharing and celebrating joys, moments, and successes together is vital not only to the health and wellbeing of families, but to the formation of collective and individual identities within the family [44].

Previous research has studied the experiences of both mothers and fathers during the postpartum, especially in the experiences of depression and mental stress [45]. In another study, it was found that mothers often expressed differences between their expectations of postpartum experiences, such as bonding, and their actual experiences [46]. It has also been previously reported parents often feel they need more support during postpartum under normal circumstances [45]. This research creates knowledge about the experiences of a group of new mothers during the COVID-19 pandemic. We can see that isolation created by public health mandates affected all participants in the study. While there were many similarities, there were also differences in how the limits and constraints of isolation affected each participant. This alerts us to the need to listen carefully to the unique relational experiences of mothers and families. Although the participants of this study were similar in many ways, consisting of birth mothers who were predominantly heterosexual, partnered white women within Nova Scotia, Canada, the findings can move beyond the local context and inform nursing practice holistically. Future studies could further explore the impact of COVID-19 isolation on the health of mothers and other family members through focus groups or observations. The postpartum time is a time of redefining family relationships, bonding, and changes in mood or mental health under the best circumstances, but our study suggests that these are heightened by mandatory public health measures of self-isolation during the COVID-19 pandemic, and informed by discursive considerations of postpartum.

The results provide deep insights into the way mothering can be understood within healthcare practices practice. Nurses and midwives are critical to influencing the way people experience their new babies. Literature suggests that supportive relationships with nurses during this period is crucial for new mothers [47,48]. We must attune ourselves as nursing professionals to recognize the complexity of experiences during the postpartum time and, in doing so, we will be able to provide more holistic service to parents both in usual times and under extreme circumstances, such as physical isolation and pandemics. By exploring both the positive and negative experiences, the blessings and the curses, of the participants, we can create an understanding that can inform nursing practice. We can develop strategies to help new parents to focus on the blessing of snuggling, bonding, and family connections, while also providing them with strategies to help with the curses.

## 5. Conclusions

This study provides a snapshot into the experiences of new mothers and their families during a pandemic, a time that was both a blessing and a curse for them. Their experiences reveal that following public health orders was neither a fully negative nor fully positive time for new families. It was a time during which complex contradictions constructed by competing social discourses created difficult dichotomies. The participants discussed the joy of family bonding and how they felt relief from the pressures of daily activities. Yet, participants also described the loss of these cherished moments and special experiences including lost opportunities to share their baby with friends and family. They also described unfulfilled expectations and hopes in terms of sharing important milestones in person versus via video chats. As part of compassionate health care practice, we should acknowledge the significance of these joys and losses to new parents. These moments of complexity need to be recognized, valued, validated, listened to, and accepted as families continue to navigate the changes related to the COVID-19 pandemic.

**Author Contributions:** Conceptualization, M.A. and S.P.; methodology, M.A. and S.P.; formal analysis, all authors.; writing, P.J.; writing—review and editing, all authors; supervision, M.A. and S.P.; project administration, M.A. and S.P. All authors have read and agreed to the published version of the manuscript.

**Funding:** This research received funding from the Dalhousie University Nursing Research Fund.

**Conflicts of Interest:** The authors declare no conflict of interest. The funders had no role in the design of the study; in the collection, analyses, or interpretation of data; in the writing of the manuscript, or in the decision to publish the results.

## References

1. Christie, J.; Poulton, B.C.; Bunting, B.P. An integrated mid-range theory of postpartum family development: A guide for research and practice. *J. Adv. Nurs.* **2008**, *61*, 38–50. [CrossRef] [PubMed]
2. Johnson, K. Maternal-Infant Bonding: A Review of Literature. *Int. J. Childbirth Educ.* **2013**, *28*, 17–22.
3. Kinsey, C.B.; Hupcey, J.E. State of the science of maternal–infant bonding: A principle-based concept analysis. *Midwifery* **2013**, *29*, 1314–1320. [CrossRef] [PubMed]
4. Bell, J.M. *Relationships: The Heart of the Matter in Family Nursing*; Sage Publications: Los Angeles, CA, USA, 2011.
5. Bell, J.M. *25th Anniversary of the Journal of Family Nursing: Significant Milestones and Top Cited Articles*; Sage Publications: Los Angeles, CA, USA, 2019.
6. Wright, L.M.; Leahey, M. *Nurses and Families: A Guide to Family Assessment and Intervention*; FA Davis: Philadelphia, PA, USA, 2005.
7. Doane, G.H.; Varcoe, C. *How to Nurse: Relational Inquiry with Individuals and Families in Changing Health and Health Care Contexts*; Wolters Kluwer Health/Lippincott Williams & Wilkins: Philadelphia, PA, USA, 2015.
8. Meeussen, L.; Van Laar, C. Feeling pressure to be a perfect mother relates to parental burnout and career ambitions. *Front. Psychol.* **2018**, *9*, 2113. [CrossRef]
9. Newman, H.D.; Henderson, A.C. The modern mystique: Institutional mediation of hegemonic motherhood. *Sociol. Inq.* **2014**, *84*, 472–491. [CrossRef]
10. Douglas, S.; Michaels, M. *The Mommy Myth: The Idealization of Motherhood and How It Has Undermined All Women*; Simon and Schuster: New York, NY, USA, 2005.
11. Brownell, C.A. Prosocial behavior in infancy: The role of socialization. *Child Dev. Perspect.* **2016**, *10*, 222–227. [CrossRef]
12. Darvill, R.; Skirton, H.; Farrand, P. Psychological factors that impact on women's experiences of first-time motherhood: A qualitative study of the transition. *Midwifery* **2010**, *26*, 357–366. [CrossRef]
13. Forster, D.A.; McLachlan, H.L.; Rayner, J.; Yelland, J.; Gold, L.; Rayner, S. The early postnatal period: Exploring women's views, expectations and experiences of care using focus groups in Victoria, Australia. *BMC Pregnancy Childbirth* **2008**, *8*, 1–11. [CrossRef]
14. Simkin, P. Just another day in a woman's life? Women's long-term perceptions of their first birth experience. Part I. *Birth* **1991**, *18*, 203–210. [CrossRef]
15. Simkin, P. Just another day in a woman's life? Part 11: Nature and consistency of women's long-term memories of their first birth experiences. *Birth* **1992**, *19*, 64–81. [CrossRef]
16. Seefat-van Teeffelen, A.; Nieuwenhuijze, M.; Korstjens, I. Women want proactive psychosocial support from midwives during transition to motherhood: A qualitative study. *Midwifery* **2011**, *27*, e122–e127. [CrossRef] [PubMed]
17. Weiss, M.E.; Lokken, L. Predictors and outcomes of postpartum mothers' perceptions of readiness for discharge after birth. *J. Obstet. Gynecol. Neonatal Nurs.* **2009**, *38*, 406–417. [CrossRef] [PubMed]
18. Dennis, C.-L. Postpartum depression peer support: Maternal perceptions from a randomized controlled trial. *Int. J. Nurs. Stud.* **2010**, *47*, 560–568. [CrossRef] [PubMed]
19. Kaunonen, M.; Hannula, L.; Tarkka, M.-T. A systematic review of peer support interventions for breastfeeding. *J. Clin. Nurs.* **2012**, *21*, 1943–1954. [CrossRef]

20. Tammentie, T.; Paavilainen, E.; AAstedt-Kurki, P.; Tarkka, M.-T. Public health nurses in Finland help to prevent postnatal depression. *Prim. Health Care* **2013**, *23*, 26–31. [CrossRef]
21. Youens, K.; Chisnell, D.; Marks-Maran, D. Mother-to-mother breastfeeding peer support: The Breast Buddies project. *Br. J. Midwifery* **2014**, *22*, 35–43. [CrossRef]
22. Price, S.L.; Aston, M.; Monaghan, J.; Sim, M.; Tomblin Murphy, G.; Etowa, J.; Pickles, M.; Hunter, A.; Little, V. Maternal knowing and social networks: Understanding first-time mothers' search for information and support through online and offline social networks. *Qual. Health Res.* **2018**, *28*, 1552–1563. [CrossRef]
23. Aston, M.; Price, S.; Monaghan, J.; Sim, M.; Hunter, A.; Little, V. Navigating and negotiating information and support: Experiences of first-time mothers. *J. Clin. Nurs.* **2018**, *27*, 640–649. [CrossRef]
24. Brage Hudson, D.; Campbell-Grossman, C.; Keating-Lefler, R.; Cline, P. New mothers network: The development of an internet-based social support intervention for African American mothers. *Issues Compr. Pediatric Nurs.* **2008**, *31*, 23–35. [CrossRef]
25. Leahy-Warren, P.; McCarthy, G.; Corcoran, P. First-time mothers: Social support, maternal parental self-efficacy and postnatal depression. *J. Clin. Nurs.* **2012**, *21*, 388–397. [CrossRef]
26. Negron, R.; Martin, A.; Almog, M.; Balbierz, A.; Howell, E.A. Social support during the postpartum period: Mothers' views on needs, expectations, and mobilization of support. *Matern. Child Health J.* **2013**, *17*, 616–623. [CrossRef] [PubMed]
27. Butler, J.P. *Giving an Account of Oneself*; Fordham Univ Press: New York, NY, USA, 2009.
28. Butler, J. Contingent Foundations: Feminism and the Question of Poststructuralism. In *The Postmodern Turn: New Perspectives on Social Theory*; Seidman, S., Ed.; Cambridge University Press: New York, NY, USA, 1994; pp. 153–171.
29. Cheek, J. *Postmodern and Poststructural Approaches to Nursing Research*; Sage Publications, Inc.: Thousand Oaks, CA, USA, 1999.
30. Foucault, M. *The Subject and Power. Afterward to H. Dreyfus & P. Rabinow (Eds.) Michel Foucault: Beyond Structuralism and Hermeneutics (pp. 208–264)*; University of Chicago Press: Chicago, IL, USA, 1983.
31. Scott, J.W. The evidence of experience. *Crit. Inq.* **1991**, *17*, 773–797. [CrossRef]
32. Aston, M. Teaching feminist poststructuralism: Founding scholars still relevant today. *Creat. Educ.* **2016**, *7*, 2251–2267. [CrossRef]
33. O'Brien, B.; Harrris, I.; Beckman, T.; Reed, D.; Cook, D. Standards for reporting qualitative research: A synthesis of recommendations. *Acad. Med.* **2014**, *89*, 1245–1251. [CrossRef]
34. Communications Nova Scotia Coronavirus (COVID-19): Restrictions and Guidance. Available online: https://novascotia.ca/coronavirus/restrictions-and-guidance/ (accessed on 23 November 2020).
35. Johnstone, B. *Discourse Analysis*, 3rd ed.; Wiley Blackwell Publishing Ltd.: Hoboken, NJ, USA, 2018.
36. Sassen, S. Women's burden: Counter-geographies of globalization and the feminization of survival. *J. Int. Aff.* **2000**, *53*, 503–524. [CrossRef]
37. West, J.M.; Power, J.; Hayward, K.; Joy, P. An exploratory thematic analysis of the breastfeeding experience of students at a Canadian university. *J. Hum. Lact.* **2017**, *33*, 205–213. [CrossRef]
38. Gholampour, F.; Riem, M.M.; van den Heuvel, M.I. Maternal brain in the process of maternal-infant bonding: Review of the literature. *Soc. Neurosci.* **2020**, *15*, 380–384. [CrossRef]
39. Aston, M. Public health nurses as social mediators: Using feminist poststructuralism to guide practice with new mothers. *Nurs. Inq.* **2008**, *15*, 280–288. [CrossRef]
40. Pascoe Leahy, C. From the little wife to the supermom? Maternographies of feminism and mothering in Australia since 1945. *Fem. Stud.* **2019**, *45*, 100–128. [CrossRef]
41. Foucault, M. *The Archaeology of Knowledge, Trans*; AM Sheridan Smith; Pantheon: New York, NY, USA, 1972.
42. Weedon, C. *Feminist Practice and Poststructuralist Theory*; Basil Blackwell: Oxford, UK, 1987.
43. Davis, B. The subject of post-structuralism: A reply to Alison Jones. *Gend. Educ.* **1997**, *9*, 271–283. [CrossRef]
44. Parse, R.R. The humanbecoming family model. *Nurs. Sci. Q.* **2009**, *22*, 305–309. [CrossRef] [PubMed]
45. Holopainen, A.; Hakulinen, T. New parents' experiences of postpartum depression: A systematic review of qualitative evidence. *JBI Database Syst. Rev. Implement. Rep.* **2019**, *17*, 1731–1769. [CrossRef] [PubMed]
46. Wardrop, A.; Popadiuk, N. Women's experiences with postpartum anxiety: Expectations, relationships, and sociocultural influences. *Qual. Rep.* **2013**, *18*, 6.

47. Aston, M.; Price, S.; Etowa, J.; Vukic, A.; Young, L.; Hart, C.; MacLeod, E.; Randel, P. The power of relationships: Exploring how public health nurses support mothers and families during postpartum home visits. *J. Fam. Nurs.* **2015**, *21*, 11–34. [CrossRef]
48. Noonan, M.; Galvin, R.; Doody, O.; Jomeen, J. A qualitative meta-synthesis: Public health nurses role in the identification and management of perinatal mental health problems. *J. Adv. Nurs.* **2017**, *73*, 545–557. [CrossRef]

**Publisher's Note:** MDPI stays neutral with regard to jurisdictional claims in published maps and institutional affiliations.

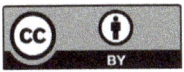

© 2020 by the authors. Licensee MDPI, Basel, Switzerland. This article is an open access article distributed under the terms and conditions of the Creative Commons Attribution (CC BY) license (http://creativecommons.org/licenses/by/4.0/).

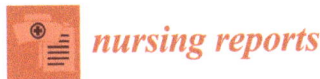 

Article

# Development and Validation of a Questionnaire to Measure Knowledge of and Attitude toward COVID-19 among Nursing Students in Greece

Athina E. Patelarou [1,*], Theocharis Konstantinidis [1], Evangelia Kartsoni [1], Enkeleint A. Mechili [2,3], Petros Galanis [4], Michail Zografakis-Sfakianakis [1] and Evridiki Patelarou [1]

1. Department of Nursing, Faculty of Health Sciences, Hellenic Mediterranean University, Estavromenos, 71140 Heraklion, Greece; harriskon@hmu.gr (T.K.); evikartsoni@gmail.com (E.K.); mzografakis@hmu.gr (M.Z.-S.); epatelarou@hmu.gr (E.P.)
2. Clinic of Social and Family Medicine, School of Medicine, University of Crete, 70013 Crete, Greece; mechili@univlora.edu.al
3. Department of Healthcare, Faculty of Public Health, University of Vlora, 9401 Vlora, Albania
4. Center for Health Services Management and Evaluation, Faculty of Nursing, National and Kapodistrian University of Athens, 15772 Athens, Greece; pegalan@nurs.uoa.gr
* Correspondence: apatelarou@hmu.gr

Received: 11 October 2020; Accepted: 12 November 2020; Published: 16 November 2020

**Abstract:** Background: During the COVID-19 pandemic, nursing students have had a key role in supporting the healthcare sector. They can join healthcare professionals in clinical practice or provide information to increase citizens' levels of knowledge and their compliance with the restriction measures. The study aimed to develop and validate a tool to measure knowledge of and attitudes toward COVID-19 among nursing students in Greece. Methods: A questionnaire was developed through theoretical research and expert consultation. A cross-sectional study was conducted among 348 undergraduate nursing students of the Department of Nursing, Hellenic Mediterranean University, recruited by convenient sampling. Validity and reliability were analyzed. Results: The Kaiser–Meyer–Olkin measure was 0.84, indicating that the sample size was adequate for factor analysis. In addition, the p-value for Bartlett's test of sphericity was <0.001, denoting that the correlation matrix was suitable for factor analysis. The construct validity of the questionnaire was determined through exploratory factor analysis (EFA), which revealed that 16 items lead to four factors: knowledge, attitude toward restriction measures, compliance with them, and volunteering. One of the key findings of this study was that participants preferred to receive information from valid sources rather than social media during the crucial period of the "infodemic". Conclusions: The questionnaire was shown to have satisfying psychometric properties and, therefore, can be used as a tool in future research in the area of nursing students' knowledge, attitudes, compliance, and volunteering during the COVID-19 pandemic.

**Keywords:** COVID-19; attitude; compliance; knowledge; nursing students; validation

## 1. Introduction

The COVID-19 pandemic is a social phenomenon; the first cases were identified in China in December 2019 and effected intense health, social, and demographic changes. The World Health Organization (WHO), on 30 December 2019, received a media statement by the Wuhan Municipal Health Commission regarding cases of 'viral pneumonia' in Wuhan, People's Republic of China, while on 30 January 2020, WHO announced a public warning regarding a health emergency of international concern [1]. Thus, on 11 February 2020, the "viral pneumonia" was named "COVID-19" and on 29 February 2020, the first considerations were published for the quarantine of individuals in the context of containment measures for the coronavirus disease [2]. By 30 September 2020, 188 countries have reported as being affected by the coronavirus, with a global number of 34 million confirmed cases, and more than one million global deaths [3]. Currently, the most affected countries worldwide are the US, India, Brazil, Russia, Colombia, Peru, and Spain [3].

The Greek government, on 10 March 2020, in response to the preventive measures against COVID-19, imposed the closure of all educational institutions and, a few days later, the suspension of arts and sports events, while from 23 March to 4 May, a confinement measure was announced accompanied by strict bans for movement [4]. Generally speaking, the Greek authorities received affirmative comments for the decision to quickly enforce restrictive measures for limiting the spread of the disease in the country [5]. In spite of the aforementioned measures, by 30 September 2020, Greece counted 18,475 confirmed cases of COVID-19 and 391 deaths [3]. Additionally, based on the local situation, restrictions were imposed in certain regions [6].

While this life-threatening pandemic rapidly spreads around the world and causes millions of deaths and observed cases, WHO highlights the threat of "another dangerous virus" called an "infodemic" [7]. This term refers to the fake news and rumors in the context of the misinformation that feeds confusion against slowing the spread of disease [7]. With respect to this phenomenon, WHO states that reducing misconceptions and confusion about the virus and dealing effectively with the vast amount of valid and invalid coronavirus information is a matter of necessity [7] because "misinformation costs lives" [8]. There is evidence showing the strong positive correlation between knowledge and attitude [9], and in the case of the pandemic, the more knowledgeable the citizens are, the more positive attitude they hold toward COVID 19-related measures and recommendations for health behavioral changes as preventive strategies [10]. Indeed, knowledge is clearly stated by researchers as the key component of evidence-based practice, not only in the area of COVID-19 but also during their training as future health professionals [11,12].

According to Nutbeam (2000), health literacy is a combination of three different domains (functional, interactive, and critical) [13]. Having a poor literacy level leads to belief in myths, unreliable information, and fiction over facts. This behavior does not impact just the believers of these stories but also their close environment and entire society [14]. During the COVID-19 epidemic, several studies have focused on health literacy. However, it still remains an underestimated public health issue [10]. In a study conducted in Vietnam, medical students were less frightened due to health literacy [15]. Another study concluded that people with poor health literacy were likely to be more confused about COVID-19 information [8]. It is clear that an increase in the general population's knowledge and health literacy is of paramount significance for managing the epidemic and for controlling and preventing its spread [16].

Health professionals, education providers, and health science students have a key role in increasing the citizens' level of knowledge, the implementation of the pandemic measures, and compliance with them [17]. Due to the lack of healthcare personnel, in many countries, final-year medical and nursing students were invited to voluntarily join the frontline healthcare workforce in the COVID-19 battle, in order to enhance health sectors during this public health crisis. In any case, researchers claim that, even if medical students are not involved in clinical practice during the COVID-19 outbreak, they play a key role in serving as information providers [17]. Therefore, it is of major importance to avoid misconceptions and myths, identify students' possible knowledge gaps, encourage them as future health providers to search, critically appraise them, and adopt the new evidence in order to make informed decisions [8,18].

To our knowledge, no fully validated tool exploring nursing students' knowledge of and attitudes toward the COVID-19 public health crisis exists. Due to a shortage of appropriate research tools for answering this research question, we aimed to develop and validate a new instrument for the purpose of this study.

## 2. Material and Methods

### 2.1. Development of Survey Questionnaire

The study questionnaire, which comprised 24 items, was constructed using reference materials, guidance, and information on COVID-19 developed by WHO, the CDC, and National Health Services (NHS). The survey covered the domains of student demographics, general awareness, information sources, knowledge, and attitude toward COVID-19, as well as level of adherence to the restriction measures. The tool was constructed with input by diverse public health professionals and professors. The first version of the questionnaire was validated by face and content validation methods by five selected experts (two nurses, one physician, and two faculty members). This was done in order to assess its readability and validity before pilot testing among ten randomly selected nursing students to confirm the clarity and acceptability [19]. Finally, all the participants' comments were incorporated and led to a new modified version of the tool with a better understanding and a more suitable order of questions. The final survey link was delivered to students via the educational platform of the institute.

### 2.2. Validation Process—Pilot Study

The questionnaire was evaluated for face validity by an interdisciplinary team of ten senior researchers (experts) in the fields of education and community nursing. Special attention was given to item construction, in order to avoid ambiguity or incomprehensibility [20]. The experts involved in the process critically scrutinized the scales on completeness and the items in terms of possible misunderstandings or ambiguities.

A pilot study with 30 students was conducted in order to estimate the face validity of the questionnaire. Students were asked to participate in the pilot study by completing an online Google Form developed for the purposes of the present study. Special attention was given to item construction to avoid ambiguity or incomprehensibility [20]. The participants carefully checked the scales on completeness and the items in terms of possible misunderstandings or ambiguities. All the items were clear and comprehensive, and finally, only a few syntax corrections were made by the researchers. All returned questionnaires had all items answered and were used for the statistical analysis.

### 2.3. Full Implementation Study

Following the validation process, a cross-sectional study was conducted in Greece during the period of total lockdown due to the pandemic (April–May 2020). Data were collected from April 27 to May 5 by using an online survey, from a convenience sample of undergraduate students who were attending distance classes organized by the university (Hellenic Mediterranean University). Participants were informed about all aspects of the study and voluntarily confirmed their willingness to participate. No personal data were recorded and all questionnaires were completed anonymously. Study approval was obtained by the Hellenic Mediterranean University ethical committee (ethical number 16/27.04.2020).

## 2.4. Statistical Analysis

The construct validity of the questionnaire was estimated with exploratory factor analysis, identifying the underlying factors. The varimax rotation method was used to identify correlations between items and construct the factors. Accordingly, the level for acceptable factor loading was set at >0.4 and for acceptable eigenvalues, set at >1. The Kaiser–Meyer–Olkin test was also used to measure the adequacy of the sample size for factor analysis, with values >0.7 considered as acceptable. Bartlett's test of sphericity was applied to estimate the covariance between the items and values <0.05 indicated that the correlation matrix was suitable for factor analysis. Internal consistency for the factors was measured with the use of the raw coefficient alpha and values >0.7 were considered as acceptable.

For each factor that emerged from factor analysis, a total score was calculated by adding the answers in the factor's items and dividing by the number of items. Thus, a total score from 1 to 5 was created, with higher values indicating greater agreement.

Continuous variables are presented as mean (standard deviation), while categorical variables are presented as numbers (percentages). The Kolmogorov–Smirnov test ($p > 0.05$) was used to test the normality assumption for the continuous variables. Bivariate analyses between demographic characteristics and total factor scores included a Student's $t$-test, Spearman's correlation coefficient, and Pearson's correlation coefficient. The Student's $t$-test was used to compare a continuous variable with a dichotomous one, while Spearman's correlation coefficient was used to correlate a continuous variable with an ordinal one. Furthermore, the correlation between two continuous variables that followed normal distribution was assessed with Pearson's correlation coefficient. Then, multivariable linear regression was performed with total factor scores as the dependent variables. Accordingly, the backward stepwise linear regression was applied and the coefficients' beta, 95% confidence intervals, and $p$-values were calculated. All tests of statistical significance were two-tailed, and $p$-values < 0.05 were considered as statistically significant. Statistical analysis was performed with the IBM SPSS 21.0 (IBM Corp. Released 2012. IBM SPSS Statistics for Windows, Version 21.0 Armonk, NY, USA).

## 3. Results

### 3.1. Demographic Characteristics

From the 451 students initially approached, 348 of them completed the questionnaire (a response rate of 77.16%) and their demographic characteristics are presented in Table 1. The mean age was 23.6 years, while the majority of students were female (84.8%), single (91.7%), and living with others during pandemic (92%) in Crete (65.5%). 55.2% lived with high-risk groups, 29.9% worked before the pandemic, and 10.9% have been working during the pandemic.

### 3.2. Factor Analysis

The Kaiser–Meyer–Olkin measure was 0.84, indicating that the sample size was adequate for factor analysis. Additionally, the p-value for Bartlett's test of sphericity was <0.001, denoting that the correlation matrix was suitable for factor analysis. The results of the exploratory factor analysis are presented in Table 2. There were four factors, including the 16 items out of the 24 questionnaire items. This four-factor model explained 50% of the questionnaire's variance. According to common sense and the meaning of items, we characterized the factors as the following: (a) COVID-19 knowledge, (b) Attitudes toward restriction measures, (c) Compliance with restriction measures, (d) Volunteering.

**Table 1.** Students' demographic characteristics.

| Items | N | % |
|---|---|---|
| Sex | | |
| Male | 53 | 15.2 |
| Female | 295 | 84.8 |
| Age [a] | 23.6 | 7.4 |
| Marital status | | |
| Single | 319 | 91.7 |
| Married | 24 | 6.9 |
| Divorced | 5 | 1.4 |
| Paternal educational level | | |
| Basic education | 113 | 32.5 |
| High school | 139 | 39.9 |
| University degree | 76 | 21.8 |
| M.Sc./Ph.D. degree | 20 | 5.7 |
| Maternal educational level | | |
| Basic education | 63 | 18.1 |
| High school | 169 | 48.6 |
| University degree | 105 | 30.2 |
| M.Sc./Ph.D. degree | 11 | 3.2 |
| City of residence during pandemic | | |
| Crete | 228 | 65.5 |
| Athens | 55 | 15.8 |
| Other | 65 | 18.7 |
| Living status | | |
| Alone | 28 | 8.0 |
| With others | 320 | 92.0 |
| Living with people at high-risk groups | | |
| Yes | 192 | 55.2 |
| No | 156 | 44.8 |
| Working status before the pandemic | | |
| Yes | 104 | 29.9 |
| No | 244 | 70.1 |
| Working status during the pandemic | | |
| Yes | 38 | 10.9 |
| No | 310 | 89.1 |

[a] mean, standard deviation.

**Table 2.** Exploratory factor analysis for the 24 questionnaire items.

| Items | Factors Derived from the Exploratory Factor Analysis | | | |
|---|---|---|---|---|
| | 1 | 2 | 3 | 4 |
| | Knowledge | Attitudes | Compliance | Volunteering |
| I am aware of COVID-19 infection symptoms. | 0.73 | | | |
| I am aware of the factors affecting COVID-19 transmission. | 0.69 | | | |
| I am aware of the correct use of protective equipment in cases of the epidemic. | 0.65 | | | |
| I know what to do if I come in contact with a confirmed case. | 0.74 | | | |
| I know which groups are at high risk for serious disease from COVID-19. | 0.64 | | | |
| I know where to search for updated evidence regarding the COVID-19 epidemic. | 0.56 | | | |
| Compliance with self-protective/restriction measures is of high importance for limiting the spread. | | 0.57 | | |
| My country announced the restriction measures in a timely manner. | | 0.79 | | |
| The measures that have been implemented in my country against COVID-19 make me feel safe. | | 0.74 | | |
| Strict compliance with restriction measures is imperative for securing public health. | | 0.69 | | |
| I personally strictly adopt the restriction measures for social isolation, and I remain at home. | | | 0.74 | |
| When I am outside my house, I keep safe distances. | | | 0.71 | |
| I perform hand hygiene according to the guidelines in my daily life. | | | 0.68 | |
| I feel able to volunteer my services in clinical practice. | | | | 0.82 |
| I would like to volunteer my services in clinical practice for the treatment of the COVID-19 epidemic. | | | | 0.82 |
| I am afraid to offer my services voluntarily in clinical practice for the treatment of the COVID-19 epidemic (reversal). | | | | 0.74 |
| My main source of information is social media (Facebook, Instagram, etc.). | | | | |
| I get informed through official organizations (National Public Health Organization, World Health Organization, CDC, etc.). | | | | |
| I search for reliable information about COVID-19 in scientific articles from bibliographic databases (e.g., PubMed). | | | | |
| I get informed about COVID-19 mainly through the media. | | | | |
| Social distancing (quarantine) can damage my health (reversal). | | | | |
| I feel able to appropriately adopt hygiene protection measures and equipment (e.g., mask, gloves). | | | | |
| Guidelines regarding hygiene rules and restriction measures are clear and there is no confusion among citizens. | | | | |
| I believe that this epidemic will significantly change our way of life from now on. | | | | |

Values express loadings.

## 3.3. Reliability Analysis

The reliability analysis for the questionnaire is presented in Table 3. According to the raw coefficient alpha and the Spearman–Brown coefficient, the questionnaire developed very good reliability. In particular, all raw coefficients alpha values and Spearman–Brown coefficients were >0.70, except one. The raw coefficient alpha for the overall instrument was 0.80 and the Spearman–Brown coefficient was 0.77. The raw coefficient alpha values for the four factors that emerged from the factor analysis ranged from 0.71 to 0.78.

Table 3. Reliability analysis for the questionnaire.

| Items | Factors Derived from the Exploratory Factor Analysis | | | | Overall Instrument |
|---|---|---|---|---|---|
| | 1 | 2 | 3 | 4 | |
| | Knowledge | Attitudes | Compliance | Volunteering | |
| Raw coefficient alpha | 0.78 | 0.71 | 0.73 | 0.78 | 0.80 |
| Spearman–Brown coefficient | 0.73 | 0.73 | 0.70 | 0.71 | 0.77 |
| Part 1 | 0.73 | 0.41 | 0.72 | 0.81 | 0.70 |
| Part 2 | 0.70 | 0.72 | 1 | 1 | 0.73 |

*3.4. Descriptive Statistics*

Descriptive statistics for the 24 questionnaire items and the four factors are presented in Table 4. Mean total scores for the four factors were above the mid-point value (= 3) of the scale, indicating high knowledge levels (mean = 4.22), positive attitudes toward restriction measures (mean = 4.14), high levels of compliance with restriction measures (mean = 4.12), and intentions of students to volunteer in clinical settings ($n$ = 3.34). Regarding other aspects of the questionnaire, students preferred to be more informed by official organizations (e.g., WHO, Centers for Disease Control and Prevention, etc.) (mean = 3.87), public media (mean = 3.35), and electronic databases (e.g., PubMed) (mean = 3.21), compared with social media (e.g., Facebook, Instagram, etc.) (mean = 2.46). Moreover, students believed that quarantine measures could have a moderate effect on their health (mean = 2.93), while the COVID-19 pandemic could change people's lives in a significant way (mean = 3.90).

*3.5. Bivariate and Multivariable Analysis*

Bivariate analyses between demographic characteristics and the factors' scores that emerged from factor analysis are shown in Table 5. There were no significant associations between demographic characteristics and COVID-19 knowledge. Students that lived with others during the pandemic had more positive attitudes toward the restriction measures ($p$ = 0.04), while females showed greater compliance with restriction measures ($p$ = 0.02). In bivariate analyses, age, marital status, maternal educational level, and working before the pandemic were associated with volunteering. However, in the multivariable linear regression analysis, only increased age was associated with increased intention to volunteer (coefficient beta = 0.02, 95% confidence interval = 0.004 to 0.03, $p$ = 0.011).

Table 4. Descriptive statistics for the 24 questionnaire items and the four factors.

| Items | Mean | SD | Median | Min | Max |
|---|---|---|---|---|---|
| I am aware of COVID-19 infection symptoms. | 4.27 | 0.6 | 4 | 3 | 5 |
| I am aware of the factors affecting COVID-19 transmission. | 4.27 | 0.7 | 4 | 2 | 5 |
| I am aware of the correct use of protective equipment in cases of the epidemic. | 4.25 | 0.7 | 4 | 2 | 5 |
| I know what to do if I come in contact with a confirmed case. | 4.14 | 0.8 | 4 | 1 | 5 |
| I know which groups are at high risk for serious disease from COVID-19. | 4.40 | 0.6 | 4 | 2 | 5 |
| I know where to search for updated evidence regarding the COVID-19 epidemic. | 3.97 | 0.8 | 4 | 1 | 5 |
| Compliance with self-protective/restriction measures is of high importance for limiting the spread. | 4.22 | 0.9 | 4 | 1 | 5 |
| My country announced the restriction measures in a timely manner. | 4.33 | 0.8 | 4 | 1 | 5 |
| The measures that have been implemented in my country against COVID-19 make me feel safe. | 3.74 | 0.9 | 4 | 1 | 5 |
| Strict compliance with restriction measures is imperative for securing public health. | 4.26 | 0.8 | 4 | 1 | 5 |
| I personally strictly adopt the restriction measures for social isolation and remain at home. | 3.97 | 0.9 | 4 | 1 | 5 |
| When I am outside my house, I keep safe distances. | 4.08 | 0.8 | 4 | 1 | 5 |
| I perform hand hygiene according to the guidelines in my daily life. | 4.32 | 0.8 | 4 | 1 | 5 |
| I feel able to volunteer my services in clinical practice. | 3.48 | 1.1 | 3 | 1 | 5 |
| I would like to volunteer my services in clinical practice for the treatment of the COVID-19 epidemic. | 3.34 | 1.2 | 3 | 1 | 5 |
| I am afraid to offer my services voluntarily in clinical practice for the treatment of the COVID-19 epidemic (reversal). | 2.78 | 1.2 | 3 | 1 | 5 |
| My main source of information is social media (Facebook, Instagram, etc.). | 2.46 | 1.2 | 2 | 1 | 5 |
| I get informed through official organizations (National Public Health Organization, World Health Organization, CDC, etc.). | 3.87 | 0.9 | 4 | 1 | 5 |
| I search for reliable information about COVID-19 in scientific articles from bibliographic databases (e.g., PubMed). | 3.21 | 1.1 | 3 | 1 | 5 |
| I get informed about COVID-19 mainly through the media. | 3.35 | 1.1 | 4 | 1 | 5 |
| Social distancing (quarantine) can damage my health (reversal). | 2.93 | 1.1 | 3 | 1 | 5 |
| I feel able to appropriately adopt hygiene protection measures and equipment (e.g., mask, gloves). | 4.40 | 0.7 | 4 | 1 | 5 |
| Guidelines regarding hygiene rules and restriction measures are clear and there is no confusion among citizens. | 3.27 | 1.0 | 3 | 1 | 5 |
| I believe that this epidemic will significantly change our way of life from now on. | 3.90 | 1.0 | 4 | 1 | 5 |
| COVID-19 knowledge | 4.22 | 0.2 | 4.2 | 3 | 5 |
| Attitudes toward the restriction measures | 4.14 | 0.6 | 4.3 | 1.3 | 5 |
| Compliance with restriction measures | 4.12 | 0.7 | 4 | 1 | 5 |
| Volunteering | 3.34 | 1.0 | 3.3 | 1 | 5 |

SD: standard deviation.

Table 5. Bivariate analysis between demographic characteristics and factors' scores that emerged from factor analysis.

| Items | Knowledge | | | Attitudes | | | Compliance | | | Volunteering | | |
|---|---|---|---|---|---|---|---|---|---|---|---|---|
| | Mean | SD | p | Mean | SD | p | Mean | SD | p | Mean | SD | p |
| Sex | | | 0.5 [a] | | | 0.5 [a] | | | 0.02 [a] | | | 0.8 [a] |
| Male | 4.2 | 0.5 | | 4.1 | 0.6 | | 3.9 | 0.7 | | 3.4 | 0.9 | |
| Female | 4.2 | 0.5 | | 4.1 | 0.6 | | 4.2 | 0.7 | | 3.3 | 0.9 | |
| Age | 0.04 [b] | | 0.5 [b] | 0.03 [b] | | 0.5 [b] | 0.05 [b] | | 0.3 [b] | 0.14 [b] | | 0.01 [b] |
| Marital status | | | 0.9 [a] | | | 0.7 [a] | | | 0.7 [a] | | | 0.03 [a] |
| Single/divorced | 4.2 | 0.5 | | 4.1 | 0.6 | | 4.1 | 0.7 | | 3.3 | 0.9 | |
| Married | 4.2 | 0.5 | | 4.1 | 0.8 | | 4.2 | 0.5 | | 3.8 | 0.8 | |
| Paternal educational level | 0.02 [c] | | 0.6 [c] | 0.04 [c] | | 0.5 [c] | 0.06 [c] | | 0.3 [c] | −0.07 [c] | | 0.18 [c] |
| Maternal educational level | −0.11 [c] | | 0.2 [c] | 0.01 [c] | | 0.8 [c] | −0.02 [c] | | 0.7 [c] | −0.14 [c] | | 0.01 [c] |
| Living status | | | 0.5 [a] | | | 0.04 [a] | | | 0.9 [a] | | | 0.8 [a] |
| Alone | 4.2 | 0.5 | | 3.9 | 0.9 | | 4.1 | 0.6 | | 3.4 | 0.9 | |
| With others | 4.2 | 0.5 | | 4.2 | 0.6 | | 4.1 | 0.7 | | 3.3 | 0.9 | |
| Living with people in high-risk groups | | | 0.9 [a] | | | 0.2 [a] | | | 0.3 [a] | | | 0.7 [a] |
| Yes | 4.2 | 0.5 | | 4.1 | 0.6 | | 4.1 | 0.7 | | 3.3 | 0.9 | |
| No | 4.2 | 0.5 | | 4.2 | 0.7 | | 4.2 | 0.6 | | 3.4 | 0.9 | |
| Working status before the pandemic | | | 0.2 [a] | | | 0.2 [a] | | | 0.7 [a] | | | 0.02 [a] |
| Yes | 4.3 | 0.5 | | 4.1 | 0.8 | | 4.1 | 0.6 | | 3.5 | 0.9 | |
| No | 4.2 | 0.5 | | 4.2 | 0.6 | | 4.1 | 0.6 | | 3.3 | 0.9 | |
| Working status during the pandemic | | | 0.3 [a] | | | 0.8 [a] | | | 0.6 [a] | | | 0.1 [a] |
| Yes | 4.3 | 0.5 | | 4.1 | 0.8 | | 4.1 | 0.5 | | 3.6 | 0.9 | |
| No | 4.2 | 0.5 | | 4.1 | 0.6 | | 4.1 | 0.5 | | 3.3 | 0.9 | |

[a] Student's t-test, [b] Pearson's correlation coefficient, [c] Spearman's correlation coefficient, SD: standard deviation, $p$: $p$-value, Bold: $p$-values < 0.05.

## 4. Discussion

The abrupt spread of the COVID-19 pandemic worldwide and the declaration of the disease as a Public Health Emergency of International Concern were bad omens for public health. Healthcare providers and health science students were always at high risk of infectious diseases and, conclusively, their knowledge of and their attitudes toward the new virus are of major importance for future interventions and health policy planning.

According to our knowledge, this is the first study to develop a tool with these dimensions investigating Greek nursing students' views during the COVID-19 confinement. In this study, which was conducted one month after the announcement of lockdown in Greece, the researchers attempted to investigate COVID-19-related knowledge, the attitude toward this new situation, the level of adherence towards the restriction measures, and volunteerism among nursing students. The developed instrument was comprehensively tested and showed satisfactory psychometrical properties, and it can be used as a valid research tool in future studies in this field. The instrument accounted for 50% of the total variance, indicating that the four factors model was statistically appropriate, including COVID-19 knowledge, attitudes toward restriction measures, compliance with restriction measures, and volunteering. Regarding the dimension of COVID-19 knowledge, we conclude that knowledge is an essential issue, as has been confirmed by several studies [21–24]. Increased awareness and promotion of positive attitudes among students are imperative to changing students' health practices and improving compliance with preventive measures. Positive attitudes and compliance with restriction measures could significantly improve the public's preventive health behaviors and the preparedness for COVID-19 [21–23,25,26]. Finally, a relatively new issue emerged from our factor analysis: the factor "volunteering". Health care students internationally volunteered to assist in hospitals due to the COVID-19 pandemic, providing crucial aid to hospital functioning and patients' care in healthcare systems [27,28].

One of the main results of this study was the students' high knowledge levels (mean = 4.22), as well as their preference to get informed by official organizations and official electronic databases compared with social media. Recent studies show the importance of the need for health science students to be well-informed regarding the symptoms of COVID-19 and prevention strategies [17]. Further, a study in Turkey regarding nursing students revealed that almost half of the respondents (48%) were well-informed about the coronavirus disease, despite the fact that knowledge was associated with an increase in their stress levels [29]. Furthermore, a study based on medical and health students in India found a lack of availability of credible knowledge, with the majority (65.17%) getting informed through social media, and a small percentage of them (11.47%) not informed regarding the pandemic [19]. Notably, there is evidence indicating that health science students have higher levels of knowledge compared with social science students [30], and also have an obligation to adopt true knowledge and disseminate valid evidence regarding the spread of the virus [17].

Literature highlights the need for students' attention to the value of the knowledge refinement process and evidence-based answers through critical appraisal of the information before applying or sharing it [31]. At the same time, authors in cooperation with public health organizations and WHO suggest frameworks, strategic partnerships, and coordinated actions for infodemic management, involving health professionals, students, researchers, and stakeholders [32–34]. As a further step, researchers claim that virus-related knowledge and health literacy are needed in order to achieve higher levels of compliance with restriction measures to control citizens' fear, resist the infodemic, and to promote citizens' trust in reliable information and recommendations [15].

Moreover, in this study, most of the participants hold a positive attitude toward restriction measures. Similarly, a national study in the United Kingdom conducted among final year medical students showed that the majority (93.6%) believed that the measures during the pandemic are necessary [35]. In contrast, in the US, 37.8% of the students presented unwillingness to comply with restriction measures, while in Cyprus, researchers showed that women and individuals over the age of 30 were more likely to implement the measures [36,37].

Additionally, the present study reveals the intentions of students to volunteer in clinical settings. This is in line with previous studies' findings in Spain, which found that a high percentage of students expressed the desire to assist nurses in providing patient care during the pandemic [38]. Internationally, nursing and medical students were willing to volunteer for certain tasks in order to assist the healthcare system and support the COVID-19 response effort [39]. Volunteerism in the period of the COVID-19 crisis, although can cause uncertainty and fear for students acting in the frontlines, is still considered a valuable lesson for their future interprofessional practice, and therefore, a high percentage of students report a willingness to get involved [28,35].

Moreover, students reported that the COVID-19 pandemic could change people's lives in a significant way, which is in line with previous findings. Similarly, a study conducted in Hong Kong showed that the vast majority of participants (97%) were worried about COVID-19 and its impact on their daily routines [40], while another study conducted in the United Kingdom reported medical students' disappointment due to the worldwide travel restriction [35].

In the present study, a portion of the participants alleged that the quarantine measures could have a moderate effect on their health (mean = 2.46). Rawls and Gibson stated that the pandemic may cause negative economic, psychological, and cultural consequences [41], as this situation affects students' psychological status and creates anxiety and fears for their future careers [38,42]. In addition, there is evidence linking social isolation with uncertainty, insecurity, and instability to students, as well as with emotional difficulties during student life [36]. Generally speaking, studies have shown that the COVID-19 pandemic and measures to control it have a great impact on individuals' quality of life and mental health, while in a study conducted in the general population of Cyprus, the psychological morbidity was associated with being a university student [42].

The present study has some strengths, as well as limitations. A possible limitation of our study is its cross-sectional study design, which does not allow us to assess possible changes in nursing students' attitudes, their levels of knowledge, or their adherence to restrictions over the different stages of the COVID-19 pandemic. On the other hand, the cross-sectional design allows researchers to use real-time data and clearly depicts the participants' knowledge and attitudes at that point in time, during the confinement. It is worth noting that to our knowledge, this is the first study to develop and validate a tool to assess nursing students' knowledge and attitudes toward COVID-19 in a university environment during the period of quarantine. Another limitation is that we did not perform a confirmatory factor analysis since we did not have a prior theory regarding the number and the structure of the factors. Thus, there is a need for further studies in this field to confirm and expand our findings.

## 5. Conclusions

The questionnaire developed proved to have satisfactory psychometric properties in terms of validity and reliability. This instrument can be used as a tool in future research among different student populations in the area of knowledge, attitudes, compliance, and volunteering during the COVID-19 pandemic.

**Author Contributions:** Conceptualization, visualization, and supervision A.E.P. & E.P.; Methodology A.E.P., P.G., E.P.; Investigation, data curation A.E.P., T.K., M.Z.-S., E.P.; formal analysis P.G.; validation P.G.; Writing—original draft A.E.P., E.K., P.G., E.A.M., E.P.; Writing—review and edit A.E.P., E.K., T.K., M.Z.-S., E.A.M., E.P. All authors have read and agreed to the published version of the manuscript.

**Funding:** This research received no external funding.

**Conflicts of Interest:** The authors declare no conflict of interest.

## References

1. World Health Organization. Director-General's Statement on IHR Emergency Committee on Novel Coronavirus (2019-nCoV). Available online: https://www.who.int/dg/speeches/detail/who-director-general-s-statement-on-ihr-emergency-committee-on-novel-coronavirus-(2019-ncov) (accessed on 30 September 2020).

2. World Health Organization. Institutional Repository for Information Sharing. Available online: https://apps.who.int/iris/handle/10665/331299 (accessed on 29 September 2020).
3. Johns Hopkins Coronavirus Resource Center. Global Map. Available online: https://coronavirus.jhu.edu/map.html (accessed on 6 October 2020).
4. European Union Agency for Fundamental Rights. Coronavirus COVID-19 Outbreak in the EU Fundamental Rights Implications. Available online: https://fra.europa.eu/sites/default/files/fra_uploads/greece-report-covid-19-april-2020_en.pdf (accessed on 23 September 2020).
5. Fouda, A.; Mahmoudi, N.; Moy, N.; Paolucci, F. The COVID-19 pandemic in Greece, Iceland, New Zealand, and Singapore: Health policies and lessons learned. *Health Policy Technol.* **2020**, *10*, 1016.
6. U.S. Embassy & Consulate in Greece. Available online: https://gr.usembassy.gov/covid-19-information/ (accessed on 30 September 2020).
7. Managing the COVID-19 Infodemic: Promoting Healthy Behaviors and Mitigating the Harm from Misinformation and Disinformation. Available online: https://www.who.int/news-room/detail/23-09-2020-managing-the-covid-19-infodemic-promoting-healthy-behaviours-and-mitigating-the-harm-from-misinformation-and-disinformation (accessed on 23 September 2020).
8. Okan, O.; Bollweg, T.M.; Berens, E.-M.; Hurrelmann, K.; Bauer, U.; Schaeffer, D. Coronavirus-Related Health Literacy: A Cross-Sectional Study in Adults during the COVID-19 Infodemic in Germany. *Int. J. Environ. Res. Public Health* **2020**, *17*, 5503. [CrossRef] [PubMed]
9. Patelarou, A.E.; Dafermos, V.; Brokalaki, H.; Melas, C.D.; Koukia, E. The evidence-based practice readiness survey: A structural equation modeling approach for a Greek sample. *Int. J.* **2015**, *13*, 77–86. [CrossRef] [PubMed]
10. Paakkari, L.; Okan, O. COVID-19: Health literacy is an underestimated problem. *Lancet* **2020**, *5*, e249–e250. [CrossRef]
11. Gemuhay, H.M.; Kalolo, A.; Mirisho, R.; Chipwaza, B.; Nyangena, E. Factors affecting performance in clinical practice among preservice diploma nursing students in Northern Tanzania. *Nurs. Res. Pract.* **2019**, *9*, 3453085. [CrossRef] [PubMed]
12. Kwiecień-Jaguś, K.; Mędrzycka-Dąbrowska, W.; Galdikienė, N.; Via Clavero, G.; Kopeć, M. A cross-international study to evaluate knowledge and attitudes related to basic life support among undergraduate nursing students—A questionnaire study. *Int. J. Environ. Res. Public Health* **2020**, *17*, 4116.
13. Nutbeam, D. Health literacy as a public health goal: A challenge for contemporary health education and communication strategies into the 21st century. *Health Promot. Int.* **2020**, *15*, 259–267. [CrossRef]
14. Spring, H. Health literacy and COVID-19. *Inf. Libr. J.* **2020**, *37*, 171–172. [CrossRef]
15. Nguyen, H.T.; Do, B.N.; Pham, K.M.; Kim, G.B.; Dam, H.T.; Nguyen, T.T.; Duong, T.V. Fear of COVID-19 scale—Associations of its scores with health literacy and health-related behaviors among medical students. *Int. J. Environ. Res. Public Health* **2020**, *17*, 4164. [CrossRef]
16. Hashemi-Shahri, S.M.; Khammarnia, M.; Ansari-Moghaddam, A.; Setoodehzadeh, F.; Okati-Aliabad, H.; Peyvand, M. Sources of news as a necessity for improving community health literacy about COVID-19. *Med. J. Islam. Repub. Iran* **2020**, *34*, 63.
17. Gohel, K.H.; Patel, P.B.; Shah, P.M.; Patel, J.R.; Pandit, N.; Raut, A. Knowledge and perceptions about COVID-19 among the medical and allied health science students in India: An online cross-sectional survey. *Clin. Epidemiol. Glob. Health* **2020**, in press. [CrossRef] [PubMed]
18. Patelarou, A.E.; Laliotis, A.; Brokalaki, H.; Petrakis, J.; Dafermos, V.; Koukia, E. Readiness for and predictors of evidence base practice in Greek healthcare settings. *ANR* **2017**, *35*, 64–70. [CrossRef] [PubMed]
19. DeVellis, R.F. *Scale Development: Theory and Applications*, 4th ed.; Sage Publications: Newbury Park, CA, USA, 2016.
20. Streiner, D.L.; Norman, G.R.; Cairney, J. *Health Measurement Scales: A Practical Guide to Their Development and Use*, 5th ed.; Oxford University Press: Oxford, UK, 2015.
21. Dardas, L.A.; Khalaf, I.; Nabolsi, M.; Nassar, O.; Halasa, S. Developing an understanding of adolescents' knowledge, attitudes, and practices toward COVID-19. *J. Sch. Nurs.* **2020**. [CrossRef] [PubMed]
22. Srichan, P.; Apidechkul, T.; Tamornpark, R.; Yeemard, F.; Khunthason, S.; Kitchanapaiboon, S.; Wongnuch, P.; Wongphaet, A.; Upala, P. Knowledge, attitudes and preparedness to respond to COVID-19 among the border population of northern Thailand in the early period of the pandemic: A cross-sectional study. *WHO South East Asia J. Public Health* **2020**, *9*, 118–125. [PubMed]

23. Adesegun, O.A.; Binuyo, T.; Adeyemi, O.; Ehioghae, O.; Rabor, D.F.; Amusan, O.; Akinboboye, O.; Duke, O.F.; Olafimihan, A.G.; Ajose, O.; et al. The COVID-19 crisis in Sub-Saharan Africa: Knowledge, attitudes, and practices of the Nigerian public. *Am. J. Trop Med. Hyg.* **2020**, *20*, 0461. [CrossRef] [PubMed]
24. Jarab, A.S.; Al-Qerem, W.; Mukattash, T.L.; Al-Hajjeh, D.M. Pharmacy and Pharm. D students' knowledge and information needs about COVID-19. *Int. J. Clin. Pract.* **2020**. [CrossRef] [PubMed]
25. Li, X.; Liu, Q. Social Media Use, eHealth literacy, disease knowledge, and preventive behaviors in COVID-19 pandemic: A cross-sectional study on Chinese netizens. *J. Med. Internet Res.* **2020**, *22*, e19684. [CrossRef]
26. Nnama-Okechukwu, C.U.; Chukwu, N.E.; Nkechukwu, C.N. COVID-19 in Nigeria: Knowledge and compliance with preventive measures. *Soc. Work Public Health* **2020**, *35*, 590–602. [CrossRef]
27. Pickell, Z.; Gu, K.; Williams, A.M. Virtual volunteers: The importance of restructuring medical volunteering during the COVID-19 pandemic. *Med. Humanit.* **2020**, 011956. [CrossRef]
28. Buckland, R. Medical student volunteering during COVID-19: Lessons for future interprofessional practice. *J. Interprof. Care* **2020**. [CrossRef]
29. Aslan, H.; Pekince, H. Nursing students' views on the COVID-19 pandemic and their perceived stress levels. *Perspect. Psychiatr. Care* **2020**, *17*, 12597. [CrossRef] [PubMed]
30. Rakhmanov, O.; Dane, S. Knowledge and anxiety levels of African university students against COVID-19 during the pandemic outbreak by an online survey. *Int. Dent. J.* **2020**, *8*, 53–56.
31. Ikhlaq, A.; Hunniya, B.E.; Riaz, I.B.; Ijaz, F. Awareness and attitude of undergraduate medical students towards 2019-novel corona virus. *Pak. J. Med. Sci.* **2020**, *36*, 32–36.
32. Zarocostas, J. How to fight infodemic. *Lancet* **2020**, *395*, 676. [CrossRef]
33. Tangcharoensathien, V.; Calleja, N.; Nguyen, T.; Purnat, T.; D'Agostino, M.; Garcia-Saiso, S.; Landry, M.; Rashidian, A.; Hamilton, C.; AbdAllah, A.; et al. Methods and results of an online, crowdsourced WHO technical consultation. *J. Med. Internet Res.* **2020**, *22*, 19659. [CrossRef] [PubMed]
34. Eysenbach, G. How to Fight an Infodemic: The four pillars of infodemic management. *J. Med. Internet Res.* **2020**, *22*, 21820. [CrossRef]
35. Choi, B.; Jegatheeswaran, L.; Minocha, A.; Alhilani, M.; Nakhoul, M.; Mutengesa, E. The impact of the COVID-19 pandemic on final year medical students in the United Kingdom: A national survey. *BMC Med. Educ.* **2020**, *20*, 206. [CrossRef]
36. Geldsetzer, P. Knowledge and perceptions of COVID-19 among the general public in the United States and the United Kingdom: A cross-sectional online survey. *Ann. Intern. Med.* **2020**, *173*, 157–160. [CrossRef]
37. Solomou, I.; Constantinidou, F. Prevalence and predictors of anxiety and depression symptoms during the COVID-19 pandemic and compliance with precautionary measures: Age and sex matter. *Int. J. Environ. Res. Public Health* **2020**, *17*, 4924. [CrossRef]
38. Ramos-Morcillo, A.J.; Leal-Costa, C.; Moral-García, J.E.; Ruzafa-Martínez, M. Experiences of nursing students during the abrupt change from face-to-face to e-learning education during the first month of confinement due to COVID-19 in Spain. *Int. J. Environ. Res. Public Health* **2020**, *17*, 5519. [CrossRef]
39. Gishen, F.; Gill, D.; Bennett, S. Covid-19—The Impact on Our Medical Students Will Be Far-Reaching. Available online: https://blogs.bmj.com/bmj/2020/04/03/covid-19-the-impact-on-our-medical-students-will-be-far-reaching/ (accessed on 13 November 2020).
40. Kwok, K.O.; Kin, K.L.; Chan, H.H.; Yi, T.Y.; Tang, A.; Wei, W.I.; Wong, Y.S. Community responses during the early phase of the COVID-19 epidemic in Hong Kong: Risk perception, information exposure and preventive measures. *Emerg. Infect. Dis.* **2020**, *26*, 1575–1579. [CrossRef] [PubMed]
41. Rawls, A.; Gibson, D. Social Interaction and presentation of self in a masked world. *ASA* **2020**, *48*, 3.
42. Rajab, M.H.; Gazal, A.M.; Alkattan, K. Challenges to online medical education during the COVID-19 pandemic. *Cureus* **2020**, *12*, 8966.

**Publisher's Note:** MDPI stays neutral with regard to jurisdictional claims in published maps and institutional affiliations.

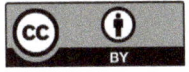

© 2020 by the authors. Licensee MDPI, Basel, Switzerland. This article is an open access article distributed under the terms and conditions of the Creative Commons Attribution (CC BY) license (http://creativecommons.org/licenses/by/4.0/).

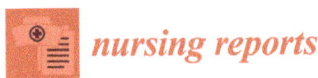 

*Commentary*

# Nurses and Doctors Heroes? A Risky Myth of the COVID19 Era

Carlo V. Bellieni

Ethics Committee of the Tuscany Region and Pediatric Intensive Care Unit, University Hospital of Siena, 53100 Siena, Italy; carlo.bellieni@ao-siena.toscana.it

Received: 29 August 2020; Accepted: 14 September 2020; Published: 28 September 2020

**Abstract:** Recent newspapers reports have named health professionals as "heroes". This is surprising, because in the last few decades, doctors and nurses have been taken into account by mass media only to describe cases of misconduct or of violence. This change was due to the coronavirus pandemic scenario that has produced fear in the population and the need for an alleged "savior". This need for health professionals seen as heroes is also disclosed by the fact that even politicians have abdicated to their role in favor of the healthcare "experts" to whom important decisions on social life during this pandemic have been delegated, even those decisions that fall outside of the specific health field. This commentary is a claim to framing the job of caregivers in its correct role, neither angel nor devil, but allied to the suffering person, that the image of "heroes" risks to overshadow.

**Keywords:** COVID-19; pandemic; medical humanities

---

Until a few months ago, the medical chronicles were full of reports showing increasing episodes of violence against doctors and nurses [1]. The newspapers used to report clinical news mainly about cases of misconduct or medical errors. Suddenly, in the shadow of the nefarious coronavirus, one reads only of healthcare heroes: On 24 March, an article appeared on the CNN site titled "The real modern heroes are the health workers", and on 24 April, on this track the BBC asked: "Will coronavirus change how we define heroes?" with reference to the efforts of COVID-19 caregivers. "From rags to riches", we would say; but careful: As it is commonly said, "all that glitters ain't gold" because there is a high risk that all this sanctification may end soon and lead again to a scenario where health professionals are unsatisfactory again. The aim of this commentary is to point out this paradox and to warn against the illusion that this really represents a correct vision of caregivers' role.

Across the centuries, physicians, due to increasing knowledge and technique, have become something like "demi-gods" for the public. This perspective has been questioned in more recent decades due to a certain emancipation of the public and the criticism toward scientists, including physicians. For nursing, it is not quite the same as with physicians, because nurses have emerged as a role more recently. In antiquity and in later centuries, persons who acted as nurses or midwives were either revered or blamed as witches. In more recent centuries, particularly with the growing influence of Florence Nightingale, nursing has moved into a more scientific sphere, obtaining a higher regard. However, in recent decades, nursing—for example, in Europe—has been struggling for recognition and has itself failed to demonstrate the potential that nurses bring to the table [2]; the public has lost interest and trust in nursing to some extent and the reasons for this decline will be explained later in this text.

In more recent years, healthcare professionals have often been in a negative light, and the reason seems evident: The assimilation of nurses and doctors to any other job by measuring costs, effects, and users' satisfaction to appreciate their efforts. The caregiver–patient relationship has been reduced to a contract, and in the absence of the "customer's satisfaction" or of the sometimes-unrealistic fulfillment of the contract clauses, many pressed legal charges. The caregiver–patient relationship has become a contractual relationship [3], as if the concepts of mutual trust and respect were an insignificant corollary: 3000 years of healthcare history based on the Hippocratic concept have been put in a closet and locked up. However, if the doctor–patient and the nurse–patient relationship has turned into a contract between an operator and a client, and if the hospitals have become "companies", mistrust skyrockets, then dissatisfaction, and eventually intolerance follow. Ivan Illich explained this well in his book Medical Nemesis [4]: Having ceased curing the person and started curing diseases, the role of doctor and nurses turns against itself in a sort of nemesis, a consequence of a society who sees everything as laws to be followed, contracts, and operating instructions, and as service of a person who got sick and wants—Illich wrote—«to find in the eyes of the doctor a reflection of his own anguish and some recognition of uniqueness of his own suffering».

In the last few weeks, this scenario has been subverted, exceeding on the other side of the coin. With the deadly threat of the coronavirus, people have felt alone, afraid, and have seen that nurses and doctors are not only "health workers", but they have, strangely enough, gone too far in this reevaluation: Now, the collective imagination identifies them as heroes. There is too much idealization in this: Doctors and nurses are not to be identified with "misconduct", but they are neither supermen and superwomen. People seem to adore them, and even politicians tend to abdicate to their decisional power in favor of doctors: "scientific experts" are, these days, asked to supply them strong certainties [5]. This discloses an initial flaw: Experts cannot give strong and definitive certainties, at least in the ultimate mode that they are asked to give, because experts respond to what they are asked for; so, if the only request is to inform politicians regarding when the quarantine shall end, they cannot answer because this answer requires considering not only health issues, but also economic and social aspects of the COVID pandemic [6,7], and also because the epidemiologist can respond about epidemiology, and the virologist or the intensivist only for their respective fields.

Delegating political issues to technicians, and in this case to healthcare experts, reflects a theme that has been widely debated in the philosophic arena. Hannah Arendt in 1958 wrote the book The Human Condition, in which she explained that for the ancient philosophers, human activity was divided into three levels: Simple manual work, and technical and political work, both a function of a higher level activity: Contemplative activity. However, the idea of contemplation has been overshadowed, and politics has lost importance in favor of technical activity. Politics has shifted "from the old questions of 'what' and 'why'" to the new question of 'how'" with "the belief that every problem can be solved and every human motivation reduced to the principle of utility; we consider everything that is given as raw material and we see nature as an immense fabric from which we can cut out what we want" [8]. Furthermore, today, political, moral, and even religious activity seem to be subordinated to the technical data, which cannot however give social or normative granitic certainties; politics is no longer a function of elevated principles or high human functions (philosophy or ethics). So we live in expectation of a definitive and far-sighted response that would arrive from a place from where it cannot come: Technique.

This is the risk of a disembodied and disenchanted Technique, aimed at the useful and not at beauty, as Enzo Tiezzi, a chemist and politician, would have liked [9]. The technician (biologist, architect, doctor, teacher, nurse) is no longer educated to look up, but simply to respond to his job/function. What is worrisome is not the finalism of technology, but the step backward that human conscience, culture, and politics takes, transforming ethics and virtues following a slavish follow-up of finalistic technical protocols. Protocols are not wrong, but they cannot show a wide and futuristic project. Gunther Anders explained that western man lives by an envy towards technology, of which he would like to be a mechanism among others, to lose unpredictability and fantasy for the benefit of a gray wellbeing and routine [10]. Additionally, Umberto Galimberti says that "we continue to think that we have technology as a tool at our disposal. It is not true; it is absolutely not true. Technique has now become the subject of the world and men have turned into apparatuses of this technique. If the technique becomes the universal canon to achieve any purpose, it is no longer an instrument but the first and pervasive purpose of existence" [11]. It is not a mere coincidence that people look for heroes in a disorienting era, and in the midst of a disorienting pandemic. Doctors are being glorified after having been under attack; but let us quote Bertoldt Brecht: "Unfortunate the country that needs heroes" [12]. Brecht did not want to mock heroes, but he pitied those who need them, because this happens when people live in silent fear a solitary, grey life, as well as when those who are responsible for politics and moral issues have abdicated to their role in favor of those who manage technology.

Today, doctors and nurses are certainly in the trenches, in contact with a bad enemy: COVID19. Many give much more than what is required by the protocols, many are encouraged to do that, and we see how much interregional and international solidarity arose in recent days [13]. However, the idealization of the caregivers as heroes is certainly unexpected and undue, as if people were looking for something decidedly more than a strong ally in the doctor: A sacred granitic security.

This heroic glorification risks to be a soap bubble: If the system does not change, this scenario of "Hallelujah" towards nurses and doctors is to be short-lived. Most doctors and nurses are unsatisfied and tired of uselessly asking for a better health system. This glorification will be a bubble if those who want to be gratified by their job will go on only being considered "employees", engaged with their patients not by trust but by a contract. Doctors and nurses need a health system where the caregiver–patient relationship is not all based on rapid and extorted information, where caregivers do not hide behind cold pages of illegible consents to be signed [14], where health workers have continuous motivations [15], and in which humanity is not overshadowed by bureaucracy, a plethora of useless clinical tests, and protocols [16]; where nurses belong to a world "that focuses on the human-universe-health process articulated in the nursing framework and theories" [2]. Let us take advantage of this transitory scenario, to reaffirm what really nurses and doctors are, what they want, and what people can realistically expect from them.

The role of the politics should no more be to transfer to the experts their own role of decision makers and coordinators of public life, because health professionals are only one group of the likely experts who can provide advice to the decision-makers. At the same time, caregivers should receive more motivation because they are not heroes, or saints; they neither are mere employees, but the images of "heroes" risk to overshadow their real role.

**Funding:** This research received no external funding.

**Conflicts of Interest:** The author declares no conflict of interest.

## References

1. Thomas, J.A.; Thomas, J.J.; Paul, A.B.; Acharya, S.; Shukla, S.; Rasheed, A.; Pratapa, S.K. Medical vandalism: Awareness and opinions; beyond the clinician's window. *J. Family Med. Prim. Care* **2019**, *8*, 4015–4020. [CrossRef] [PubMed]
2. Barrett, E.A.M. Again, what is nursing science? *Nurs. Sci. Q.* **2017**, *30*, 129–133. [CrossRef]
3. Bellieni, C.V. Consumerism: A threat to health? *J. R. Soc. Med.* **2018**, *111*, 112. [CrossRef]
4. Illich, I. *Medical Nemesis*; Boyars, M., Ed.; Pantheon Books: London, UK, 1976.
5. This Is Who Americans Trust About Coronavirus Information. Available online: https://www.washingtonpost.com/politics/2020/03/20/were-all-anxious-about-pandemic-who-do-americans-want-hear/ (accessed on 15 September 2020).
6. Van Gelder, N.; Peterman, A.; Potts, A.; O'Donnell, M.; Thompson, K.; Shah, N.; Oertelt-Prigione, S. COVID-19: Reducing the risk of infection might increase the risk of intimate partner violence. *EClinicalMedicine* **2020**, *21*, 100348. [CrossRef] [PubMed]
7. Tummers, J.; Catal, C.; Tobi, H.; Tekinerdogan, B.; Leusink, G. Coronaviruses and people with intellectual disability: An exploratory data analysis. *J. Intellect. Disabil. Res.* **2020**, *64*, 475–481. [CrossRef] [PubMed]
8. Arendt, H. *The Human Condition*; University of Chicago Press: Chicago, IL, USA, 1958.
9. Tiezzi, E. *La Bellezza e la Scienza*; Raffaello Cortina: Milan, Italy, 1998; ISBN 978-8870785197.
10. Anders, G. *The Outdatedness of Human Beings 1. On the Soul in the Era of the Second Industrial Revolution*; Rivages: Paris, France, 1956.
11. Galimberti, U. *Se la Tecnica Distrugge la Natura*; Feltrinelli: Milan, Italy, 2006.

12. Brecht, B. Life of Galileo. In *Collected Plays: Five*; Bertolt Brecht: Plays, Poetry and Prose Ser; Willett, J., Manheim, R., Eds.; Willett, J., Translator; Methuen: London, UK, 1980.
13. Smith, G.D.; Ng, F.; Li, W.H.C. COVID-19: Emerging compassion, courage and resilience in the face of misinformation and adversity. *J. Clin. Nurs.* **2020**, *29*, 1425–1428. [CrossRef] [PubMed]
14. Bellieni, C.V.; Coradeschi, C.; Curcio, M.R.; Grande, E.; Buonocore, G. Consents or waivers of responsibility? Parents' information in NICU. *Minerva Pediatr.* **2018**. [CrossRef]
15. Mathew, R. Rammya Mathew: Why are doctors so unhappy? *BMJ* **2020**, *368*, m100. [CrossRef] [PubMed]
16. Schwartz, B. *Why We Work*; Simon and Schuster Inc.: New York, NY, USA, 2015.

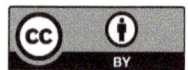

© 2020 by the author. Licensee MDPI, Basel, Switzerland. This article is an open access article distributed under the terms and conditions of the Creative Commons Attribution (CC BY) license (http://creativecommons.org/licenses/by/4.0/).

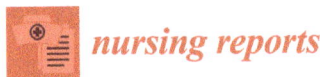 

Review

# Nursing Surge Capacity Strategies for Management of Critically Ill Adults with COVID-19

Abbas Al Mutair [1,2,*], Anas Amr [3], Zainab Ambani [4], Khulud Al Salman [5] and Deborah Schwebius [1]

1. Research Center, Dr. Sulaiman Al Habib Medical Group, Riyadh 91877, Saudi Arabia; dg.schwebius@gmail.com
2. Nursing School, University of Wollongong, Wollongong, NSW 2522, Australia
3. Patient Safety Center, Riyadh 9264, Saudi Arabia; aamr@spsc.gov.sa
4. Nursing College, King Saud Ben Abdulaziz University for Health Sciences, Al-Hofuf 32641, Saudi Arabia; ambaniz@ksau-hs.edu.sa
5. Nursing Department, Al-Jaber Hospital for Ear, Nose, Throat and Eye, Ministry of Health, Al-Hofuf 36422, Saudi Arabia; kaalsalman@moh.gov.sa
* Correspondence: abbas.almutair@drsulaimanalhabib.com

Received: 24 August 2020; Accepted: 4 September 2020; Published: 8 September 2020

**Abstract: Background:** There is a vital need to develop strategies to improve nursing surge capacity for caring of patients with coronavirus (COVID-19) in critical care settings. COVID-19 has spread rapidly, affecting thousands of patients and hundreds of territories. Hospitals, through anticipation and planning, can serve patients and staff by developing strategies to cope with the complications that a surge of COVID-19 places on the provision of adequate intensive care unit (ICU) nursing staff—both in numbers and in training. Aims: The aim is to provide an evidence-based starting point from which to build expanding staffing models dealing with these additional demands. **Design/Method:** In order to address and develop nursing surge capacity strategies, a five-member expert panel was formed. Multiple questions directed towards nursing surge capacity strategies were posed by the assembled expert panel. Literature review was conducted through accessing various databases including MEDLINE, CINAHL, Cochrane Central, and EMBASE. All studies were appraised by at least two reviewers independently using the Joanna Briggs Institute JBI Critical Appraisal Tools. **Results:** The expert panel has issued strategies and recommendation statements. These proposals, supported by evidence-based resources in regard to nursing staff augmentation strategies, have had prior success when implemented during the COVID-19 pandemic. **Conclusion:** The proposed guidelines are intended to provide a basis for the provision of best practice nursing care during times of diminished intensive care unit (ICU) nursing staff capacity and resources due to a surge in critically ill patients. The recommendations and strategies issued are intended to specifically support critical care nurses incorporating COVID-19 patients. As new knowledge evidence becomes available, updates can be issued and strategies, guidelines and/or policies revised. **Relevance to Clinical Practice:** Through discussion and condensing research, healthcare professionals can create a starting point from which to synergistically develop strategies to combat crises that a pandemic like COVID-19 produces.

**Keywords:** COVID-19; coronavirus 2019; ICU surge capacity; nursing surge capacity and strategies

---

## 1. Introduction

The recent viral outbreak initiated from Wuhan, China, has now crossed all borders and has spread into more than 224 countries [1]. The outbreak is caused by a novel strain of coronavirus which is very much similar to the SARS-CoV that resulted in the SARS outbreak [2]. Initially, this new coronavirus was named as 2019-nCoV and then was renamed as Severe Acute Respiratory Syndrome Corona Virus-2 (SARS-CoV-2) by the International Committee on Taxonomy of Viruses (ICTV) [1]. The World Health Organization (WHO) has termed COVID-19 for the disease associated with the infection caused by SARS-CoV-2 [3–5]. The coronavirus has been the focus of global attention after its first report in Wuhan, China, in December 2019. COVID-19 has rapidly spread all over the globe [6]. According to the WHO, as of July 13th, 2020, there were 12,880,565 confirmed cases of COVID-19 including 568,573 reported deaths globally [6].

SARS-CoV-2 transmission of the virus from human to human has become evident and documented in multiple published studies [7]. The mode of transmission for COVID-19 virus was initially thought to occur through droplets of saliva or discharge from the nose when an infected person coughs, sneezes, or speaks [8]. Recent studies have shown that the virus may remain suspended in the air, in the form of aerosols, for upwards of several hours [8]. However, the WHO maintains that these studies do not replicate typical cough conditions as they were produced with high-powered jet nebulizers and they have not altered their recommendations as of the date of this article submission [9]. Although maintaining at least one-meter of distancing is recommended by the WHO, it has been suggested by a recent study published in *The Lancet*, that more protection can be had if that distance is extended to two meters or more if possible. The avoidance of large gatherings, the wearing of masks, wearing of eye protection and regular hand-washing or use of alcohol-based hand rub is important to stop the transmission cycle and minimize the risk of infection [8]. Until now, there are no approved specific vaccines or treatments for COVID-19 [7]. Maintaining at least one-meter distance among individuals and regular hand-washing or using alcohol-based hand rub is important to stop the transmission cycle and minimize the risk of infection [10]. The most common symptoms of COVID-19 include fever, dry cough, and tiredness [7]. An infected person may develop some less common symptoms such as pain, sore throat, loss of taste or smell, headache, and diarrhea [7]. In critical cases, serious symptoms may appear as difficulty breathing, chest pain, and loss of speech or movement [7]. The foremost problem with COVID-19 is that a major proportion of infected persons do not exhibit or experience symptoms and hence serve as asymptomatic carriers. COVID-19 virus can transmit from symptomatic and asymptomatic carriers to other people and cause the disease [10].

Frontline healthcare workers in general, and nursing staff more specifically, as the backbone of any healthcare system, face additional burdens and hazards as they respond to the current COVID-19 pandemic. These burdens include exposure to pathogens, physical and psychological distress, fatigue, long working hours, and burnout [11]. The COVID-19 pandemic denotes a unique challenge to intensive care services. During a pandemic, the principal difficulties surround the preparation of intensive care units (ICU) and healthcare workers for the expected surge in caseload [11]; likely, complicated by workforce challenges including potential difficulty in maintaining standard staffing ratios [11]. In fact, frontline workers tend to get more severely ill than patients and it is not based on expectation of their ages [12]. This could be due to higher viral load exposure but also the high level of stress acting to depress the immune systems of overtaxed frontline healthcare workers [12]. Healthcare workers may experience severe symptoms and lose their ability to work due to admission or death, or they may experience mild symptoms and go under self-isolation for 14 days or more [12]. In both cases, healthcare facilities are expected to lose a considerable number from their manpower and functionality at this critical time [12]. The COVID-19 pandemic has placed a huge strain on health systems due to the increasing number of patients requiring acute and critical health care, staff, hospital beds, supplies, and resources [12].

To deal with this crisis, some countries developed plans and guidelines for crisis management [3]. The management is targeting the scarcity of staff, space, beds, and supplies [3]. Some of these plans were made by the national (governmental) level such as inviting all healthcare professionals to re-join the workforce, relaxing some of the licensing requirements, and accelerating credentialing processes to rapidly incorporate healthcare workers into working in hospitals [11]. Other plans were made at the hospital levels such as developing triage protocol to reallocate human and medical resources to equitably meet the needs of patients [13,14]. Triage process often starts by inventory of potential ICU resources, such as ventilatory capacity in the hospital, and then follows an algorithm for screening and admission [13]. Periodic patient assessment is necessary to check if there is any change in patients' needs in order to transfer, admit, or discharge patients [14]. Triage protocols may also be developed at a regional level to allow for communication and resource sharing among all hospitals in one region [14]. This strategy gives more opportunities for better utilization of resources [14].

The goal of nursing surge capacity is to find wise ways to augment and extend the hospital workforce; to allocate healthcare resources in an ethical, rational, and organized method to do the greatest good for the greatest possible number of patients [14]. In order to combat the complications that the pandemic threatens to level of care, a decision was made to develop nursing surge capacity recommendations and strategies for management of critically ill patients with COVID-19 in the ICU. The objectives of these strategies are to provide guidance and recommendations in order to help nursing administrators and leaders to prepare for a COVID-19 pandemic in ICU.

## 2. Methods

### 2.1. Data Sources

The search strategy aimed to find published studies in MEDLINE, CINAHL, Cochrane Central, and EMBASE from December 2019 through March 2020 (Figure 1). The keywords used were: *COVID-19, coronavirus 2019, ICU surge capacity, nursing surge capacity,* and *strategies*. The filters applied included "humans", "last 10 years", and "English language". The unpublished studies were searched in ProQuest and MEDNAR.

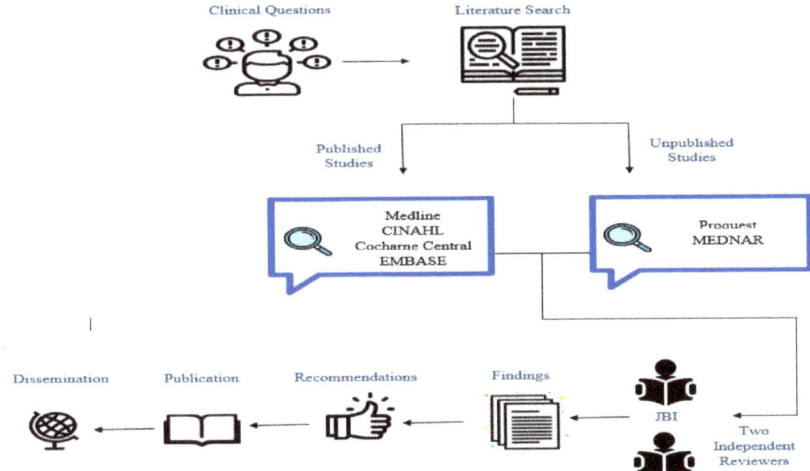

**Figure 1.** Literature searching and recommendations' development framework.

### 2.2. Quality Assessment of Extracted Data

Initially, all titles and abstracts were screened independently by at least two reviewers. All full texts of the studies which passed through the initial stage were retrieved and assessed against the review inclusion criteria in detail. These eligible studies were again appraised by at least two reviewers independently using the Joanna Briggs Institute JBI Critical Appraisal Tools [15]. The JBI appraisal has different checklists to be applied against different study designs. The instrument consists of 10 items that assess the methodological quality of a study and determines the extent to which a study has addressed the possibility of bias in its design, conduct, and analysis. The results of the JBI appraisal have been taken into full account and used to inform the synthesis and interpretation of the results of the recommendations (Figure 1).

A total of 220 studies were retrieved. After reading the titles and abstracts, 150 studies were excluded. After reading the full articles, a total of 53 articles were excluded and 17 articles were included which met the inclusion criteria (Figure 2). All identified publications were collated and fed into Endnote X10 software. The evidence-based strategies issued are to support critical care nurses to manage critical patients in the intensive care unit during the COVID-19 pandemic. Four recommendations and rationales were issued by the expert panel based on evidence.

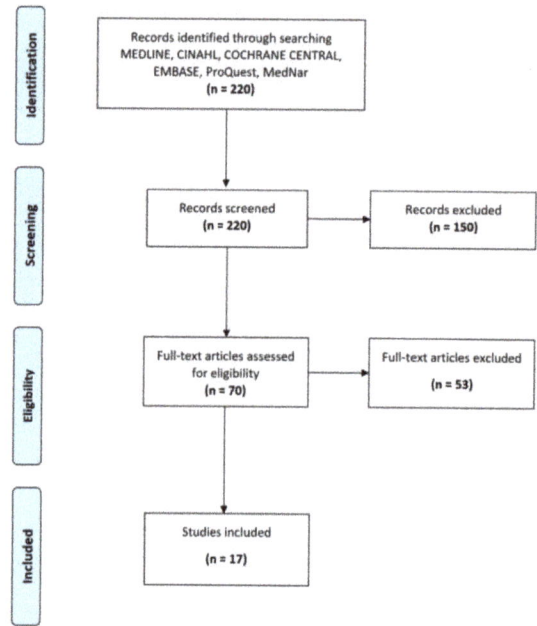

**Figure 2.** Flow diagram.

## 3. Strategies to Meet Nursing Surge Capacity during the COVID-19 Pandemic

### 3.1. Recommendation 1: Regular Patient-to-Nurse Ratio

When able to, recommend nursing staffing (1:1 or 1:2) in the ICU during the COVID-19 pandemic to provide high-quality patient care, improve safety, have fewer complications, and better outcomes (Figure 3). This should be followed until such time that the surge is felt. At that time, progression to Recommendation 2 will be made.

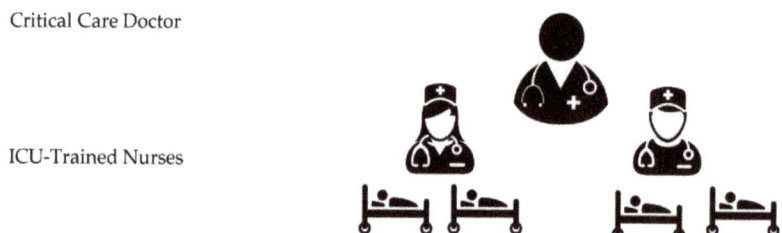

**Figure 3.** Standard ICU staffing model. (1 ICU-trained nurse: 2 patients).

Rationale

Matching patient needs with adequately trained nurses and maintaining safe patient-to-nurse ratio is essential to ensure the provision of safe and high-quality patient care. As such, nurse staffing ratios in critical care units is an important aspect when planning care [16]. The literature on nursing ratios in ICU has confirmed the relationship between ICU nurse staffing and patient outcomes. The reviewed studies confirm that a higher number of registered nursing staff to patient ratio (1:1 or 1:2) is highly associated with improved patient safety and better outcomes [13]. In the U.S. and Canada, the nurse-to-patient ratio in ICU stays close to (1:1.5) at both time points. Western Europe and Latin America had lower nurse staffing, especially at night, with an overall ratio of (~1:1.8) [17]. Note that this is the preferable situation when applicable or during non-pandemic times.

Additionally, critically ill patients require the care of nurses who have specialized knowledge and skills and who are given enough time to provide that care safely. Appropriate staffing ensures effective pairing of patient/family needs with the assigned nurse's knowledge, skills, and abilities. In fact, evidence confirms that the likelihood of serious complications and mortality rates increase when fewer registered nurses (RNs) are assigned to care for patients [13,18,19]. Similarly, a considerable amount of research indicates healthy work environments and better patient outcomes when a higher percentage of patient care tasks are provided by RNs [20].

*3.2. Recommendation 2: Finding Alternate Staff from Internal and External Resources to Support ICU Staff during Crisis Time*

Rationale

Most countries that have already been hit hard by COVID-19, attempted to increase the supply of healthcare. Having care directed by trained and experienced ICU nurses is an effective way to provide high-quality care for critically ill patients [21]. However, during crisis times, the number of ICU nurses cannot accommodate a large number of patients. Additional personnel can be identified internally through the scale-back of elective and non-urgent services in the hospital. As elective surgeries are placed on hold, nurses from areas like the Surgical ICU, Endoscopic units, Step-down units, Post Anesthesia Care Unit (PACU), and Pre-Op become available for ICU staffing needs. These nurses should be the first choice to augment ICU staffing and expand ICU beds during pandemics such as COVID-19, as their skills are most readily transferable, thereby having the potential to increase the critical care capacity of the hospital in the safest way possible. To expand the staffing capacity further, hospitals may consider external searching resources to identify and recruit ICU nurses who had transitioned to ambulatory care settings and other nurses from community care settings to support ICU staff during the crisis [7]. Additionally, other qualified medical professionals can be recruited to safely manage the care of mechanically ventilated patients. Anesthesiologists and physicians who have ventilator management experience are potential resources to supplement ICU care teams. With minimal orientation, they can easily support respiratory therapists and nurses to achieve safe ventilatory support to those requiring it [7]. Other potential caregiver support could include students in medical, nursing, and other health education programs who are nearing the end of their studies. Many would be suitable for providing services to patients or helping to respond to public concerns through telephone hotlines [21].

*3.3. Recommendation 3: Implement a Team-Based Approach (Tiered Staffing Strategy or Care Team Model) to Manage Critically Ill Patients*

A Team-Based Approach Outlines Care Being Provided by Teams of Healthcare Professionals for Groups of Patients (Figures 4–6).

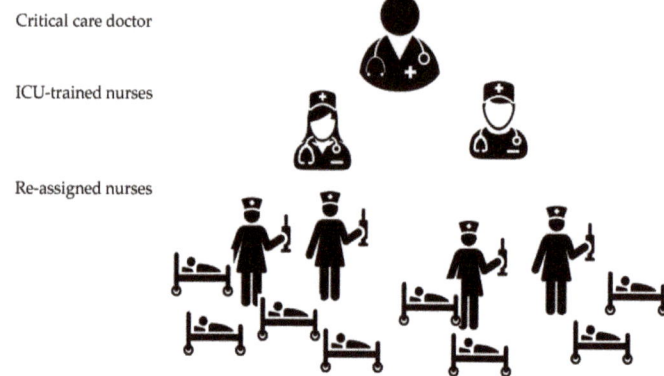

**Figure 4.** ICU tiered staffing strategy for COVID-19 pandemic; (1 ICU-trained nurse: 2 re-assigned nurses: 4 patients). This model can be expanded on a needs basis as pandemic scales up.

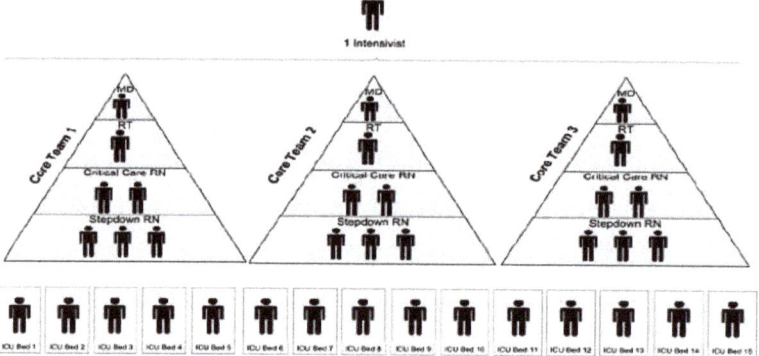

**Figure 5.** Model of ICU care teams.

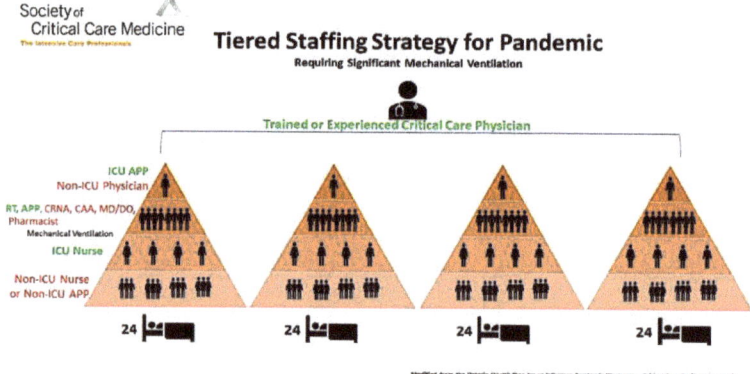

**Figure 6.** Expanded application of tiered staffing strategy for pandemic.

The team is led by an ICU physician who works with a respiratory therapist trained in critical care and 2 ICU nurses who supervised 3 step-down nurses. Each team provides care for 15 patients [12].

In this model, one experienced ICU physician oversees 4 teams composed of ICU physicians, respiratory therapist, and nurses supported by other hospital professionals to take care of 24 patients each [10].

3.3.1. Rationale

To overcome the anticipated shortage of ICU staff during the COVID-19 pandemic, hospitals are recommended to adopt a team-based approach. In the Ontario Health Plan for an Influenza Pandemic Care Team Approach, and the Society of Critical Care Medicine (SCCM) Tiered Staffing Strategy for a Pandemic are recommended models for ICU staff augmentation strategies during pandemics such as COVID-19. Both strategies have similar concepts and applications. They focus on the utilization of non-experienced healthcare workers to work in collaboration (in teams) with experienced staff to increase the capacity of care for critically ill patients. This strategy demonstrated to work effectively in pandemic situations [7,21].

The tiered staffing strategy combines experienced ICU nurses with reassigned hospital nurses. Instead of the regular care delivery model where each ICU nurse provides care for one to two patients (Figure 2), in this strategy, each ICU-trained nurse will supervise and direct other two re-assigned nurses who have useful skills but lack experience in the ICU setting to ultimately provide care for four critically ill patients. ICU physician(s) trained in critical care or those who regularly manage ICU patients will oversee all nurse teams (Figure 3) [12,13,21,22].

As the situation unfolds, teams can be expanded to care for more patients such as six or eight or more as required. Tiered staffing models are not set standards and each hospital must determine the best combination of staff based on their resources [11,23,24]. Combining experienced and non-experienced ICU-trained nurses will help to ensure adequate levels of care and not overwhelm ICU-trained staff. When implementing the current strategy and combining inexperienced team members, it is recommended to maintain effective communication among the team. This can be achieved through utilizing different ways such as team huddles at the start of each shift and at regular intervals, such as every 4 hours, to discuss team assignments, patient care goals, and red flags that should be reported immediately to the team leader [25]. This will ensure effective communication and allows each team member to discuss his/her patients' needs and get the experts' opinion. If a physical huddle is difficult, virtual huddles can be applied to enhance patients' safety and to keep all team members aware of all updates and changes in the unit [25].

3.3.2. Applications of a Team-Based Approach

The report of the Ontario Health Plan for an Influenza Pandemic presented an example of a tiered strategy and called it Care Team Model (Figure 4). In this model, healthcare workers who have useful skills but lack experience in critical care can work in teams supervised by experienced staff and collectively care for a larger group of patients. In place of an individual specialized nurse caring for one to two patients, a team of mixed experienced nurses provides the care for a group of patients. This is possible because in combination, they have the complete skills set and pertinent experience required to care for expanded patient numbers. In this example, one intensivist can supervise three teams, each composed of one physician, one respiratory therapist and two ICU nurses who supervised three step-down nurses. Each one of the 3 teams will take care of 5 patients and the 3 teams together will provide care to 15 patients [10,11]. The care team model focuses on the provision of care by a team of healthcare workers. Teams would be created with feedback loops and operate under this designated hierarchy and guided by expected job functions and responsibilities. This model has proven to be effective in past emergencies [10,11,15,16].

The SCCM presented an expanded example of the applications of tiered staffing strategy for pandemics with a larger number of healthcare workers and larger capacity for care provision (Figure 5). It suggests that one ICU-experienced physician oversees the care of 4 teams, and each team provides care for 24 patients. Each one of these teams is supervised by an ICU physician or non-ICU physician such as an anesthesiologist, pulmonologist, surgeon, or hospitalist, who does not frequently perform ICU care but has some ICU training. Each team is composed of an experienced respiratory therapist and other clinicians such as physicians, nurse anesthetists, or pharmacists who are experienced in managing ventilated patients. There are four ICU nurses in each team; each nurse is responsible for supervising the other three re-assigned nurses and each re-assigned nurse will care for two patients. Ultimately each team will provide care for 24 patients and the four teams together will provide care for 96 patients [16]. This strategy is an alternative strategy that may be implemented as ICU-trained nurses fall ill and ICU-trained nurses become less available to care for patients.

*3.4. Recommendation 4: Training Model for ICU Tiered Staffing Strategy for COVID-19 Pandemic*

Illustrated in this model (Figure 7) is a team composed of two ICU nurses; each nurse trains one re-assigned nurse and together they provide care for two critically ill patients. Training should only be added for the re-assigned nurse to care for two patients (hopefully, at least one of which is ventilated) under the direction of an ICU-trained nurse. This will orient the re-assigned nurse as well as orient the ICU-trained nurse as to what tasks and responsibilities will be assigned, divided, and shared. In the training, ventilator management should be the main focus, including modalities, high PEEP considerations, O2 saturations, ABG interpretation, suctioning, proning, sedation, paralytics, and pain control, though sedation vacations must be reviewed by medical staff as to risk versus benefit.

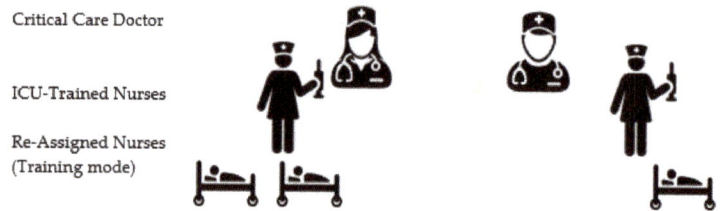

**Figure 7.** Training preparation for tiered staffing strategy for COVID-19 pandemic preparation.

Rationale

A significant number of critically ill patients will be admitted to intensive care units during the COVID-19 pandemic. Staffing will be further strained by the threat of experienced ICU staff nurses becoming ill [26]. During the COVID-19 pandemic, it is anticipated that the projected shortfall of well-trained ICU nurses will impact the care of critically ill ventilated patients. Consequently, the focus should not be only to increase the numbers of mechanical ventilators but must also address the number of trained critical care nurses required to care for mechanically ventilated COVID-19 patients, alongside non-COVID-19 patients requiring ICU care [25,26]. Assigning hospital nurses to work immediately in ICU during crisis time without enough training may put the nurse and patients at high risk. Therefore, planning for appropriate nursing staff prior to such a pandemic is required. Augmenting critical care nursing staff is one innovative way to scale up staffing capacity during a pandemic. Individual healthcare organizations must modify their strategies thereby aligning ICU staffing with their patient needs and with available resources [25,26]. In this strategy, consideration should be made to have already chosen and delegated non-ICU-trained nurses to be stationed in the ICU and be assigned to an ICU nurse in order to form a controlled baseline training prior to the actual surge. This will establish roles and responsibilities and form the foundation to build an expanding team when a surge becomes evident.

## 4. Conclusions

In anticipation of COVID-19 demands upon nursing staff and subsequent potential weakening of care levels in the provision of patient care, specifically in the ICU setting, a panel was formed to raise and answer critical concerns. The nursing surge capacity of critically ill patients with COVID-19 in the ICU was addressed through searching available evidence. Substantiation was retrieved from a variety of databases inclusive of published and unpublished studies. The retrieved studies were then reviewed by a minimum of two reviewers independently using JBI critical appraisal tools. The recommendations in the recent guidelines covered ICU nursing surge capacity strategies. We recommend that hospitals implement the evidence-based strategies that have been shown to be effective such as a team-based approach, and to establish other innovative strategies for ICU nursing staff surge capacity in the COVID-19 pandemic. As new evidence presents itself, further updates of the guideline will be issued.

**Author Contributions:** A.A.M.–Conception, manuscript preparation; A.A.–Conception; Z.A.–Manuscript preparation; K.A.S.–Manuscript preparation; D.S.–Manuscript preparation. All authors have read and agreed to the published version of the manuscript.

**Funding:** This research received no external funding.

**Acknowledgments:** Authors acknowledge Sulaiman Al Habib Research Center that supported this research.

**Conflicts of Interest:** The authors declare no conflict of interest.

## References

1. Alhazzani, W.; Al-Suwaidan, F.; Al Aseri, Z.; Al Mutair, A.; Alghamdi, G.; Rabaan, A.; Algamdi, M.; Alohali, A.; Asiri, A.; Alshahrani, M.; et al. The saudi critical care society clinical practice guidelines on the management of COVID-19 patients in the intensive care unit. *Saudi Crit. Care J.* **2020**, *4*, 27–44. [CrossRef]
2. Wu, Z.; McGoogan, J.M. Characteristics of and important lessons from the coronavirus disease 2019 (COVID-19) outbreak in China: Summary of a report of 72 314 cases from the Chinese Center for Disease Control and Prevention. *JAMA* **2020**, *323*, 1239–1242. [CrossRef] [PubMed]
3. Livingston, E.; Bucher, K. Coronavirus disease 2019 (COVID-19) in Italy. *JAMA* **2020**, *323*, 1335. [CrossRef] [PubMed]
4. Milton, D.K.; Fabian, M.P.; Cowling, B.J.; Grantham, M.L.; McDevitt, J.J. Influenza virus aerosols in human exhaled breath: Particle size, culturability, and effect of surgical masks. *PLoS Pathog.* **2013**, *9*, e1003205. [CrossRef] [PubMed]
5. World Health Organization. Corona Virus Disease (COVID-19) Dashboard. Available online: https://covid19.who.int (accessed on 13 July 2020).
6. World Health Organization. Rational Use of Personal Protective Equipment for Coronavirus Disease 2019 (COVID-19) Interim Guidance 27 February 2020. Available online: https://apps.who.int/iris/bitstream/handle/10665/331215/WHO-2019-nCov-IPCPPE_use-2020.1-eng.pdf (accessed on 5 April 2020).
7. World Health Organization. Coronavirus. Available online: https://www.who.int/health-topics/coronavirus#tab=tab_1 (accessed on 16 July 2020).
8. Chu, D.K.; Akl, E.A.; Duda, S.; Solo, K.; Yaacoub, S.; Schünemann, H.J.; Chu, D.K.; Akl, E.A.; El-harakeh, A.; Bognanni, A.; et al. Physical distancing, face masks, and eye protection to prevent person-to-person transmission of SARS-CoV-2 and COVID-19: A systematic review and meta-analysis. *Lancet* **2020**, *395*, 1973–1987. [CrossRef]
9. World Health Organization. Advice on the Use of Masks in the Context of COVID-19. Available online: https://www.who.int/publications/i/item/advice-on-the-use-of-masks-in-the-community-during-home-care-and-in-healthcare-settings-in-the-context-of-the-novel-coronavirus-(2019-ncov)-outbreak (accessed on 7 September 2020).
10. Society of Critical Care Medicine. United States Resource Availability for COVID-19. Available online: https://sccm.org/getattachment/Blog/March-2020/United-States-Resource-Availability-for-COVID-19/United-States-Resource-Availability-for-COVID-19.pdf?lang=en-US (accessed on 7 September 2020).
11. Aragon Penoyer, D. Nurse staffing and patient outcomes in critical care: A concise review. *Crit. Care Med.* **2010**, *38*, 15211528. [CrossRef] [PubMed]
12. Ontario Health Plan for an Influenza Pandemic Care. Critical Care During a Pandemic. Available online: http://www.cidrap.umn.edu/sites/default/files/public/php/21/21_report.pdf (accessed on 7 September 2020).
13. Maves, R.C.; Downar, J.; Dichter, J.R.; Hick, J.L.; Devereaux, A.; Geiling, J.A.; Kissoon, N.; Hupert, N.; Niven, A.S.; King, M.A.; et al. Triage of scarce critical care resources in COVID-19—An implementation guide for regional allocation: An expert panel report of the task force for mass critical care and the American College of Chest Physicians. *Chest* **2020**, *158*, 212–225. [CrossRef]
14. Chung, W.; Sohn, M. The impact of nurse staffing on in-hospital mortality of stroke patients in Korea. *J. Cardiovasc. Nurs.* **2018**, *33*, 47–54. [CrossRef] [PubMed]

15. The University of Toronto Interdepartmental Division of Critical Care Medicine Working Group. Management Principles of Adult Critically Ill COVID-19 Patients. Available online: https://criticalcare.utoronto.ca/file/180/download?token=E8_KA4WU (accessed on 23 March 2020).
16. Murthy, S.; Gomersall, C.D.; Fowler, R.A. Care for critically Ill patients with COVID-19. *JAMA* **2020**, *323*, 1499–1500. [CrossRef]
17. Ajao, A.; Nystrom, S.V.; Koonin, L.M.; Patel, A.; Howell, D.R.; Baccam, P.; Lant, T.; Malatino, E.; Chamberlin, M.; Meltzer, M.I. Assessing the capacity of the US health care system to use additional mechanical ventilators during a large-scale public health emergency. *Disaster Med. Pub. Health Prep.* **2015**, *9*, 634–641. [CrossRef]
18. Kleinpell, R.M.; Grabenkort, W.R.; Kapu, A.N.; Constantine, R.; Sicoutris, C. Nurse practitioners and physician assistants in acute and critical care: A concise review of the literature and data 2008–2018. *Crit. Care Med.* **2019**, *47*, 1442–1449. [CrossRef]
19. McHugh, M.D.; Ma, C. Hospital nursing and 30-day readmissions among medicare patients with heart failure, acute myocardial infarction, and pneumonia. *Med. Care* **2013**, *51*, 52–59. [CrossRef] [PubMed]
20. Cho, E.; Chin, D.L.; Kim, S.; Hong, O. The relationships of nurse staffing level and work environment with patient adverse events. *J. Nurs. Scholarsh.* **2016**, *48*, 74–82. [CrossRef] [PubMed]
21. American College of Chest Physicians. Surge Priority Planning COVID-19: Critical Care Staffing and Nursing Considerations. Available online: http://www.chestnet.org/Guidelines-and-Resources/Resources/Surge-Priority-Planning-COVID-19-Critical-Care-Staffing-and-Nursing-Considerations (accessed on 7 September 2020).
22. Scott, D.; Irfan, U.; Kirby, J. The Next Coronavirus Crisis Will Be A Shortage of Doctors and Nurses. Available online: https://www.vox.com/2020/3/26/21192191/coronavirus-us-new-york-hospitals-doctors-nurses (accessed on 29 March 2020).
23. Society of Critical Care Medicine. Critical Care Statistics. Available online: https://www.sccm.org/Communications/Critical-Care-Statistics (accessed on 7 September 2020).
24. Driscoll, A.; Grant, M.J.; Carroll, D.; Dalton, S.; Deaton, C.; Jones, I.; Lehwaldt, D.; McKee, G.; Munyombwe, T.; Astin, F. The effect of nurse-to-patient ratios on nurse-sensitive patient outcomes in acute specialist units: A systematic review and meta-analysis. *Eur. J. Cardiovasc. Nurs.* **2017**, *17*, 6–22. [CrossRef] [PubMed]
25. Kleinpell, R.M. ICU workforce: Revisiting nurse staffing. *Crit. Care Med.* **2014**, *42*, 1291–1292. [CrossRef] [PubMed]
26. North Carolina Healthcare Foundation. Strategies to Support Nursing Surge Capacity during Biological Event. Available online: https://www.ncbon.com/vdownloads/coronavirus/nursing-surge-capacity-resource.pdf (accessed on 20 July 2020).

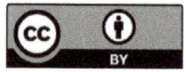

© 2020 by the authors. Licensee MDPI, Basel, Switzerland. This article is an open access article distributed under the terms and conditions of the Creative Commons Attribution (CC BY) license (http://creativecommons.org/licenses/by/4.0/).

MDPI
St. Alban-Anlage 66
4052 Basel
Switzerland
www.mdpi.com

*Nursing Reports* Editorial Office
E-mail: nursrep@mdpi.com
www.mdpi.com/journal/nursrep

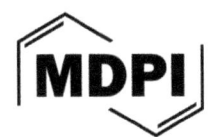

Disclaimer/Publisher's Note: The statements, opinions and data contained in all publications are solely those of the individual author(s) and contributor(s) and not of MDPI and/or the editor(s). MDPI and/or the editor(s) disclaim responsibility for any injury to people or property resulting from any ideas, methods, instructions or products referred to in the content.

www.ingramcontent.com/pod-product-compliance
Lightning Source LLC
LaVergne TN
LVHW070726100526
838202LV00013B/1177